ALLE · ZEIT · WACH · 1842

M. Aebi, P. Regazzoni (Eds.)

Bone Transplantation

With 125 Figures and 30 Tables

Springer-Verlag Berlin Heidelberg New York
London Paris Tokyo

PD Dr. Max Aebi

Klinik und Poliklinik für Orthopädische Chirurgie,
Inselspital, CH-3010 Bern

PD Dr. Pietro Regazzoni

Kantonsspital Basel, Departement für Chirurgie,
Spitalstr. 21, CH-4031 Basel

ISBN-13:978-3-642-83573-5 e-ISBN-13:978-3-642-83571-1
DOI: 10.1007/978-3-642-83571-1

Library of Congress Cataloging-in-Publication Data.
Bone transplantation / M. Aebi, P. Regazzoni (eds.).
p. cm. Includes index.
ISBN-13:978-3-642-83573-5 (U.S.)
1. Bone–Transplantation. 2. Homografts. I. Regazzoni, P. (Pietro), 1944– . II. Aebi, M. (Max)
[DNLM: 1. Bone and Bones–transplantation. 2. Transplantation, Homologous. WE 190 B712]
RD123.B65 1988 617'.4710592–dc 19 DNLM/DLC

Softcover reprint of the hardcover 1st edition 1989

Typesetting: Brühlsche Universitätsdruckerei, Giessen

2124/3020-543210 – Printed on acid-free paper

Preface

This book is the result of an international symposium on bone transplantation, the first of its kind, held in Berne, Switzerland, on May 14–16, 1987. This symposium brought together some of the most outstanding experts – from all over the world, principally from North America and Europe – in the clinical bone transplantation and in basic research. It was an unique opportunity to summarize in a few days the state of the art in this field and to bring clinicians who carry out some research related to their work together with basic scientists. The clinician can on the one hand profit from the basis researcher's knowledge and on the other stimulate the researcher to share the orthopedic surgeon's interest in osteoarticular allografts. The book, like the symposium, contains two types of contributions:

1. Papers from invited experts who have often dedicated a significant part of their professional life to the subject of bone transplantation. Knowledge which would otherwise be scattered among original papers from many different sources, some of it less firmly established and therefore less well known, is thus collected together in one volume, so that the reader does not have to weed out a mass of less important material. These chapters may for a certain time act as a textbook on bone transplantation, but inevitably will eventually be superseded by new findings.
2. Descriptions of current research in all the main subjects covered in the state-of-the-art papers. To give all the contributors the opportunity to have their work published, this part takes the form of short communications, giving the reader an overview of current activity in bone transplantion research. It may be that some important topics are "underweighted" here; if this should be the case, however, the reader who needs more detailed information will be well served by the extensive bibliographies.

It was never our intention with this volume to present only one consistent approach to osteoarticular transplantation; rather the views reproduced accurately reflect the diversity of thinking and of research directions in this important area of orthopedic surgery and in related disciplines.

If the book stimulates more scientists to embark upon research into osteoarticular transplantation and arouses the interest of biologists, immunologists, and bone physiologists, an important goal has been reached.

The editors are indebted to all those who supported the symposium and the book, especially the Maurice E. Müller Foundation, Switzerland, and the Research Department of Sandoz Switzerland Ltd. We are particulary grateful to the staff of Springer-Verlag for their tireless cooperation and in editing and formatting the many contributions. We also wish to thank all the authors who dedicated so much time and energy to providing the manuscripts for the symposium and for this book.

Bern and Basel, October 31st, 1988

M. Aebi
P. Regazzoni

Table of Contents

Bone Alternatives

Introduction to Update on Osteochondral Allograft Surgery

M. R. Urist

Bone Research Laboratory, University of California at Los Angeles, Los Angeles, California 90024, USA

Progress in the surgery of bone transplantation requires understanding the unsolved problem of cell differentiation, with special reference to induced bone cell differentiation. Such knowledge as we have to share with each other on induced bone formation comes from two very recently investigated experimental systems. One consists of implants of bone matrix in muscle and subcutis. The other comes from explants of neonatal muscle connective tissue outgrowths in vitro. Both are more consistently reproducible in rodents than in long-lived dogs, monkeys, and human beings. Nevertheless, in the session on bone alternative, we have an unusual opportunity to review and discuss applications of experimentally induced bone cell formation for repair of bone defects. A potential pitfall of basic research is to extrapolate observations on rodents to bone repair problems in long-lived species.

The interplay of six circumstances determines the success of the bone graft operation: (a) the viability and proliferative capacity of the host bed; (b) the viability of the graft; (c) the volume or size of the defect in the host bed to be repaired; (d) the bone morphogenetic protein (BMP) content of the graft or implant, including the surface of the host bed; (e) the species involved with particular reference to the metabolic activity index (MAI); and (f) homostructural function of the donor tissue. An allogeneic graft is a transplant between individuals of the same species but of disparate genotype. An autogeneic graft is a transplant from one part to another of the same individual.

Host Bed. The location of the host bed in the skeleton determines proliferative capacity of osteoprogenitor cells and perivascular connective tissue cells competent to respond to BMP. This is associated with blood flow and with bone marrow activity (especially bone marrow stoma), which is characteristic of each bone or part of each bone of the human skeleton. The most obvious indicator of the viability and proliferative activity of the host is the rate of fracture healing. Failure of bone grafts is most frequent in host bone bed with the lowest rates of fracture healing.

Viability of the Bone Graft. The rate of healing and success of the operation is determined by the viability of the graft. Since nearly 95% of bone cells of a graft do not survive transplantation, most successful bone grafts are transplanted from the cancellous tissue of the host iliac or are used as a microvascular transplant from the rib or fibula. In both instances, the autogeneic graft is recommended to avoid the delayed immune responses of the host to allogeneic tissue. The larger the host bed defect, the greater the requirements for autogeneic transplantation.

Bone Transplantation
Eds.: M. Aebi, P. Regazzoni

The smaller the bone defects, the more justifiable and effective the use of freeze-dried allogeneic bone. In a small defect in an area of highly vascular, rapidly healing host bone, it is almost unjustifiable to transplant autogeneic bone from the iliac crest.

Volume of the Host Bed to be Engrafted. The rate of incorporation of a bone graft is directly proportional to the size or volume of the bone defect in the host bed that is being grafted. The larger the bone defect, the longer the period of time necessary for incorporation and the greater the complications of pathological fracture or nonunion. The larger the area of the defect, the lower the ratio of surface of bone bed to surface area of graft or implant to be incorporated. For this reason, the selection of a graft with a large internal surface area, such as the spongiosa of the crest of the ilium, becomes important. The larger the defect in the host bed, the higher the requirements for internal fixation and for absolute contact compression between the graft and the host bed.

Bone Morphogenetic Protein, Content, or Activity. The BMP activity of the host bed and the bone graft or implant induces perivascular connective tissue cells of the host bed to enter into a bone morphogenetic pathway of development. BMP recruits supplemental cell populations of the host bed and thereby augments the process of incorporation of the bone graft. The evidence of augmentation is the repair of large bone defects with bridges of new bone formation induced by BMP in polylactic polyglycolic acid copolymer delivery systems. Without any bone graft or preexisting cells, an implant of BMP in a muscle pouch or subcutaneous space in rodents induces bone formation. The perivascular connective tissue cells of the muscle are induced to enter an osteogenetic pathway of development, which otherwise would not occur in the lifetime of the individual.

Species Specificity and Metabolic Activity Index. the capacity to repair fractures, incorporate bone grafts, and respond to BMP is correlated with MAI. Heart rate, blood flow, basal metabolic rate, respiratory rate, and body temperature are some of the elements that comprise the MAI of the species. The dog has a MAI of 1.5 relatively close to that of man, 1.0. The laboratory mouse and rat have MAI levels of 15.6 and 5.15, respectively. For this reason, the dog provides the best experimental test system for substitutes for bone grafts. However, for rapid bioassay work, the mouse and rat are economically essential to save time and to reduce the costs of research on BMP.

Homostructural Function of a Bone Graft. Transplantation of a bone graft, either autogeneic or allogeneic, into a large bone defect restores the continuity of the bone with homostructural material. When a large defect from an incision of a bone tumor is repaired with a bone graft, the donor tissue performs the function of a "spacer." Even if the space is bridged by external fixation devices or by internal fixation with contact compression, the donor tissue may not be incorporated or replaced by host bed derived bone in the lifetime of the individual. It is only when the graft is resorbed and invaded by blood vessels and connective tissue ingrowths from the host that fatigue fractures of the graft occur. The fracture occurs at the interface between the living and dead tissue. No nonviable substance is known to perform as efficiently as bone tissue itself. For this reason, there are

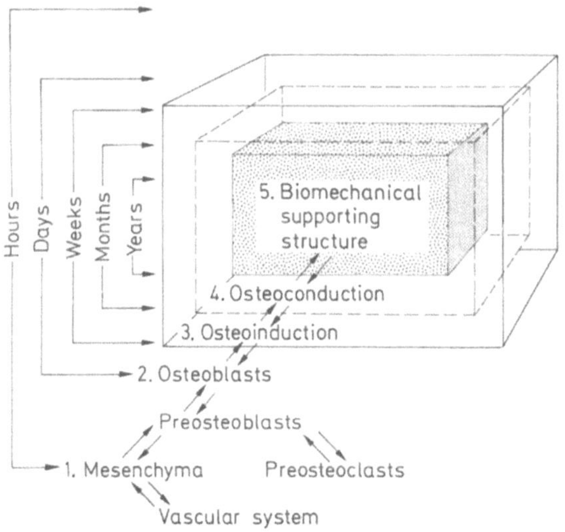

Fig. 1. Diagrammatic representation of the six circumstances of the incorporation of a bone graft, illustrating the three-dimensional relationship and time sequences. The end-point is reached when the inert biomechanical structure of donor tissue is completely encased in remodeled lamellar bone deposits of the recipient

presently no known synthetic substitutes for the homostructural function of a bone graft (Fig. 1).

Bone Alternatives

There are no alternatives superior to fresh warm autogeneic bone for general clinical application. However, this fact does not dissuade us in the search for alternatives, because bone is one of the only mammailian tissues for available experiments on induced cell differentiation. In this field, new methods are constantly being devised, and old observations are frequently rediscovered to have new meaning. The motivating force of research on bone alternatives is the need for new information with clinical potential. Many of the experiments reported in this symposium have clinical application as well as academic information. Consequently, in research on induced bone formation, the difference between fundamental and applied research is irrelevant.

The most important consideration in understanding alternatives to autogeneic bone is the obligate requirement to induce the host bed to recapitulate embryonic developmental processes. For this reason, alternatives with denatured BMP, i.e., a massive implant of nonviable bone-frozen, lyophilized, and sterilized either by irradiation or autoclaving – are limited in function to osteoconduction. Bone devoid of BMP is so slowly resorbed that it is an obstacle to the ingrowth of host bone. The host must resorb a large part of the donor before it can be replaced by living bone or incorporated in the host bed. Alternatives which transfer BMP are implanted with the assumption that a large bone defect is surrounded by perivascular connective tissue cells with the embryonic potential. These cells are the target tissue for BMP and must be competent to adopt a bone morphogenetic pathway of development. Kreichbergs and Köhler demonstrated that by autoclaving and reimplanting autogeneic bone, including dead tumor, the implant serves as a spacer. The autogeneic spacer becomes attached to the host bed at its margins by the growth of bone by extension from he host bed. Bereiter et al. reached a similar conclusion with the use either of anorganic bovine bone or of synthetic calcium phosphates in rabbits. Katthagen and Mittelmeier first treated bone defects in rats, rabbits, and dogs and later 800 patients with bone defects prepared with a composite or malleable mixture of xenogeneic bovine collagen and sintered hydroxyapatite particles; the mixture of xenogeneic collagen and hydroxyapatite granular is ceramic (Collapat); spongy bone from which the organic material was extracted (Pyrost) is also being treated.

Albert et al. implanted pulverized demineralized dog bone matrix into muscle pouches for periods of 18–135 days to determine the composition of the products of induced bone formation. Thorngren et al. injected a homogenate of bone matrix and autogeneic bone marrow. To compare the effects of autogeneic cancellous bone for repair of a segment of rabbit segmental defects, Bettex-Galland and Burger described the histophysiology of relationships between osteoclastic resorption and angiogenesis in induced formation of bone ossicles in rats. Thieleman and Etter and Holz et al. focused on species differences in response of the recipient of allogeneic implants and observed the influence of cyclosporine for immunosuppression; observations in rats could not be extrapolated to dogs, sheep, and man because species differences were associated with different levels of osteoinductivity or immunoreactivity, or both, to bone matrix proteins.

Rueger et al. observed that in bone defects in rats, implants of a composite of calcium phosphate and bone matrix gelatin increased bone yield five-fold; bone matrix gelatin was highly immunogeneic in xenogeneic recipients and is not an acceptable bone alternative to autogeneic bone for clinical application.

Munting and Delloye made a survey of factors which extinguish and factors which preserve the osteoinductive activity in bone matrix of rats, rabbits, and dogs. Meenen et al. investigated the incorporation of porous hydroxyapatite ceramic in rabbits, including bone remodeling in drill holes in the distal ends of the femur. Lindholm and Ragni implanted demineralized allogeneic rabbit bone matrix in posterolateral spinal fusions and interbody fusions of the lumbar spine in rabbits to compare the response to synthetic hydroxyapatite in these experimental systems. Hydroxyapatite produced bony fusion only when it was implanted as a composite with bone marrow.

Differing from the foregoing description of purely theoretical experimental research, the session organized by Ganz and Gilbert consisted of practical surgical procedures of transplantation of vascularized and nonvascularized autografts. Gilbert demonstrated the highly effective results of reconstruction of posttraumatic large bone defects with vascularized autografts; vascularized autografts were successful even in patients with congenital pseudarthrosis. Weiland resected and then successfully replaced septic lesions with healthy vascularized autografts. Ganz demonstrated revascularization of joints with pediculed autografts. Answering the enourmous challenges of bone defects from resection of large bone tumors, Capanna et al. demonstrated a successful Ernest-Lexer–type nonvascularized bone autograft.

Observing that the excision of large autografts from the iliac crest often creates serious complications and unexpected disability, Grob emphasized the importance of research aimed at finding substitutes for massive autografts. DeBoer and Wood outlined the problems and statistical results of transfer of vascularized fibular autografts. Milinkovich et al. observed the rapid incorporation of vascularized pedicular rib grafts. To validate the objective of preservation of circulation in pedicle bone grafts, Klingmüller and Schwetlick demonstrated an angiogram of the host bed. Judet et al. described osteonecrosis bone defects in the femoral head, successfully treated by free vascularized grafts.

Further evidence of the practicality of modern-day bone allograft surgery is found in the work of Capanna and of Gross. Gross demonstrated long-term follow-up results of bone allografts for repair of bone defects in the proximal end of the femur to fulfill the requirements of revision arthroplasty. Massive replacement of the joints by osteoarticular allografts in tumor excision surgery are also presented with a long-term follow-up report by Tomford et al. Muschler et al. investigated the combination of bone and bone substitutes for repair of tumor excision defects. Gross emphasized the practicality of replacement of osteochondral defects for traumatic lesions of relatively small areas of joint surfaces. Radojevich et al. filled defects in the acetabulum in total hip arthroplasty operations with allografts. Ceroni et al. repaired bone deficiencies for total hip arthroplasties with fresh bone allografts. Weill et al. implanted autoclaved, sterilized, allogeneic bone in the proximal end of the femur for a total hip arthroplasty without cement. Johnson and Urist demonstrated augmentation of autogeneic bone grafts with home BMP for reconstruction of segmental defects ranging from 3 to 17 cm in length. Ueno implanted sintered autoclaved bone for osteoconductive effects. One of the largest experiences on record of freeze-dried allografts for nontumorous orthopedic constructive procedures with long-term statistics and follow-up examinations was presented by Mnaymneh et al. One hundred massive osteoarticular preserved allografts with equally long term results were presented by Waber et al. Delloye et al. described an experience with cryopreserved osteoarticular allografts. Alho et al. described successful results with allogeneic, osteoarticular defects implanted in knee joint surfaces. Delepine et al. described a comprehensive approach to reconstructive surgery with allografts for replacement of large defects from malignant bone tumors. In a further contribution these authors observed the variable influences of chemotherapy on the incorporation of allografts for patients with reconstructive surgery for malignant bone tumors. Winkelmann and Jürgens reviewed the effects of both pre- and postoperative chemotherapy on incorporation of bone grafts. Aho et al. compared the results of experimental and clinical allografts relative to proportions, size, and repair of bone tumor excisions.

Peltonen et al. reviewed the results of the new principle of osteotomy and distraction in experimental and clinical bone defects. De Pablos et al. reviewed bone lengthening with the excision of large segmental bone defects.

As briefly outlined here, a wide selection of problems of bone regeneration are presently under investigation. The problem of repair of large bone defects is studied by correlated observations on animals and patients with old infections, tumor resections, nonunited fractures, and congenital disorders. In this conference, in the clinic as in the laboratory, more unanswered questions were raised than could be answered in the short span of 3 days. The sessions on free papers were especially valuable for revealing centers of research activity that would otherwise hardly come to the attention of clinicians. Spectacular cases treated by vascularized organ transplants of whole knee joints, and massive nonvascularized bone allografts represent new standards for successful end results. However, the enthusiasm of the 1- to 2-year follow-up reports are being tempered with the knowledge of the long-term sequelae, such as pathological fractures, low-grade infections, ankylosis, unexplained pain, etc. In this respect, modern-day surgery of massive bone defects resembles the search for the limits of space exploration. Bone graft surgeons are searching for the limits of the capacity of the body to regenerate bone. Even the most fundamental question of factors regulating bone cell differentiation are not understood. We are uncertain about whether bone is a two- or three-cell tier system of cell differentiation. The mesenchymal cell is the inner; the osteoprogenitor cell or committed stem population is the middle; the osteoblast is the outer tier. The question is, therefore, whether BMP is an osteopoietic comparable to erythropoietin in regulation of bone marrow cell differentiation at the second as well as the first level of cell differentiation. Does an embryonic-type mesenchymal become a committed cell with limited potential for development? Experience with patients with head injuries and paraplegics developing heterotopic bone formations shows that the potential for developing bone is much greater than our knowledge of controlling and directing the process of regeneration. The problem to be solved is determining how the body localizes and regulates bone formation. The challenge is to find the answer to these questions, in laboratories and operating rooms, and to explore new leads toward treatment of disabled people.

Drs. Aebi and Regazzaoni have found exactly the right format for the symposium on bone transplants by opening with established workers in the field and by ending with free papers from both experienced clinicians and investigators who are exploring bold approaches to unsolved problems of induced bone cell differentiation.

Early Research on Bone Transplantation

H. de Boer

De Wever Hospital, H. Dunantstraat 5, 6419 PC Heerlen, The Netherlands

The reconstruction of large skeletal defects presents a challenging problem to the orthopedic community. The treatment of these defects has evolved significantly during the past two decades [14]. The recent, increased demand for bone grafts for reconstruction in limb salvage surgery for bone tumors and for reconstruction of failed arthroplasties has renewed interest in bone graft surgery. The types of grafts clinically available for use are nonvascularized auto- and allografts. Allografts (formerly homografts) are taken from a different individual of the same species, whereas autografts are harvested from the same individual. Xenografts (formerly heterografts) are grafts from a different species and are rarely used [58, 59]. Cellular elements in allografts are dead, due to processes that are used to diminish the immune response [50, 98]. Fairly convincing data support the concept that only a few cells on the surface of autografts survive, most undergoing necrosis [37, 82, 87].

Bone autografts, allografts, and even vascularized bone autografts are currently used in almost every orthopedic center throughout the world. Only autografts can be used for microvascular reconstructions because the immunological problems associated with allografts prevents satisfactory vascularization. Transplantation of bone, which depends upon fundamental facts of bone structure and growth, has been the subject of many experimental and clinical studies. In 1668 the Dutch surgeon Job van Meekeren [72] described the first bone graft procedure (Fig. 1). This graft, taken from a dog's skull, was used for the successful repair of a traumatic defect in a soldier's cranium. Because of this seemingly barbaric method of treatment the patient was excommunicated. He later asked the surgeon to remove the graft so that he could be returned to the good graces of the Church – but by that time the graft had taken.

Today, we know that three physiological functions may be attributed to bone grafts [12, 23, 100]. First, osteoinduction can occur in the process of inducing bone formation locally by the recruitment of cells which have a potential for bone formation [60, 64, 100–103]. Secondly, bone grafts may serve for osteoconduction, providing a framework for bone deposition [9, 30, 38, 82]. And finally, bone grafts may provide a source of bone-forming cells [1, 8, 85]. Each grafting technique may be responsible for one or several of these functions to varying degrees.

The Dutch scientist Anton van Leeuwenhoek was the first to describe bone structure [63] (Fig. 2). In his letter dated June 1, 1674, addressed to the publisher of *Philosophical Transactions*, van Leeuwenhoek wrote: "I reviewed the shin bone of a calf, in which I found several little holes, passing from without inwards; and

Bone Transplantation
Eds.: M. Aebi, P. Regazzoni

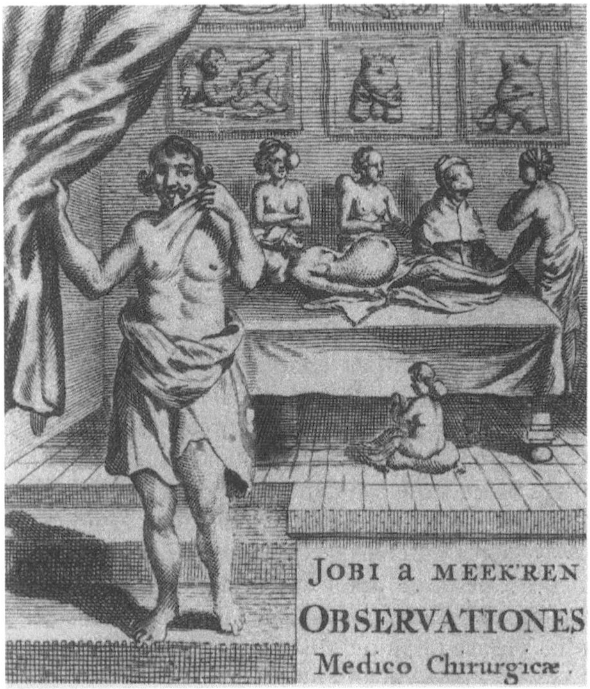

Fig. 1. Title page from Job van Meekeren's work [72]

I then imagined, that this bone had divers small pipes going long ways" [63]. Today these pipes are known as haversian canals [49]. As described by Chase and Herdon [29], Duhamel, who published his work in 1742, is generally credited with the first scientific investigations into the problem of osteogenesis. However, it was the Dutch scientist de Heyde had published his work about experimental observations made on frogs 60 years earlier [51]. De Heyde concluded that callus was formed by calcification of the blood clot around the broken bone ends.

A century after Duhamel's work, and following many less well-known works and discussions on the subject, came the great work of his fellow countryman, the Frenchman Ollier (Fig. 3), entitled "Traité expérimental et clinique de la régénération des os" [77]. This classic surgical work was so thorough that its conclusions from experiments on rabbits and young dogs were to attain an almost unassailable position. Ollier showed that autografts can be viable, and he recognized that separate living bone fragments without periosteum could live and grow in a suitable environment [47]. In Russia, experimental work was carried out by Penski, who, according to Aho [2], in 1893 was the first to perform an allogenic joint transplantation in an animal [2].

Since the beginning of this century, not only experimental but also clinical observations have been made on the behavior of transplanted bone. Working independently, Barth [9] in Germany and Curtis [30] in the United States published works on bone transplantation. Barth described *schleichenden Ersatz*, the absorp-

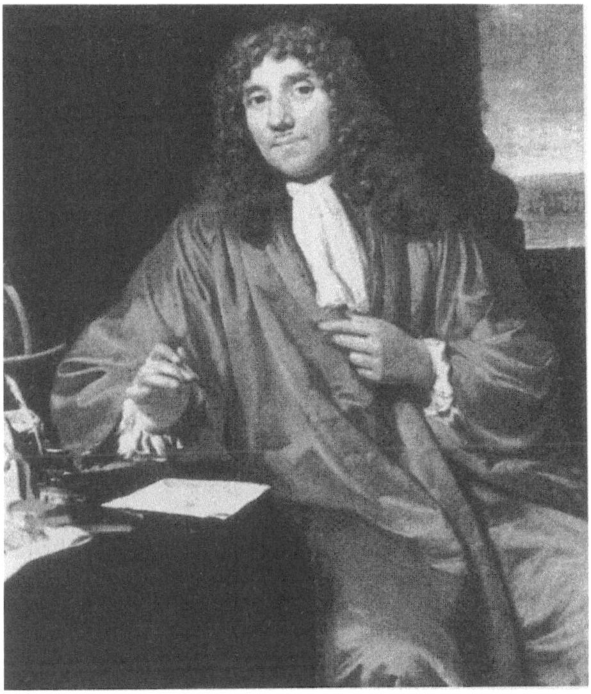

Fig. 2. Anton van Leeuwenhoek. Publication in *Philosophical Transactions* in 1674 on the structure of bone [63]

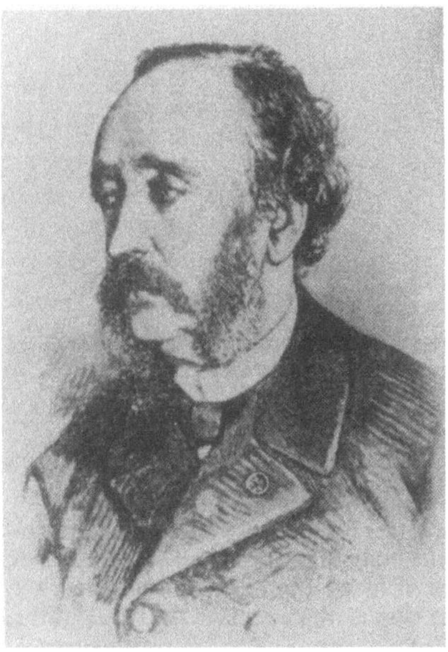

Fig. 3. L. Ollier published his work „Traité expérimental et clinique de la régénération des os" in 1867 [77]

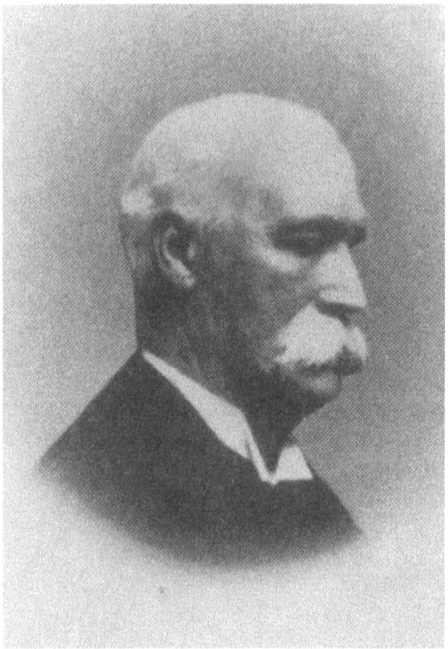

Fig. 4. W. Macewen performed the first allograft in 1880 [68]

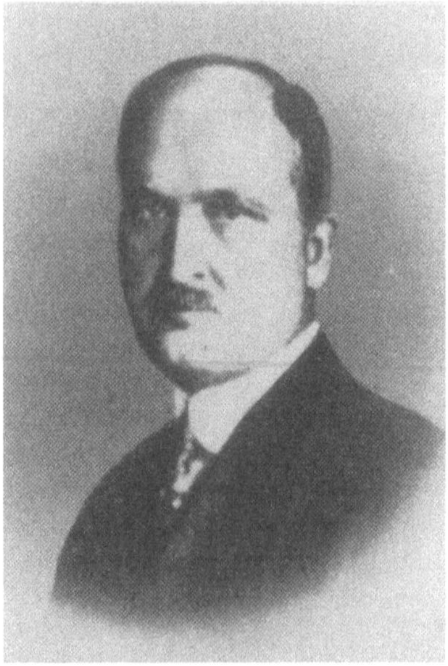

Fig. 5. F. H. Albee published his book on bone graft surgery in 1915 [4]

tion of dead tissue in the bone graft and the formation of new bone, which grew into the graft from the surrounding living bone. Curtis noted that:

> The Haversian canals, moreover, afford easy avenues for the growth of granulation tissue, and in some cases it has been observed that the bone turns a rosy hue within a short time after implantation, apparently by absorption of blood, two factors which probably explain why ossification so soon takes place in the tissues which replace the bone graft as it is absorbed.

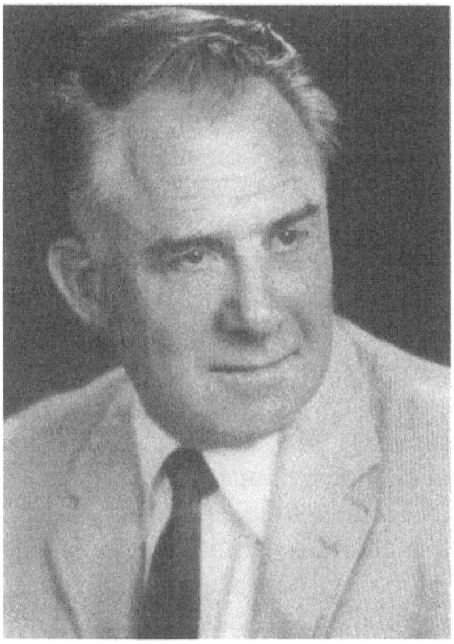

Fig. 6. M. Vrist studied osteogenic induction extensively and has separated a bone morphogenetic protein

This process was later called "creeping substitution" by Phemister [82].

The first clinical autograft had already been performed in 1820 by von Walter in Germany. He replaced parts of the skull surgically removed after trepanotomy [105]. The first allograft was performed in 1880 by Macewen from Scotland (Fig. 4). He successfully reconstructed an infected humerus of a 4-year-old boy with a graft obtained from the tibia of a child with rickets [68]. But it was only after Albee's work on bone graft surgery (Fig. 5), published in the United States in 1915, that the transplantation of bone began to be performed more frequently [4].

Since that time, numerous publications have appeared with discussions on the fate of transplanted bone and the regenerative power of its various constituents [20, 47, 82]. Whether bone-forming cells are provided by host or graft remains a topic of controversy. In the 1930s some investigators believed that bone arose by metaplasia from the surrounding connective tissue, while others believed that it arose only from tissues associated with bone [60, 64]. Urist (Fig. 6) and his colleagues introduced the theory of osteoinduction. They suggested that a chemical mediator from the bone graft could induce bone formation by recruitment of cells with potential for bone formation [100–103]. The current understanding of the histologic fate of nonvascularized auto- and allografts following transplantation is similar to the view originally presented by Barth and Curtis [9, 30], except that the theory of induction offers promising possibilities for further investigation.

Bone Grafts Currently Used

The vast majority of bone autografts are used to augment fracture healing or to reconstruct small skeletal defects. Recently, allografts, consisting of cancellous or cortical parts or of a massive bone and stored in a bone bank, have renewed interest in reconstruction of larger skeletal defects. This topic has been the subject of numerous clinical and experimental investigations since the experiments described by Lexer in 1908 and 1925 [65, 66]. Cadaver allografts stored in established bone banks have provided a good supply of bone. Since the report of Inclan in 1942 [54], the banking program has been described in several recent publications [35, 39, 96].

In recent decades, several studies have discussed the clinical usefulness of allograft reconstruction, however careful analyses of the results suggest that numerous problems remain unsolved [25, 45, 69, 73, 74, 80]. Fresh allografts are associated with a marked immune response that is primarily cellular, but there is also a humoral component [10, 17, 24, 28, 44, 62, 86, 89]. Several studies have investigated methods to diminish this immune response [11, 36, 95], but controversy still exists regarding the nature and significance of the immune response evoked by bone and cartilage. There is also discussion as to how recipient immune mechanisms operate in affecting the end result of the allotransplantation system [40]. The best methods for preserving segments, and also the best method of cryopreservation of cartilage, have not yet been fully established [21, 48, 61, 95, 97]. Because of attempts to reduce the immunogenicity of allografts, cellular elements undergo necrosis [23, 50, 98]. Thus an allograft serves only as an inert scaffold to which soft tissues can be attached, providing structural strength and, if necessary, an articulation [3, 104].

The techniques and results of adequate resection of bone tumors and subsequent reconstruction of large bone defects with allografts have been reported in several large series [45, 69, 74, 80]. The processes of vascularization, resorption, new bone formation, and remodeling of the allograft reconstruction of large skeletal defects can take more than 2 years [38]. Nonunion between the allograft and the recipient bone, infection, resorption of bone, and fractures of the graft are possible complications [25, 45, 69, 73, 74, 79]. Transplantation of a bone segment which remains vascularized or is immediately revascularized has been suggested as a means to reduce these complications.

A bone graft with an intact pedicle of blood supply remains viable and can unite directly with the recipient bone without having to be revascularized and replaced by creeping substitution. Since these grafts act as living bone struts, their mechanical strength is probably better than a nonvascularized graft. Furthermore, because of their intact vasculature these grafts may be more resistant to bacterial infection, and antibiotic access to the wound and bone segments is unimpeded.

The concept of transplanting a living vascularized bone graft is not new. In 1893 Curtis [30] stated in his classic paper "that calcified bone was at present the most practical material for use in the ordinary cases, while we are waiting the ideal of the future: the insertion of a piece of living bone which will exactly fill the gap and will continue to live without absorption." This had already been attempted by Phelps [81], who in 1891 had connected a piece of bone from a dog as an interposition graft in a defect of the tibia of a boy. After the operation, the boy and the dog were attached to each other for 2 weeks. The graft failed and was removed after 5 weeks.

Huntington has been given credit for first describing a pedicular transfer of the ipsilateral fibula into the tibia in 1905 [53]. Davies described a pedicular graft of the anterior part of the iliac crest based on the tensor fasciae latae, which was used as a live strut for hip fusion [33]. Recently Chacha described the technique of various pedicular bone grafts, which can be applied in clinical situations by any orthopedic specialist without the need for elaborate and highly specialized expertise [27]. The use of a pedicular graft is limited by the extent to which the length of the soft tissue pedicle allows rotation to the recipient site.

Publication of Carrel's [26] results in transplantation of blood vessels, organs, and limbs heralded the birth of vascular surgery. However, until microvascular surgery began to flourish in the 1960s with the development of the operating microscope, improvement of microsurgical instruments and suture material, vascularized bone grafts – the "future" that Curtis spoke of in 1893 – did not become a reality [6, 55]. The work of Östrup and Fredrickson [78], from Sweden, stimulated this new type of bone transplantation; they described an experimental distant transfer of free, living rib grafts by microvascular anastomoses in dogs. Taylor, from Australia, reported the first free vascularized fibular graft in 1975 [91]. He reconstructed a traumatic tibial defect with a fibula from the opposite leg in April 1974; revascularization was accomplished with microvascular anastomosis. The actual first free vascularized fibular transfer probably took place in Japan. Using this technique, Ueba from the Orthopedic Department of the University Hospital of Kyoto reconstructed a pseudoarthrosis of the ulna in December 1973 [99]. This case was published in the Japanese journal for orthopedic trauma surgery as a follow-up report in 1983.

This new technique of bone transplantation has become an accepted method of reconstruction of certain bony defects and recalcitrant nonunion [15, 91, 92, 106–114]. Such skeletal defects can be the result of trauma, infection, or tumor resection. Additional indications for vascularized bone transfer that have been suggested congenital pseudarthrosis of the tibia or forearm [5, 16, 84, 108], congenital hypoplasia of the radius [83], extensive anterior spinal fusion [52], limb-lengthening procedures [76], and avascular necrosis of the femoral head withouth its collapse [41, 43, 56]. The technique involves the isolation of a large segment of bone on its nutrient artery and vein pedicle. The graft is totally detached from its origin and reattached at a remote recipient site. The blood supply to the graft is restored by anastomosis of the nutrient artery and vein of the bone graft to appropriate recipient site vessels. This procedure should ensure the viability of cells within the transferred bone segment that may directly aid in the processes of bone healing and remodeling [7, 18, 19, 34, 78]. Thus, reconstruction of a large defect may be accomplished by a mode of healing similar to that of a segmental fracture, rather than the usual, more lengthy processes of graft incorporation [7, 31, 82, 93].

The spectrum of available donor bones in which the circulation may be restored by microvascular anastomosis includes segments of rib [22, 32, 88], fibula [90–92, 106–114], iliac crest [92, 107, 109, 111], part of radius or ulna [13, 67], portion of scapula [94], and metatarsal bones [75]. Situations occasionally arise during an ablative surgical procedure or trauma in which composite tissue, which would otherwise be discarded, may serve as vascularized tissue transfer for distant reconstruction [111]. Meals and Lesavoy reported a vascularized free radius transfer for clavicle reconstruction concurrent with below elbow amputation [71]. The three donor bones which have been used most frequently for free vascularized transfer are the rib, iliac crest, and fibula. Although the rib was the first free bone graft used clinically, its application in orthopedics is limited, and vascularized rib transfer has mainly been used for mandibular reconstruction [70, 88]. In general, the iliac crest free transfer is more useful for shorter (under 10 cm) defects, particularly when it is desirable to include a generous amount of accompanying skin or muscle [107, 110]. The iliac crest may also be used in situations in which a certain amount of sculpturing of the bone segment is necessary to match a complex defect at the recipient site.

The fibula is best suited for reconstruction of long bones of the extremities. Its diameter matches almost exactly that of the radius and the ulna, and it may fit snugly into the medullar cavity of the humerus, femur, and tibia [92]. Due to its high proportion of cortical bone and its triangular cross-section, it may be superior to the rib or iliac crest in resisting angular and rotational stress. The fibula, when used as a free vascularized tissue transfer, is based on the peroneal vascular pedicle, which supplies both its periosteal and endosteal circulation [19, 90, 91]. The technique of harvest is well described, and bone of up to 35 cm in length can be obtained [42, 107]. Preoperative arteriography may be indicated particularly in posttraumatic, postirradiation, or congenital cases to evaluate the anatomy of the donor as well as the recipient site vessels. It is furthermore possible to design a flap that includes a cuff of muscle, an attached muscle flap, or an accompanying skin flap. If a skin island (buoy flap) is able to be combined with the bone transfer, this can be used to achieve cover of the transferred bone or to act as a valuable monitor to the blood circulation through the graft [115]. The fibular is readily accessible and can be harvested from most patients simultaneously with the preparation of the recipient defect [57]. For all these reasons, therefore, as well as for the remarkably limited donor site morbidity, the fibula is probably the most suitable bone for vascularized transfer to reconstruct large skeletal defects.

Recently, the combination of an allograft and a vascularized graft was introduced, a technique which provides both immediate strength and viability for the reconstruction of large skeletal defects [12, 46]. Although several reconstructive methods are available, the problem of large skeletal defects remains a challenging one. The current state of knowledge of the histologic fate of auto- and allografts following transplantation is similar to the original views presented by Barth [9] and Curtis [30], although the theory of induction is a promising field for further investigation [100–103].

Acknowledgements. The author thanks Mrs. Jolanda Hofman for assistance in preparing the manuscript.

References

1. Abbott LC, Schottsteadt ER, de Saunders JB, Bost FC (1947) The evaluation of cortical and cancellous bone grafting material. A clinical and expermental study. J Bone Joint Surg [Am] 29A:381

2. Aho AJ (1973) Allogenic joint transplantation in the dog. Ann Chir Gynaecol Fenniae 62:226
3. Aho AJ (1985) Half-joint transplantation in human bone tumours. Int Orthop (SICOT) 9:77
4. Albee FH (1915) Bone graft surgery. Saunders, Philadelphia
5. Allieu Y, Gomis R, Yoshimura M, Dimeglio A, Bonnel F (1981) Congenital pseudarthrosis of the forearm – two cases treated by free vascularized fibular graft. J Hang Surg 6A:475
6. American Replantation Mission to China (1973) Replantation surgery in China. Plast Reconstr Surg 52:476
7. Arata MA, Wood MB, Cooney WP (1984) Revascularized segmental diaphyseal bone transfers in the canine. J Reconstr Microsurg 1:11
8. Axhausen G (1907) Histologische Untersuchungen bei Knochentransplantationen am Menschen. Dtsch Z Chir 91:388
9. Barth A (1893) Über histologische Befunde nach Knochenimplantationen. Arch Klin Chir 46:409
10. Bassett CAL (1962) Current concepts of bone formation. J Bone Joint Surg [Am] 44A:1217
11. Bassett CAL (1972) Clinical implication of cell function in bone grafting. Clin Orthop 87:49
12. Bieber EJ, Wood MB (1986) Bone reconstruction. Clin Plast Surg 13:645
13. Biemer E, Stock W (1983) Total thumb reconstruction: one stage thumb reconstruction using an osteo-cutaneous forearm flap. Br J Plast Surg 36:52
14. de Boer HH (1988) The history of bone grafts. Clin Orthop 226:26
15. de Boer HH (1988) Free vascularized fibular transfer. PhD thesis, University of Leiden
16. de Boer HH, Verbout AJ, Nielsen HKL, van der Eijken JW (1988) Free vascularized fibular graft for tibial pseudarthrosis in neurofibromatosis. Acta Orthop Scand 59:425
17. Bonfiglo M, Jeter WS, Smith CL (1955) The immune concept. Its relation to bone transplantation. Ann NY Acad Sci 59:417
18. Bos KE (1979) Bone scintigraphy of experimental composite bone grafts revascularized by microvascular anastomoses. Plast Reconstr Surg 64:353
19. Bos KE (1980) Transplantation of revascularized autologenous bone, an experimental study. Thesis, University of Amsterdam, 1980
20. Brooks B, Hudson WA (1920) Studies in bone transplantations. An experimental study of the comparative success of autogenous and homogenous transplants of bone in dogs. Arch Surg 1:284
21. Brown JB (1940) Preserved and fresh homotransplants of cartilage. Surg Gynecol Obstet 70:1079
22. Buncke HJ, Furnas DW, Gordon L, Achauer BM (1977) Free osteocutaneous flap from a rib to the tibia. Plast Reconstr Surg 59:799
23. Burchardt H (1983) The biology of bone graft repair. Clin Orthop 174:28
24. Burwell RG (1963) Studies in the transplantation of bone. The capacity of fresh and treated homografts of bone to evoke transplantation immunity. J Bone Joint Surg [Br] 45B:386
25. Campbell CJ (1972) Homotransplantation of a half or whole joint. Clin Orthop 87:146
26. Carrel A (1908) Results of the transplantation of blood vessels, organs and limbs. JAMA 51:1661
27. Chacha PB (1984) Vascularized pedicular bone grafts. Int Orthop (SICOT) 8:117
28. Chalmers J (1959) Transplantation immunity in bone homografting. J Bone Joint Surg [Br] 41B:160
29. Chase SW, Herndon CH (1955) The fate of autogenous and homogenous bonegrafts. J Bone Joint Surg [Am] 37A:809
30. Curtis BF (1893) Cases of bone implantation and transplantation for cyst of tibia, osteomyelitis cavities and ununited fractures. Am J Med Sci 106:30

31. Cutting CB, McCarthy JG (1983) Comparison of residual osseous mass between vascularized and non vascularized onlay bone transfers. Plast Reconstr Surg 72:672
32. Daniel RK (1977) Free rib transfer by microvascular anastomoses. Plast Reconstr Surg 59:737
33. Davies JB (1954) The muscle-pedicle bone graft in hip fusion. J Bone Joint Surg [Am] 36A:790
34. Doi K, Tominaga S, Shibata T (1977) Bone grafts with microvascular anastomoses of vascular pedicles. J Bone Joint Surg [Am] 59A:809
35. Doppelt SH, Tomford WW, Lucas AD, Mankin HJ (1981) Operational and financial aspects of a hospital bone bank. J Bone Joint Surg [Am] 63A:244
36. Enneking WF (1957) Histological investigation of bone transplants in immunologically prepared animals. J Bone Joint Surg [Am] 39A:597
37. Enneking WF, Burchardt H, Puhl JJ, Piotrowski G (1975) Physical and biologic aspects of repair in dog cortical bone transplants. J Bone Joint Surg [Am] 57A:232
38. Enneking WF, Eady JL, Burchardt H (1980) Autogenous cortical bone grafts in the reconstruction of segmental skeletal defects. J Bone Joint Surg [Am] 62A:1039
39. Friedlaender GE, Mankin HJ (1981) Bone banking: current methods and suggested guidelines. In: Murray D (ed) AAOS instructional course lectures, vol 30. Mosby, St Louis pp
40. Friedlaender GE, Mankin HJ, Sell KW (1981) Osteochondral allografts. Little, Brown, Boston
41. Fujimaki A, Yamauchi Y (1983) Vascularized fibular grafting for treatment of aseptic necrosis of the femoral head. Microsurgery 4:17
42. Gilbert A (1979) A free transfer of the fibula shaft. Int J Microsurg 2:100
43. Gilbert A, Judet H, Judet J, Ayatti A (1986) Microvascular transfer of the fibula for necrosis of the femoral head. Int Orthop (SICOT) 9:885
44. Goldberg VM, Heiple KG (1983) Experimental hemi-joint and whole-joint transplantation. Clin Orthop 174:43
45. Gross AE, Lavoie MV, McDermatt P, Marks P (1985) The use of allograft bone in revision of total hip arthroplasty. Clin Orthop 197:115
46. Gross AE, McKee N, Farine I, Czitrom A, Langer F (1984) Reconstruction of skeletal defects following en bloc excision of bone tumours. Current concepts of diagnosis and treatment of bone and soft tissue tumours. Springer, Berlin Heidelberg New York, pp 163
47. Groves EWH (1917) Methods and results of transplantation of bone repair of defects caused by injury or disease. Br J Surg 5:185
48. Hagerty RF, Braid HL, Bonner WM Jr, Hennigar GR, Lee WH Jr (1967) Viable and nonviable human cartilage homografts. Surg Gynecol Obstet 125:485
49. Havers C (1691) Osteologia nova, or some new observations of the bones. S Smith, London
50. Heiple KG, Chase SW, Herndon CH (1963) A comparative study of the healing process following different types of bone transplantation. J Bone Joint Surg [Am] 45A:1593
51. de Heyde A (1684) Anatomia Mytuli, Subjecta centuria observatorium. Janssonio Waesbergios, Amsterdam
52. Hubhard LF, Herndon JH, Buonanno AR (1985) Free vascularized fibula transfer for stabilization of the thoracolumbar spine. Spine 10:891
53. Huntington TW (1905) Case of bone transference. Use of a segment of fibula to supply a defect in the tibia. Ann Surg 41:249
54. Inclan A (1942) The use of preserved bone graft in orthopaedic surgery. J Bone Joint Surg [Am] 24A:81
55. Jacobson JH, Suarez EL (1960) Microsurgery in small anastomoses of small vessels. Surg Forum 11:243
56. Judet H, Gilbert A, Judet J (1981) Essai de revascularisation de la tête fémorale dans les nécroses primitives et post-traumatiques. Rev Chir Orthop 67:261
57. Jupiter JB, Bour CJ, May JW (1987) The reconstruction of defects in the femoral shaft with vascularized transfers of fibular bone. J Bone Joint Surg [Am] 69A:365

58. Kingma JJ (1960) Results of transplantation with preserved calf bone. Arch Chir Neerl 12:221
59. Kingma MJ (1967) Deep frozen calf bone. In: Delchel MJ (ed) Dixième congres de la Société Internationale de Chirurgie Orthopédique et la Traumatologie. Les publications Acta Medica Bruxelles, Paris, p 666
60. Lacroix P (1947) Organizers and the growth of bone. J Bone Joint Surg [Am] 29A:292
61. Langer F, Czitrom AA, Pritzker KP, Gross AE (1975) The immunogenicity of fresh frozen allogenic bone. J Bone Joint Surg [Am] 57A:216
62. Langer F, Gross AE (1974) Immunogenicity of allograft articular cartilage. J Bone Joint Surg [Am] 56A:297
63. van Leeuwenhoek A (1674) Microscopical observations about blood, milk, bones, the brain, spittle, cuticula, sweat, fat and tears. Philos Trans R Soc Lond 9:125
64. Levander G (1934) On the formation of new bone in bone transplantation. Acta Chir Scand 74:425
65. Lexer E (1908) Über Gelenktransplantation. Med Klin 4:815
66. Lexer E (1925) 20 Jahre Transplantationsforschung in der Chirurgie. Arch Chir 138:251
67. Lovie MJ, Duncan GM, Glasson DW (1984) The ulnar artery forearm flap. Br J Plast Surg 37:486
68. Macewen W (1881) Observations concerning transplantation on bone. Proc R Soc Lond 32:232
69. Mankin HJ, Doppelt SH, Tomford WW (1983) Clinical experience with allograft implantation. The first ten years. Clin Orthop 174:69
70. McKnee DM (1978) Microvascular bone transplantation. Clin Plast Surg 5:283–292
71. Meals RA, Lesavoy MA (1987) Vascularized free radius transfer for clavicle reconstruction concurrent with below elbow amputation. J Hand Surg [Am] 12:673
72. van Meekeren J (1668) Heel- en geneeskonstige aanmerkingen. Commelijn, Amsterdam
73. Mnaymneh W, Malinin T, Head W, Bora F, Burkhalter W, Ballard A, Zych G, Reyes F (1986) Massive osseous and osteoarticular allograft in nontumorous disorders. Contemp Orthop 13:13
74. Mnaymneh W, Malinin T, Makley T, Dick H (1985) Massive osteoarticular allografts in reconstruction of extremities following resection of tumors not requiring chemotherapy and radiation. Clin Orthop 197:76
75. O'Brien B MC (1979) Microvascular osteocutaneous transfer using the groin flap and iliac crest and the dorsalis pedis flap and second metatarsal. Br J Plast Surg 32:188
76. Olerud S, Hendriksson T, Engkvist O (1983) A free vascularized fibular graft in lengthening of the humerus with the Wagner apparatus. J Bone Joint Surg [Am] 65A:110
77. Ollier L (1867) Traité experimental et clinique de la régénération des os. Victor Mason et Fils, Paris
78. Östrup LT, Frederickson JM (1974) Distant transfer of a free living bone graft by microvascular anastomoses. An experimental study. Plast Reconstr Surg 54:274
79. Pap K, Krompecher S (1961) Arthroplasty of the knee: experimental and clinical experiences. J Bone Joint Surg [Am] 43A:523
80. Parrish FF, (1973) Allograft replacement of all or part of the end of a long bone following excision of a tumor. Report of twenty-one cases. J Bone Joint Surg [Am] 55A:1
81. Phelps AM (1891) Transplantation of tissue from lower animals to man. Med Records 39:221
82. Phemister DB (1914) The fate of transplanted bone and regenerative power of its various constituents. Surg Gynecol Obstet 19:303
83. Pho RWH (1979) Free vascularized fibular transplant for replacement of the lower radius. J Bone Joint Surg [Br] 61B:362
84. Pho RW, Levack B, Satku K, Patradul A (1985) Free vascularized fibular graft in the treatment of congenital pseudarthrosis of the tibia. J Bone Joint Surg [Br] 67B:64

85. Ray RD (1972) Vascularization of bone grafts and implants. Clin Orthop 87:43
86. Rodrigo JJ, Fuller TC, Mankin HJ (1976) Cytotoxic HLA-antibodies in patients with bone and cartilage allografts. Trans Orthop Res Soc 1:131
87. Schenk R, Willinegger H (1964) Histologie der primären Knochenheilung. Langenbecks Arch Klin Chir 308:440
88. Serafin D, Villareal-Rios A, Georgiade N (1977) A rib containing free flap to reconstruct mandibular defects. Br J Plast Surg 30:263
89. Siffert RS, Barash ES (1961) Delayed bone transplantation: an experimental study of early host-transplant relationships. J Bone Joint Surg [Am] 43A:407
90. Taylor GI (1977) Microvascular free bone transfer. Orthop Clin North Am 8:425
91. Taylor GI, Miller GDH, Ham FJ (1975) The free vascularized bone graft. A clinical extension of microvascular techniques. Plast Reconstr Surg 55:533
92. Taylor GA (1983) The current status of free vascularized bone grafts. Clin Plast Surg 10:185
93. Teissier J, Bonnel F, Allieu Y (1985) Vascularization, cellular behavior and union of vascularized bone grafts: experimental study in the rabbit. Ann Plast Surg 14:494
94. Teót L, Bosse JP, Moufarrige R, Papillon J, Beauregard G (1981) The scapula crest pedicle bone graft. Int J Microsurg 3:257
95. Tomford WW, Mankin HJ (1983) Investigational approaches to articular cartilage preservation. Clin Orthop 174:22
96. Tomford WW, Doppelt SH, Mankin HJ, Friedlaender GE (1983) 1983 Bone bank procedures. Clin Orthop 174:15
97. Tomford WW, Duff GP, Mankin HJ (1985) Experimental freezepreservation of chondrocytes. Clin Orthop 197:11
98. Turner J, Bassett CAL, Pate JW, Sawyer PN (1955) An experimental comparison of freeze-dried and frozen cortical bone graft healing. J Bone Joint Surg [Am] 37A:1197
99. Ueba Y, Fujikawa S (1983) Nine years follow-up of a vascularized fibular graft in neurofibromatosis. A case report an literature review (in Japanese). Orthop Traum Surg 26(5):595
100. Urist MR (1953) The physiological basis of bone graft surgery, with special reference to the theory of induction. Clin Orthop 1:207
101. Urist MR (ed) (1980) Fundamental and clinical bone physiology. Lippincott, Philadelphia
102. Urist MR, Delange RJ, Finerman GA (1983) Bone cell differentiation and growth factors. Science 220:680
103. Urist MR, McLean FC (1952) Osteogenic potency and new-bone formation by induction in transplants to the anterior chamber of the eye. J Bone Joint Surg [Am] 34A:443
104. Vokov MV, Mamaliev A (1976) Use of allogenous articular bone implants as substitutes for autotransplants in the adult patients. Clin Orthop 144:192
105. Von Walter P (1821) Wiedereinheilung der bei der Trapanation ausgebohrten Knochenscheibe. Journal der Chirurgie und Augen-Heilkunde 2:571
106. Weiland AJ, Kleinert HE, Kutz JE, Daniel RK (1979) Free vascularized bone grafts in surgery of the upper extremity. J Hand Surg [Am] 4:129
107. Weiland AJ (1984) Vascularized bone transfer. Instr Course Lect 33:446
108. Weiland AJ, Daniel RK (1980) Congenital pseudarthrosis of the tibia: treatment with vascularized autogenous fibular grafts. A preliminary report. John Hopkins Med J 147:89
109. Weiland AJ, Daniel RK (1982) Vascularized bone grafts. In: Green DP (ed) Operative hand surgery. Churchill Livingstone, New York, pp 877
110. Weiland AJ, Morre JR, Daniel RK (1983) Vascularized bone autografts: experience with 41 cases. Clin Orthop 174:87
111. Wood MB, Cooney WP (1984) Vascularized bone segment transfers for management of chronic osteomyelitis. Orthop Clin North Am 15:461
112. Wood MB, Cooney WP, Irons GB (1984) Posttraumatic lower extremity reconstruction by vascularized bone graft transfer. Orthopedics 7:255

113. Wood MB, Cooney WP, Irons GB (1985) Skeletal reconstruction by vascularized bone transfer: indications and results. Mayo Clin Proc 60:729
114. Wood MB (1987) Upper extremity reconstruction by vascularized bone transfers: results and complications. J Hand Surg [Am] 12A:422
115. Yoshimura M, Shimarrura K, Yoshinobu I, Yarnauchi S, Ueno T (1983) Free vascularized fibular transplant. J Bone Joint Surg [Am] 65A:1295

Biology of Bone Auto- and Allografts

Biology of Cortical Bone Graft Incorporation

H. Burchardt

Pennsylvania Regional Tissue Bank, 814 Cedar Avenue,
Scranton, Pennsylvania 18505, USA

Bone transplantation has been a common surgical procedure since the early 1900s when it was used to unite fractures, fuse joints, and repair skeletal defects. The use of autogenous bone grafts for skeletal reconstruction has changed little since that time, and the incidence of success has remained high. To understand the reasons for the success of this surgical procedure, the interacting biomechanisms of bone graft repair need to be reviewed: the correct application of transplantable bone tissues is based on knowing the biological sequences that occur from the time of transplantation to the incorporation and secondary remodeling of the graft. This presentation discusses the biological and physical characteristics of autogenous cortical bone transplantation repair as studied in an experimental model and, secondarily, makes some correlations to autogenous cortical segmental grafts in man [7, 8].

When autogenous cortical bone transplantation is performed, the bone and some of its periosteum are placed into the new site. Due to vascular severance, the bone becomes necrotic, except for some cells that may survive by diffusion of nutrients. In order for the transplant to function both physically and physiologically, the transplant must be revascularized, become united to the host, and be internally repaired by creeping substitution.

Despite these well known generalities, three fundamentally related questions needed to be addressed with respect to the segmental cortical autograft: (a) How and why is a graft weakened in time? (b) What is the relationship between graft repair and its physical strength? and (c) Is there a pattern to the graft repair process? To answer these questions, skeletally mature dogs were used as the experimental animal because of their similarity to man: man and dog have a similar microarchitecture of bone which influences the mechanism of repair; both have an epiphyseal closure mechanism which correlates with the influence of skeletal metabolic activity on the reparative process; and they have been shown to be immunogenetically similar since they are outbred species.

The fibula was chosen as the site of experimentation, because: (a) it provided a pure segment of cortical bone; (b) a segment could be excised and reinserted as an autogenous transplant, an internal control, or exchanged as an allograft in a simple reproducible fashion; (c) no internal fixation was required; (d) the animals could resume unrestricted activity within hours of transplantation, thus minimizing disuse osteoporosis; and (e) specimens could be evaluated radiographically, tested physically, and studied histologically to determine the amounts or the pattern of repair.

Bone Transplantation
Eds.: M. Aebi, P. Regazzoni

The surgical bone graft procedure involved a subperiosteal dissection: the segment is cut, inverted, and then replaced into the same skeletal defect. All wounds were closed in four layers using 2-0 chromic. Groups of dogs were maintained at various intervals of time from 2 to 96 weeks. Each dog was maintained in indoor/outdoor runs, and throughout all intervals of time each dog received tetracycline on a daily basis to label all new bone forming sites. In addition, each animal was X-rayed once every 2 weeks to define the radiographic appearance of repair and to identify any complications, such as fatigue failure, nonunion, or union occurring after 16 weeks of transplantation.

At the appropriate intervals of time, from 2 weeks to 96 weeks, the animals were sacrificed and the mechanical strength of the autografted segments were evaluated by rapid torsional loading to failure. Subsequently, the grafts were assessed for repair, using ultraviolet light for new bone formation as it was accumulated in the grafts and microradiography for cross-sectional areas and internal porosity.

The early stages of cortical graft repair have been shown to be characterized by an inflammatory response marked by vascular buds infiltrating the transplant bed, with the exposed surfaces of the transplant bathed in nutrients [1, 2, 4, 6]. By the 2nd week, the inflammatory characteristics have diminished greatly, fibrous granulation tissue becomes increasingly dominant in the transplant bed, and osteoclastic activity becomes a prominent feature. Within the confines of the transplant, osteocytic autolysis proceeds with necrosis delineated by vacant lacunae. Following the initial inflammatory response and angioneogenesis, the necrotic tissue in the narrow spaces of the haversian canal is gradually removed by invading macrophages [3, 5, 9]. An ingrowth of capillaries and, to a lesser degree, an expansion of remaining viable transplant endothelial cells occurs with the simultaneous repopulation of the marrow spaces by accompanying primitive mesenchymal tissues.

In our temporal studies with dog cortical bone transplants, resorption at 2 weeks after transplantation was found to be significantly greater than that of normal bone, increased until the 6th week, and then gradually declined to nearly normal levels at the end of 1 year [7] (Fig. 1). Spatial analyses of the transplant repair processes showed resorption to be preferentially directed to peripherally located necrotic haversian systems and the interstitial lamellae during the first 2 weeks. By the 4th week, however, resorptive activity of the cortical interior enlarged the haversian cavities with the use of a fistlike arrangement of osteoclasts, or a cutting cone. Insignificant removal of necrotic interstitial lamellae was noted, hence the resorptive activity was largely confined to pretransplanted haversian systems. When the appropriate cavity size was attained, resorption ceased, and osteoblasts appeared and refilled the spaces.

The initiation of the appositional phase of repair occurred approximately 12 weeks after transplantation and sealed off the remaining necrotic material from further osteoclastic encroachment (Fig. 2). Additional spatial studies suggested that creeping substitution of cortical bone grafts progresses transversely and parallel to the long axis of the transplanted segment. Thus, repair was found initially to be greater at the graft-host junction, and it then migrated to the midregion between the graft-host junctions.

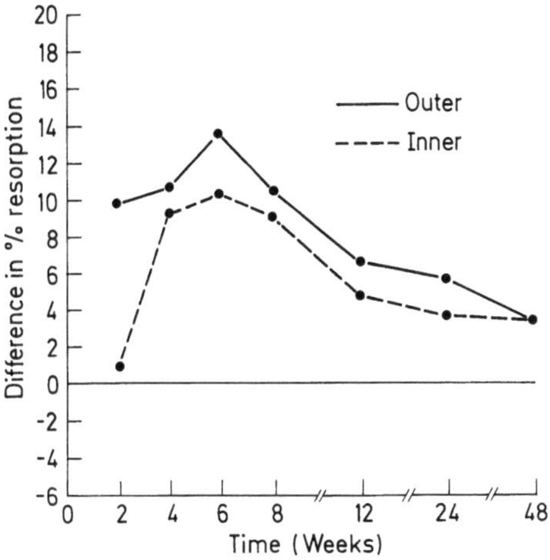

Fig. 1. Resorption of bone in inner and outer zones. The biological repair of cortical transplants is initially characterized by resorption and secondarily by apposition. During the first 2 weeks resorption in the dog fibular model is significantly elevated and peaks at 6 weeks. It then decreases and levels off, although at the end of 1 year, it is still significantly greater than normal. Note that the initial resorptive process is initiated at the periphery rather than in the interior of the graft. Once revascularization has occurred within the graft, internal resorption mirrors the activity measured at the periphery.

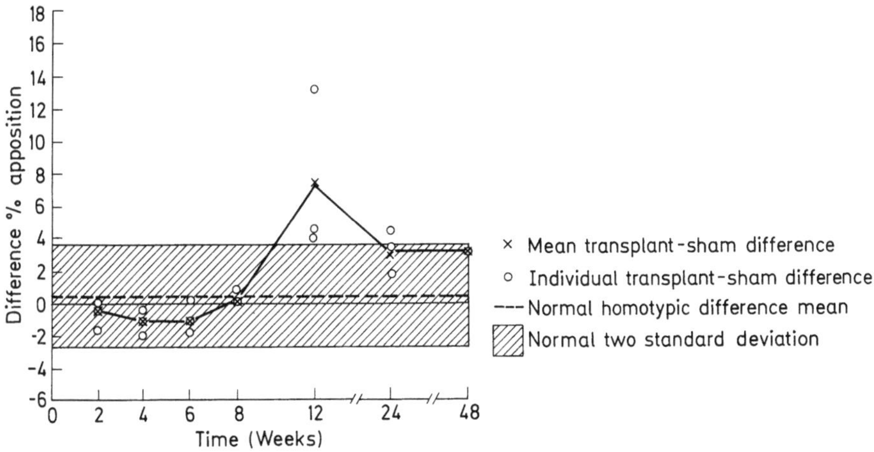

Fig. 2. Apposition of new bone in the cortical fibular graft. Appositional activity is depressed in the first 8 weeks; by the 12th week there is a rapid increase of its activity, which can be correlated with the consolidation of the graft-host junction. This subsequently decreases but remains in the upper range of normal from 24 to 48 weeks. In terms of spatial activity, apposition is equally distributed throughout the cortical graft and does not exhibit a peripheral versus an internal activity pattern as seen with resorption. *Cross-hatched area* represents ± 2.0 SD differences

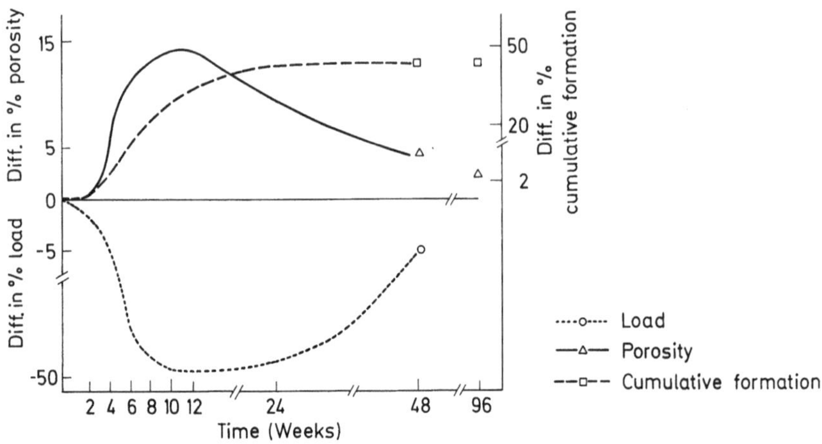

Fig. 3. The cumulative biological effects of repair and the biomechanical strength of dog segmental cortical grafts in time over 2 years. During the first 4 weeks, the biomechanical strength of the graft (*lower curve*) decreases slightly, although remaining well within normal ranges (0%–5%). Thus, the mere inertness of a graft does not significantly contribute to the weakness of a cortical graft. However, by the 6 week there is a rapid decrease in strength, which is maintained for approximately 6 months. By the end of 1 year, the strength of the graft is returned to normal, and by 2 years it is completely normal relative to the internal opposite side control and nongrafted fibula. The internal graft porosity (*solid upper curve*) is normal during the first 2 weeks, which correlates with the peripheral resorptive pattern seen in Fig. 1. It then rapidly increases as resorptive activity occurs within the cortical material and attains a peak in 6–12 weeks. This is followed by a gradual decrease for the remainder of the study, although at 48 and 96 weeks porosity within the graft is still three to four times greater than normal. The composite graph of cumulative new bone formation (*broken upper curve*) therefore illustrates that the return of cortical graft strength is associated with an incompleteness of graft repair. Porosity is three to four times greater than normal at 1 and 2 years, and less than 50% of the transplant is viable, as seen by the cumulative tetracycline-labeled new bone formation values. Hence, one may safely conclude that the incompleteness of repair is not of clinical significance since the mechanical properties of the graft are normal

The admixture of necrotic and viable bone in the cortical graft remains basically unaltered once the catabolic and anabolic stages of repair have been completed, although minor changes may in time increase the proportion of new bone to necrotic tissue. In the experimental studies with the dog fibula, the proportion of viable new bone necrotic old bone increased from 2 weeks to 6 months after transplantation; however, between 6 months and 2 years, it remained unaltered (Fig. 3). This incompleteness of cortical graft repair represents a major difference between cortical and cancellous grafts: cancellous grafts tend to be completely repaired in time, whereas cortical grafts tend to remain as admixtures of necrotic and viable bone.

Two qualifying features also were found with the dog cortical bone transplant studies: (a) the initiation of the appositional phase coincided with a consolidated graft-host junction and therefore suggested that physiologic stress may play a role in bone formation; and (b) the rate, amount, and completeness of repair were found to be greater in dogs that had more active physiologic remodeling of the skeleton than in those with less activity. This second variable in transplant repair is analogous to the clinical situation in which a child is better and more completely able to repair a skeletal injury in time than in an adult.

It is important to understand that the biomechanical strength of the bone transplant can be correlated with the process of its repair. Thus, cortical grafts are initially repaired by osteoclastic activity, which not only causes a loss of bone mass but also induces mechanical weakening through stress enhancement, with a concomitant decrease in the transplant's radiodensity. The mechanical weakening of the cortical transplant is therefore a function of the change in the graft's internal porosity: a change which is caused by the cumulative effects of increased osteoclastic and decreased osteoblastic activities. Thus, experimental bone transplants are shown to be approximately 40%–50% weaker than normal bone from 6 weeks to 6 months after transplantation, as the porosity of the transplant increases approximately 15%. By the end of the first year following transplantation, the porosity was nearly (and by the end of the second, completely) normal and mechanical strength and roentgenographic densities equal to those of normal bone (Fig. 3).

It is important for clinician and patient to understand the biomechanical changes that occur as an effect of creeping substitutional repair in order to anticipate or protect the segmental transplants at the critical time when the resorptive phase has outstripped the appositional phase. It is not known precisely when these critical reparative phases occur in humans, but the time of their appearance probably varies as a function of age, physiologic repair capacity, and the type, size, and location of the transplant.

To correlate the experimental findings with clinical radiographic observations, human cortical graft materials were collected over a period of time at the university of Florida [8]. In a number of patients, ultraviolet light and microradiographic evaluation were performed similar to the studies in the dog model.

Ultraviolet light photography, microradiography, and hematoxylin and eosin (H&E) histological evaluations showed that the mechanism of cortical bone graft repair in man and dog is the same. The only apparent and significant difference between the two species was the length of time required for the repair process to be complete: the repair process takes twice as long in humans.

Extrapolation of the biologic data to the physical strength characteristics of human cortical grafts suggests that a human autograft should lose about one-half of its strength during the first 6 months, persist for another 6 months, and be slowly reversed during the 2nd year. In time, the admixture of viable and necrotic bone in both species approximates the strength of normal bone. The validity of this extrapolation of the biologic information to physical characteristics is reinforced by the observation that, in man, fatigue failure occurs between 6 and 18 months post-transplantation, and that thereafter fatigue failures are very infrequent.

As a final consideration for the mechanism of repair in segmental cortical bone grafts in patients, it was shown that rigid immobilization influences or promotes graft-host union; protection of the graft must be considered during the stage in which porosity may be significantly elevated; and, lastly, clinicians need to consider the geometry (size, shape, and quantity) of the transplant relative to the area grafted and the function that it should serve.

References

1. Abbott LC, Schottstaedt ER, Saunders JB et al. (1947) The evaluation of cortical and cancellous bone as grafting material: a clinical and experimental study. J Bone Joint Surg [Am] 29:381
2. Albee FH (1923) Fundamentals in bone transplantation: experiences in three thousand bone graft operations. JAMA 81:1429
3. Anderson KJ, LeCocq JF, Abeson WH et al. (1964) End-point results of processed heterogenous, autogenous and homogenous bone transplants in the human: a histological study. Clin Orthop 33:220
4. Arora BK, Lastain DM (1964) Sex chromatin as a cellular label of osteogenesis by bone grafts. J Bone Joint Surg [Am] 46A:1269
5. DeBruyn PPH, Kabisch WT (1955) Bone formation by fresh and frozen autogenous and homogenous transplants of bone, bone marrow and periosteum. Am J Anat 96:375
6. Deleu J, Truets J (1965) Vascularization of bone grafts in the anterior chamber of the eye. J Bone Joint Surg [Am] 47:319–329
7. Enneking WF, Burchardt H, Prehl JJ et al. (1975) Physical and biological aspects of repair in dog cortical bone transplants. J Bone Joint Surg [Am] 57A:232
8. Enneking WF, Eady J, Burchardt H (1980) Autogenous cortical bone grafts in the reconstruction of segmental skeletal defects. J Bone Joint Surg [Am] 62A:1039
9. Richany SF, Sprinz H, Kraner K et al. (1965) The role of the diaphyseal medulla in the repair and regeneration of the femoral shaft in the adult cart. J Bone Joint Surg [Am] 47A:1565

Fate of Vascularized Bone Grafts

A. J. Weiland

Greater Chesapeake Hand Specialists, Wye Financial Center, 1400 Front Avenue, Lutherville, Maryland 21093, USA

Introduction

Advances in the field of microsurgery over the past decade have made it possible to provide a continuing circulation to bone grafts used in the reconstruction of extremities with massive segmental bone loss following trauma or secondary to tumor resection. In order to appreciate the significance of transferring segmental autogenous bone grafts on vascular pedicles in reconstructive surgery, the surgeon must have an understanding of the methods traditionally used and, more importantly, their historical development.

The clinical application of free vascularized bone grafts has raised many questions concerning the various factors affecting survival of whole bone segments transferred to distant recipient sites with reconstitution of blood supply by microvascular anastomoses. Over the past 9 years, our laboratory investigations have attempted to evaluate the effect of ischemia time on osteocyte and osteoblast survival, the effect of different storage media and perfusion techniques, the significance of preserving the medullary versus the periosteal circulation, and the role of bone scintigraphy in evaluating viability of these grafts. Additional protocols have evaluated the feasibility of performing vascularized epiphyseal plate transfers; and studies comparing vascularized bone autografts, conventional autografts, and fresh allografts have been performed. Over the past 2 years, efforts have concentrated on performing vascularized bone allograft transplantations in a genetically defined model.

Early Development

The introduction of bone grafting techniques in the late nineteenth century by Barth [8] led to their use in the treatment of nonunions [1, 16, 26, 45], arthrodesis of joints, the filling of bone cavities secondary to infection, replacement of bone loss secondary to trauma and following tumor resection, and, finally, the replacement of joint surface [25, 29, 35, 58, 61, 62, 65, 75–77, 85, 91, 105]. The various techniques employed have evolved into the following: (a) massive autogenous corticocancellous bone obtained from the ilium, tibia, or fibula [1, 16]; (b) transference of whole bone segments [26, 51]; (c) allograft bone transplants [34, 61, 65, 75–77, 103]; and (d) free vascularized bone grafts [94–98, 106–108].

Bone Transplantation
Eds.: M. Aebi, P. Regazzoni

Autogenous Bone Grafts

There is little doubt that autogenous transplants are better tolerated by the host than other types of bone grafts [2, 38, 47, 52, 64, 80]. However, the mechanisms involved in bone formation by autogenous grafts are still unresolved. Basically, two concepts have evolved. One theory is that new bone formation results from the functional activity of osteogenic cells which survive in the graft [39]. However, based on observations of bone formation by these grafts, including the fact that only a small percentage of osteocytes and osteoblasts survive transplantation, several authors have proposed another mechanism which may be referred to as the "metaplasia theory" [9, 52, 57, 58, 86, 87, 103]. This theory includes the hypothesis that bone transformation occurs under the influence of osteogenic-inducing substances which diffuse from the transplant site into the host's connective tissue [35]. Most investigators now agree that both mechanisms are involved.

Since surviving cells in autogenous grafts are entirely dependent upon nourishment from the surrounding bed directly after transfer, the superiority of autogenous cancellous bone grafts (directly related to their open structure, which facilitates diffusion of nutrient substances necessary for osteocyte and osteoblast survival) is readily appreciated. In addition, this open structure permits ingrowth of vessels from the host bed which carry undifferentiated mesenchymal cells that subsequently differentiate into osteogenic cells. Dense, cortical bone acts as a barrier to diffusion, thereby inhibiting cell survival. Since the vast majority of cells in autogenous grafts do not survive transplantation, they must be replaced and repaired by new bone.

The replacement of dead bone by new, living bone was described by Barth in 1895 [8] and Marchand in 1900 [67] as "creeping substitution" (*schleichender Ersatz*). This process indicates the penetration of newly formed bone directly into the old bone and requires simultaneous removal of the old bone and deposition of new bone at the site of contact. The term "creeping substitution" was introduced in the English literature by Phemister in 1914 [78]. The ultimate incorporation of autogenous grafts requires an adequate circulation in the recipient bed upon which new bone formation can occur in the presence of cells with an osteogenic capacity.

Allograft Bone Transplants

Although it has been shown repeatedly that allografts and xenografts are not as effective in providing an environment conductive to osteogenesis as fresh autogenous bone, the use of autogenous grafts has obvious limitations based on the amount of bone available to reconstruct large defects and their ability to replace articular surfaces [47]. The techniques of massive resection of bone tumors and subsequent reconstruction of large bone defects with allograft transplantation have been reported by Ottolenghi [75], D'Aubigne et al. [34], Mankin et al. [65], Lexer [59–62], Parrish [76, 77], and Volkov [104]. The complications associated with these procedures include nonunion between the graft and the recipient bone, resorption, collapse of articular segments, and fracture of the graft in addition to prolonged immobilization of 8–24 months required for incorporation of the graft.

In an attempt to reduce the immunogenicity of allografts, several investigators have demonstrated a reduction in antigenic properties in freeze-dried allografts [24, 32, 47–49]. This process, however, while resulting in a reduction in the antigenicity of the allograft, kills the osteoprogenitor cells in the graft. Allografts are reported to be inferior to autografts during the early stages of repair due to the cellular response of the host tissue as well as to the impairment of vascularization of the graft [38].

Pedicle Bone Grafts

As early as 1905, Huntington recognized the advantages of utilizing a bone graft with its own nutrient blood supply intact as a vascularized bone graft in the reconstruction of large tibial defects [51]. In most cases, there is little doubt that the ideal bone graft is an autogenous graft which remains organized and alive, and which defies resorption and maintains its original size and structural characteristics.

Since an unimpaired microcirculation is the indispensable basis for the continued life and function of all bone cells, it is obvious that this can only be achieved by preservation or immediate reconstitution of the primary blood supply to the bone graft. This concept of a vascularized "living" bone graft is not a new one. Regional osteomusculocutaneous flaps have been used as vehicles for sections of rib or clavicle, and composite island flaps containing underlying rib have been transferred on long, intact vascular pedicles.

Blood Supply of Cortical Bone

Several groups of arteries are usually described as being engaged in the blood supply to cortical bone. Well-defined nutrient arteries penetrate the cortex through the nutrient foramen and nutrient canal. After entering the diaphysis, the nutrient artery divides into ascending and descending branches to become the medullary arteries. These vessels have radially oriented branches which supply the diaphyseal cortex by further branching in a longitudinal direction [99]. Epiphyseal and metaphyseal arteries are found at the ends of long bones and supply their respective areas. Finally, the bones are surrounded by a periosteal vascular bed emerging from the vessels which supply the neighboring muscles. From the studies of Trueta and Caladias [101],Rhinelander [81], and Johnson [54], it is evident that the flow of blood through cortical bone depends predominantly on an intact medullary blood supply while the periosteal arteries play a minor role in direct cortical nutrition. Under normal circumstances, arterial blood flow passes centrifugally from the medullary system into the cortical arterioles and into the periosteal system [18]. Venous drainage most likely occurs in a centripetal direction [99], although this point is somewhat controversial. In pathologic or ischemic situations, blood flow may be reversed; a centripetal, periosteal supply then assumes the role of a collateral circulatory system [18].

Microsurgery

Carrell's classic paper on "Results of the Transplantation of Blood Vessels, Organs, and Limbs," published in 1908, heralded the birth of vascular surgery. He observed that:

> The idea of replacing diseased organs by sound ones, of putting back an amputated limb, or even of grafting a new limb on a patient having undergone an amputation is doubtless very old. The performance of such operations, however, was completely prevented by the lack of method for uniting vessels and, thus, reestablishing a normal circulation through the transplanted structure. The feasibility of these grafts depended on the development of the technique [28].

Following World War II, the first vascular stapling machine was developed in Russia by Androsov [6]. Various mechanical devices were designed and tested (Holt and Lewis [50]; Nakayama et al. [69]; Eadie and DeTakats [37]. Jacobson and Suarez pioneered microvascular surgery by demonstrating the value of the operating microscope in 1960 [53]. Salmon and Assimocopoulos [88], Buncke and Schultz [21–23], and Cobbett [30] were responsible for the improvement in instrumentation and early experimental work in free vascularized tissue transfer [3–5]. The first clinically successful transfer of an island flap by microvascular anastomoses was reported by Daniel and Taylor in 1973 [33]. In the ensuing years, the scope of free tissue transfer has expanded rapidly to include free muscle transfers [66, 93].

Taylor in 1975 reported the first clinically successful free bone graft with microvascular anastomoses in which a fibular segment was transferred from the contralateral leg to reconstruct a large tibial defect [94, 95]. Similarly, vascularized rib grafts were used for treatment of a nonunion of a mandible following radical resection of a tumor [89]. Free osteocutaneous flaps consisting of the rib and overlying soft tissue have been transferred by Buncke [21] and O'Brien [74], and Taylor has reported on the one-stage repair of a compound leg defect with an osteocutaneous flap from the groin [98]. Weiland, Daniel, and Riley have extended the application of free vascularized bone grafts to the treatment of malignant or aggressive bone tumors [106, 107]. The advantages of transferring segmental autogenous bone grafts on vascular pedicles for the treatment of upper extremity lesions have also been reported [108].

Vascularized Bone Grafts

The preceding sections have attempted to convey an appreciation of the traditional methods of bone grafting and to provide some insight into the microcirculation of bone and the emergence of the field of reconstructive microsurgery. In selected patients, free vascularized bone grafts offer significant advantages over conventional methods of treatment since a massive segment of bone along with its accompanying nutrient vessels can be detached from its donor site and transferred to a distant recipient site with preservation of the nutrient blood supply by microvascular anastomoses to recipient vessels. With the nutrient blood supply preserved, osteocytes and osteoblasts in the graft can survive, and healing of the graft to the recipient bone is facilitated without the usual replacement of the graft by "creeping substitution". Thus, the surgeon can achieve more rapid stabilization of bone fragments separated by a large defect without sacrificing viability. This is especially significant when the defect is situated in a highly traumatized or irradiated area with significant scarring and relative avascularity precluding incorporation of conventional bone grafts.

The fibula, rib, and iliac crest, with the latter incorporated into a free osteocutaneous flap from the groin, are the free bone transfers which have been employed most frequently as vascularized bone grafts. The medullary vascular supply to the fibula arises as a branch of the peroneal artery and enters the fibula in the proximal one-third of the bone. The venous drainage closely parallels the arterial supply and occurs through the venae comitantes of the peroneal artery and medullary sinusoidal system. The medullary vascular supply to the rib arises as a nutrient branch of the posterior intercostal artery, but recent experimental evidence from our laboratoy suggests that it is not necessary to preserve the nutrient blood supply to the rib, and that vascularized rib transfers survive equally on their periosteal or medullary blood supply [105]. While a comparable nutrient blood flow to the iliac crest does not exist, Taylor and Watson [98] have demonstrated with injection studies of the superficial circumflex iliac artery that adequate blood flow to the osseous portion of the osteocutaneous groin flap may be present. However, there is some question as to the validity of these studies, and Taylor most recently has been basing this flap on the deep circumflex iliac artery, with more favorable evidence both experimentally and clinically that the nutrient blood flow to the bone is significantly better than with the superficial circumflex iliac arter [96, 97].

Clinical Experience

Since 1975 we have performed vascularized bone grafts in 96 patients (87 free fibular transfers and 9 osteocutaneous groin flaps). There has been no significant postoperative donor site morbidity in any patient. Patients underwent bone scanning from 24 to 48 h postoperatively and again 6 weeks following surgery. The scans revealed uptake in the graft in each patient. Arteriograms performed 6 weeks postoperatively in the first eight free fibular transfers showed patent anastomoses in seven cases. Eight of the patients who had vascularized fibular grafts ultimately underwent amputation because of failure of the wound to heal, while one of the patients with an osteocutaneous groin flap required amputation because of flap failure. Many of the patients in this series would have been subjected to amputation if the techniques of vascularized bone transfers were not available since conventional techniques had, in most instances, been exhausted.

Laboratory Investigations

Personal involvement with the clinical application of vascularized bone grafts and pertinent questions raised by orthopedic colleagues regarding the biological behavior of these grafts prompted the design of experimental protocols over the past 9 years to examine the fate of vascularized bone grafts.

A summary of experience to date and discussion of its significance will follow. We found the rib to be useful as an experimental model in our early studies because it is formed by enchondral bone formation and has essentially the same characteristics as long bones in terms of the nutrient blood supply [31, 100]. Therefore, in five of the studies the canine rib was employed as the vascularized bone graft model while the fibula was used in the remaining protocols, except for the two studies with vascularized bone allograft transplantation, in a genetically defined rat model in which whole knee transplants were performed to a heterotopic site.

Effects of Different Storage Media and Perfusion. The question of whether or not to perfuse grafts in microvascular composite tissue transfers has not yet been solved to satisfaction, although most authors [43, 63, 68, 69] regard this as unnecessary and even dangerous, with risk of mechanical damage and increased endothelial edema to the vessels supplying the graft. The aim of this investigation was to evaluate the effect of three different storage media and graft perfusion on osteocyte and osteoblast survival in free composite bone grafts revascularized by microvascular anastomoses. Evaluation of graft survival at 2 weeks demonstrated that storage of the graft in chilled (+5 °C) physiological sodium chloride or Collins-Terasaki solution resulted in greater survival of osteocytes and osteoblasts than with storage in chilled BGJb solution or in room temperature air. Both chilled sodium chloride and Collins-Terasaki solution are superior to BGJb solution and storage of composite bone grafts in room air in terms of graft survival when revascularized by microvascular anastomoses. In addition, perfusion of vascularized grafts with various storage media resulted in significantly poorer graft survival when compared to the nonperfused specimens [10]. These findings could be explained by endothelial damage secondary to perfusion. Bone graft viability was assessed by fluorochrome bone labeling, microradiography, and routine histology.

Effects of Prolonged Ischemia Time. The clinical application of free vascularized bone grafts in the treatment of large segmental defects of long bones often requires an ischemia time of 3–6 h before circulation of the graft is reestablished. Puranen [79] has shown that conventional bone grafts undergo massive osteocyte death after 1 h exposure to room air or 2–3 h after storage in physiological sodium chloride solution. Other authors have published conflicting data [27, 42]. The aim of this study was to investigate the effect of prolonged ischemia time on osteocyte and osteoblast survival in bone grafts revascularized by microvascular anastomoses [11]. Bone viability was evaluated by using histological techniques as well as fluorochrome bone labeling. Our experiment showed that the bone marrow, the osteocytes, and the osteoblasts could survive completely up to 25 h of ischemia when stored in a chilled (+5 °C) Collins-Terasaki solution.

Importance of Medullary versus Periosteal Circulation. Different opinions exist as to whether the entire cortex of long bone in the normal situation is supplied exclusively by medullary arteries or by a combination of both medullary and periosteal arteries. Trueta and others have shown that the outer third of the cortex is dependent upon the periosteal blood supply, which flows in a centripetal fashion, while medullary arteries with a centrifugal blood flow supply the inner two-thirds

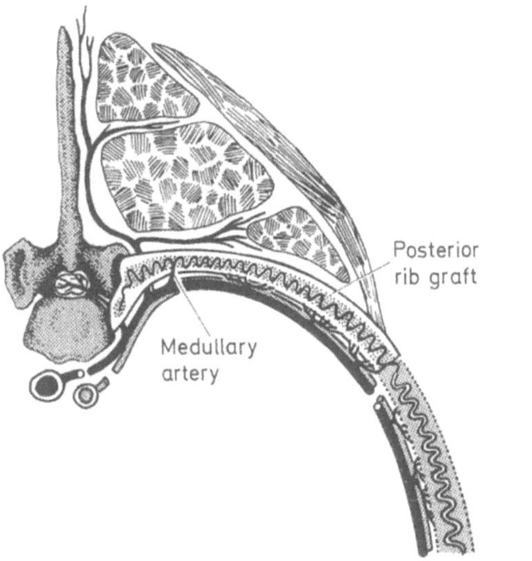

Fig. 1. Posterior rib graft

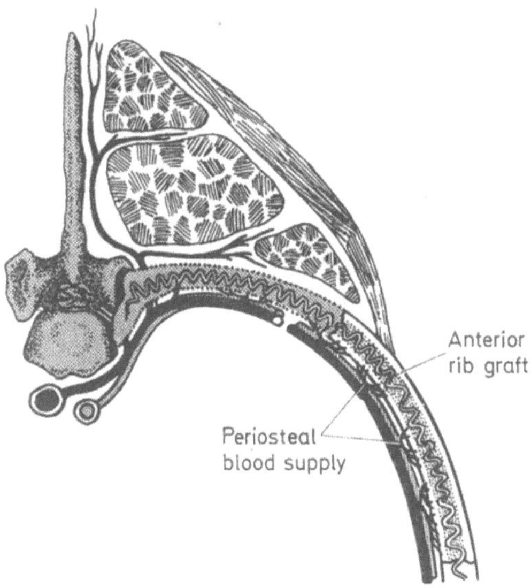

Fig. 2. Posterior lateral segmental graft

[41, 54, 82–84, 101]. On the other hand, Brookes et al. [18, 19], concluded that the blood flow throughout the compact bone is centrifugal, predominantly depending upon an intact medullary blood supply.

Two different types of vascularized rib grafts are presently used in clinical practice and as experimental models for investigations on free microvascular bone transfer: the posterior rib graft, including both medullary and periosteal blood supply to the bone (Fig. 1), and the posterior lateral segmental graft, supplied by periosteal vessels alone (Fig. 2). Complete survival of bone after successful revascularization of the posterior type of graft is well established, but this graft has the disadvantage of a complicated dorsal dissection which has limited clinical use. Instead, many microsurgeons have utilized the posterior lateral rib segment, which is easy and safe to excise although its viability and adequate microcirculation has not yet been confirmed.

In nine large dogs, the viability and vascularity of bone after transfer of the two types of bone grafts were compared by histological methods, fluorochrome bone labeling, microangiography, and technetium scintigraphy [13]. The grafts were transferred to the subcutaneous fat tissue in the groin where blood supply was reconstituted by microvascular anastomoses to local donor vessels. The results suggest that a bone transplant with revascularization of periosteal vessels only established a collateral circulation to medullary vessels, and that there is no difference in viability of the two kinds of grafts. This study demonstrated that the preservation of the periosteal blood supply alone can result in bone graft survival even when the graft is placed in a poorly vascularized bed.

In a parallel study, bone grafts with an intact medullary and periosteal blood supply were compared to bone grafts with only a periosteal supply intact with respect to the graft's ability to participate in healing towards recipient bone investigated in 21 adult mongrel dogs [12]. It was demonstrated that bone grafts with both medullary and periosteal blood supplies survived completely but were partially resorbed with time. The bone resorption observed can be explained by a relative hyperemia and hyperoxia in the posterior rib grafts. High oxygen concentration has been shown to cause bone resorption in vitro and supports the observation of Brookes et al., that hyperemia causes cancellous bone formation in cortical bone [20, 40, 90].

Periosteally supplied bone grafts demonstrated less resorption but showed, in some grafts, bone marrow necrosis and partial loss of osteocytes. Osteoblasts survived equally well in both groups. No difference in the ability to participate in healing to a recipient bone defect could be demonstrated although microangiograms revealed significant differences in the medullary vasculature at the host-graft junctions in these two types of grafts.

The question of whether to preserve the medullary blood supply when transferring whole bone segments by microvascular anastomoses is significant with respect to possible donor site selection. These studies have shown that bone grafts with an intact medullary and/or periosteal supply will survive transplantation and participate in healing to a recipient defect equally well.

Value of Bone Scintigraphy in Assessing Bone Graft Viability. Bone scintigrams have been used to evaluate the fate of autogenous and allogenous grafts both clinically [15, 56] and experimentally [17, 55, 92, 100]. More recently, scintigrams involving technetium 99 diphosphonate have been used to evaluate the survival of free revascularized bone grafts [7, 21, 36, 44, 46, 105, 106]. Clinical experience has, however, raised doubts about the validity of bone scintigraphy as a method for evaluating whether or not a bone is completely revascularized.

The aim of this study was to investigate the uptake of ^{99m}Tc methylene diphosphonate anastomoses (Fig. 3), in conventional autogenous bone grafts (Fig. 4), and periosteal grafts (Fig. 5) placed in different recipient beds [14].

The value of bone scintigraphy in the assessment of anastomotic patency and bone cell viability in free bone grafts revascularized by microanastomoses was evaluated in 27 dogs. The dogs were divided into three different groups, and scin-

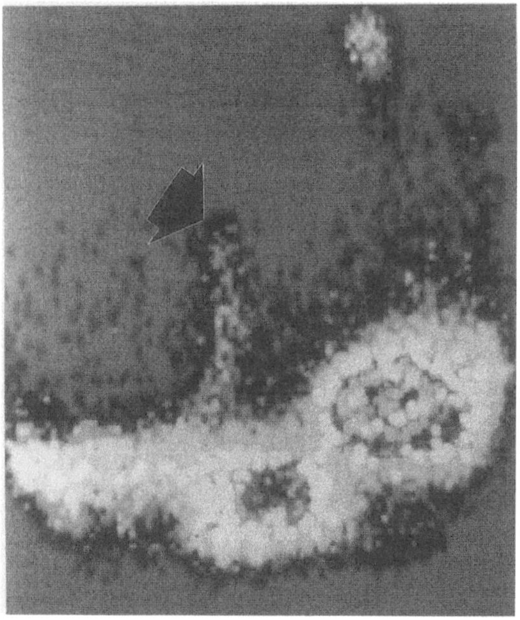

Fig. 3. Vascularized graft

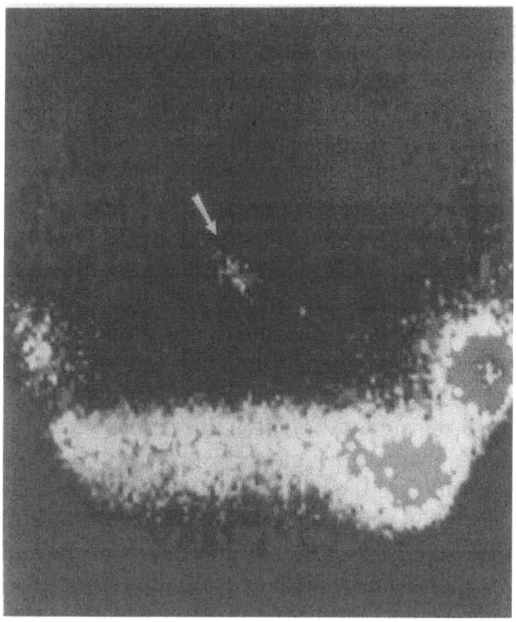

Fig. 4. Nonvascularized graft

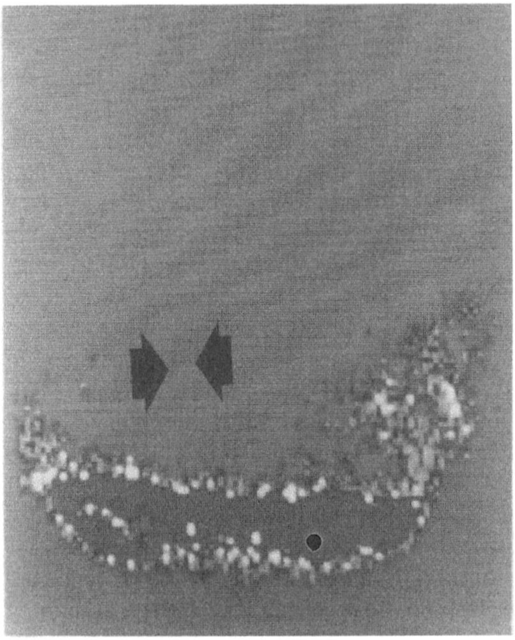

Fig. 5. Periosteal graft

tigraphy was carried out using technetium-labeled methylene diphosphonate in composite bone grafts revascularized by microvascular anastomoses, conventional autogenous bone grafts, and periosteal grafts placed in different recipient beds. The viability of the different grafts was evaluated by histologic examination and fluorescent microscopy after triple labeling with oxytetracycline on the 1st postoperative day, alizarin complexone on the 4th postoperative day, and DCAF on the 11th postoperative day. A positive scintiscan within the 1st week following surgery indicated patent microvascular anastomoses, and histological study and fluorescent microscopy confirmed that bone throughout the graft was viable. A positive scintiscan 1 week after surgery or later does not necessarily indicate microvascular patency or bone cell survival because new bone formed by creeping substitution on the surface of a dead bone graft can result in this finding.

This study demonstrated that bone scintigraphy is often unreliable when it is used to determine the viability of bone grafts. This may be especially true when positive scintiscans are considered to indicate the viability of massive allografts in view of our finding that a thin sleeve of new bone on the cortical surface of the dead graft can result in a positive scintiscan although the major portion of the graft is not viable. Scintiscans are equally unreliable in evaluating free vascularized bone grafts if they are performed later than 1 week postoperatively. However, if it is performed within the 1st week, a positive scintiscan indicates microvascular patency and the probability that osteocytes and osteoblasts are alive. If an early scintiscan is negative, patent microvascular anastomoses are unlikely.

Microvascular Epiphyseal Plate Transplantation. Clinical transplantation of nonvascularized epiphyseal growth plates (Fig. 6) has given variable and usually un-

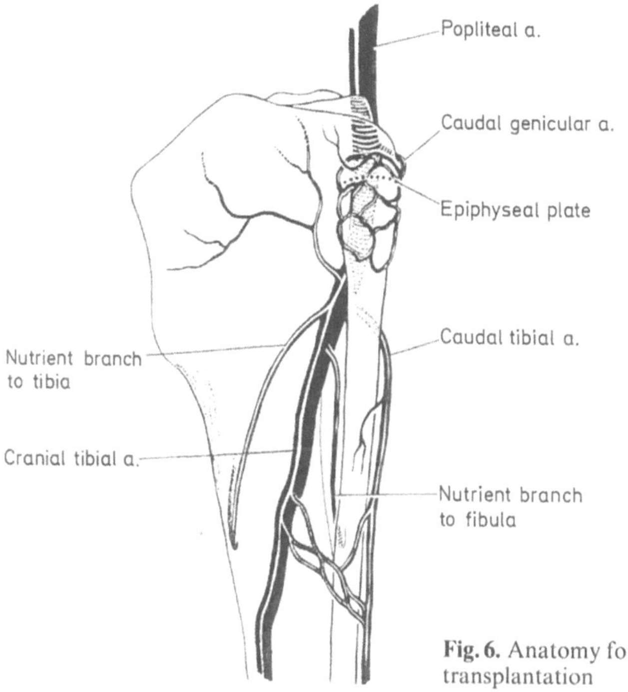

Fig. 6. Anatomy for epiphyseal plate transplantation

satisfactory results. The ability to perform vascularized epiphyseal plate transplantation to correct growth disturbances resulting from congenital deformity, trauma, infection, or following tumor excision in the growing child would have significant application in reconstructive surgery of the musculoskeletal system. To create a model for epiphyseal growth plate transplantation by microvascular technique, a well-defined donor site was established. Dissection of latex-injected adult and juvenile dogs established the vascular supply to the proximal canine fibula. By isolating 7 cm of proximal fibula on the popliteal vessels, the nutrient supply to the epiphysis, metaphysis, and diaphysis is retained. This model preserves the nutrient arterial supply to the fibula originating from the cranial tibial artery, the caudal tibial artery, and the small blood vessels from these to the epiphysis. Perfusion of the graft through the defined vascular pedicle was confirmed using ^{141}Ce-labeled microspheres. The results showed a perfusion of the established graft which was as great or greater than the control, unoperated side. It was concluded from this preliminary study that the technique described for isolation can be used for developing a model for vascularized transplantation of growth cartilage in canines [72].

To evaluate the feasibility of transplanting vascularized epiphyseal plates while maintaining normal growth in the recipient site, 22 puppies from known, large breeds were divided into one control and three experimental groups of four animals each and one long-term group of six animals [70]. The control group underwent insertion of a radiopaque marker in the fibular metaphysis bilaterally; in addition, a fibular osteotomy was performed on one side. In the experimental groups, a fibular switch was carried out selecting one fibula as the vascularized graft and the other as a nonvascularized graft. Both groups were evaluated using serial roentgenograms, histology, fluorescent bone labeling, and microangiography. At each of the time periods of 1 week, 6 weeks, 3 months, 6 months, and 7 months postoperatively, animals from each group were sacrificed. Continuous growth was observed in the vascularized epiphyseal transplants and the controls with no statistical difference noted, whereas the nonvascularized transplants exhibited considerably less or no growth. Vascularized transplants demonstrated an average of 21.2 mm increase in length while nonvascularized transplants showed 6.6 mm. Histology, fluorochrome bone labeling, and microangiography confirmed continued viability of the vascularized epiphyseal transplants in contrast to the nonvascularized transplants.

While this experiment has shown that it is possible to transplant a physis containing a vascularized graft from its normal site to the contralateral, mirror-image counterpart while maintaining normal growth capacity, the application of this technique clinically is minimal. Further investigations to determine how a transplanted growth plate reacts when transferred to a heterotopic anatomical site with altered stress loads are necessary before microvascular transfer of epiphyseal plates can be considered clinically applicable.

Heterotopic Microvascular Growth Plate Transplantation. The short-term response of the proximal fibular epiphysis to heterotopic microvascular transfer was evaluated in eight puppies of a pointer/foxhound cross and compared to orthotopically transferred controls. Autoradiographs of the physes cultured in [^{3}H]thymidine indicated continued proliferation of the growth cartilage in all revascularized transfers at the time of death 6 weeks postoperatively. However, the nonvascularized orthotopic controls did not incorporate the radioactive labels. Fluorescent bone labels were incorporated in parallel bands in the metaphyseal bone demonstrating linear bone growth in the vascularized transfers. Additional evidence for the viability of the transferred growth cartilage was obtained with histologic sections stained with hematoxylin and eosin and safranin-O. Roentgenograms and volume measurements showed a tendency towards hypertrophy of the heterotopic transfers [73].

To further evaluate the long-term reconstructive potential of heterotopic microvascular transplantation of skeletal growth plates, the distal radius was resected in two series of puppies of a known, large breed and substituted with a microsurgically revascularized transplant from the proximal fibula. Evaluation was conducted through serial roentgenograms, goniometric registration of joint mobility, volume measurements, histology, and fluorescent bone labeling. In the first series, development of neuropathic-like destruction of the weight-bearing graft ensued in the majority of the animals. In the second series, prolonged protection from weight-bearing inhibited this destruction and resulted in hypertrophy of the revascularized epiphyseal end of the transplant but clearly reduced longitudinal growth, with only one transplant exhibiting longitudinal growth that exceeded 50% of the value for the control.

This experiment demonstrated that heterotopically transplanted skeletal growth plates possess a capacity for hypertrophy under the influence of increased loads but a clearly reduced capacity for longitudinal growth. Whether this adaptability is sufficient to allow microvascular transplantation of growth plates to become a clinically useful procedure remains unknown. Further investigation concerning transplanted epiphyses and their reaction to altered loads is indicated, in addition to studies concerning the possible programmed growth inherent in physes in different anatomical locations prior to the clinical application of vascularized epiphyseals transfers [71].

Comparison of Autografts, Fresh Allografts, and Free Vascularized Bone Grafts. An experimental model was developed to compare the efficacy of free vascularized bone grafts, conventional segmental autografts, matchstick autografts, and fresh segmental allografts in terms of their ability to reconstruct a 7-cm segmental diaphyseal defect in the canine femur (Fig. 7) [109]. Forty-five, adult mongrel dogs were studied and followed for 6–12 months prior to sacrifice. This evaluation included radiologic assessment of graft incorporation and hypertrophy, histology, and biomechanical testing. These studies indicated that microsurgically revascularized autografts were superior to all other groups in terms of early incorporation, hypertrophy, and the highest mechanical strength to failure. Union of the graft to the recipient femur was achieved by 6 months in 25 of 26 autografts, and no difference in union rate was seen within the autograft group. However, only two of five allografts achieved bony union during this time interval. Arteriography, microangiography, fluorochrome and histologic studies all supported the concept that microsurgically revascularized grafts, when successful, maintain their viability. However, the premise that all osteocytes survive in a successfully revascularized bone graft is open to question. While decalcified sections showed

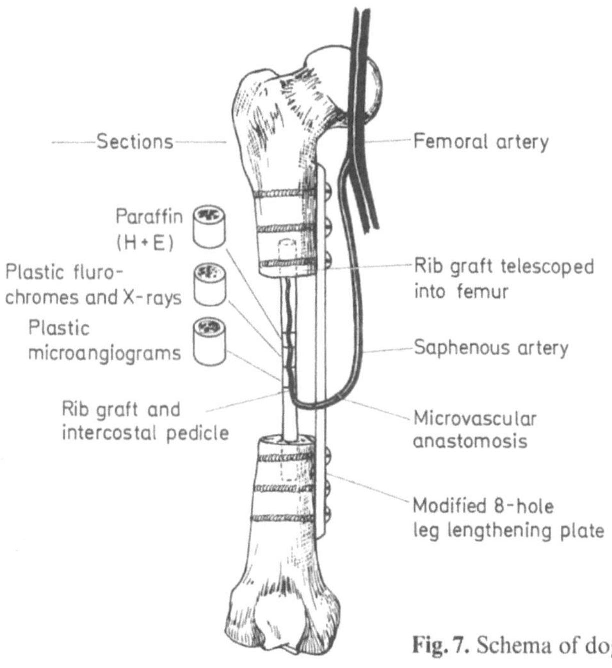

Fig. 7. Schema of dog model

that all microsurgically revascularized grafts maintain normal viability in the central marrow and cancellous portions when compared to the other three groups, the viability of cortical bone in the vascularized autograft was less clear. Undecalcified fluorochrome sections suggested that circulation was not preserved in portions of the cortex. Revascularization of the nonvascularized autograft was complete at 6 months while, in the avascular allograft, the process was not complete at 6 months.

The animal model employed in this study enabled us to evaluate the efficacy of avascular autografts, avascular matchstick autografts, fresh or vascular block allografts, and microsurgically revascularized autografts in the reconstruction of a 7-cm segmental bone defect created in the dog femur. Of the three most commonly used bone grafting techniques employed to reconstruct massive bone defects, the avascular autograft and the avascular matchstick autograft are clearly superior to the avascular allograft. The two types of avascular autografts behave similarly while the allografts were inferior with respect to delayed or absent incorporation and frequent bone resorption. The autografts revascularized by microsurgical techniques demonstrated a high rate of vascular patency and bone survival especially in the central portions of the graft. Vascularized grafts were more successful than the other three types in terms of early bone union, hypertrophy, and mechanical strength to failure.

Vascularized Bone Allograft Transplantation in a Genetically Defined Rat Model. A heterotopic subcutaneous model for experimental vascularized bone allograft transplantation has been developed (Figs. 8, 9). This model uses genetically defined rats and allows serial assessment of graft viability. The reliability of this model has been proven by successful isograft transplantation.

This model was used to study the effect of matching at the major histocompatibility complex on vascularized bone allograft survival. Whereas grafts transplanted across a minor histocompatibility barrier survived until sacrifice, grafts transplanted across a major histocompatibility barrier were victims of an acute rejection process between 1 and 2 weeks. This study therefore showed genetic disparity to be a critical determinant of vascularized bone allograft survival. It indicates that primary vascularized bone allografts are as susceptible to rejection as heart and kidney allografts. For these reasons, it can be anticipated that genetic matching will be important in clinical vascularized bone allograft transplantation.

The model used in this study should be useful for obtaining further fundamental immunologic information concerning vascularized bone allograft transplantation.

A Histological and Histochemical Analysis of the Acute Rejection of Vascularized Bone Allografts. Using a proven reliable, genetically defined rat model, a systematic, detailed histological and histochemical analysis of the acute rejection of vascularized bone allografts was performed. A total of 160 grafts including vascularized and nonvascularized isografts, vascularized and nonvascularized allografts transplanted across a strong histocompatibility barrier, and vascularized bone allografts transplanted across a weak histocompatibility barrier were performed; specimens were harvested at intervals up to 12 weeks.

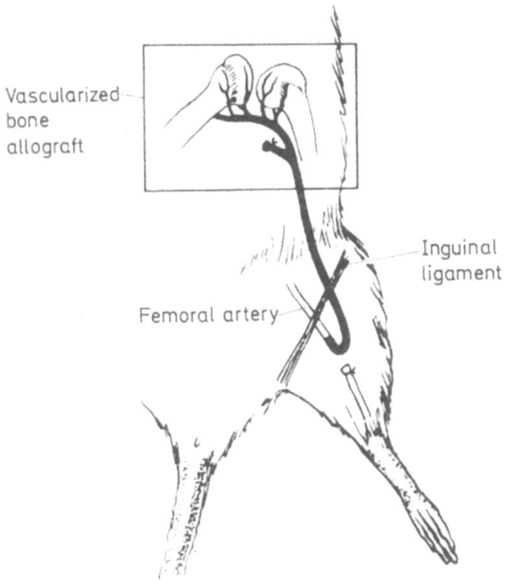

Fig. 8. Heterotopic model for vascularized rat knee allograft transplantation

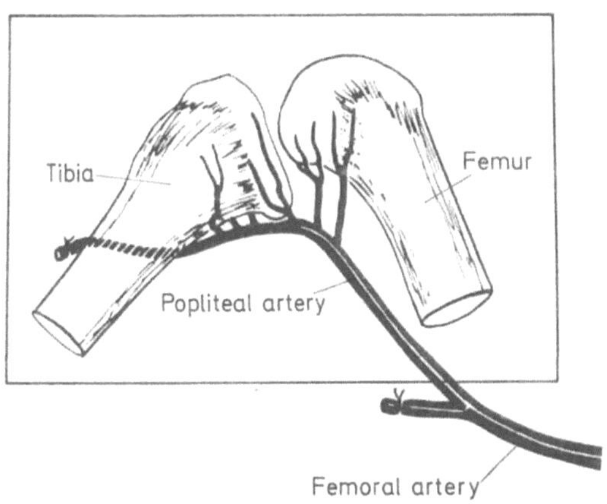

Fig. 9. Vascularized rat knee allograft

Vascularized bone allografts transplanted across a strong histocompatibility barrier showed evidence of rapid rejection. This was manifested at 1 week by massive extravasation and fibrin deposition in the marrow and cessation of all osteocyte activity and microcirculatory flow despite patency of the major vascular pedicle (Figs. 10–12). Transplants across a weak histocompatibility barrier were victims of a less intense rejection process and allowed the investigators to watch the rejection process unfold. In these grafts, osteoprogenitor cells in the growth plate and the marrow were early targets showing damage by 1 week. Early osteoprogenitor cell loss resulted in arrest of the process of endochondral ossification. Arrest of this process together with persistent cartilage viability and proliferation resulted in a giant growth plate. Osteocyte loss in other areas of the graft occurred later and only in the areas where the microcirculation had been lost. These data

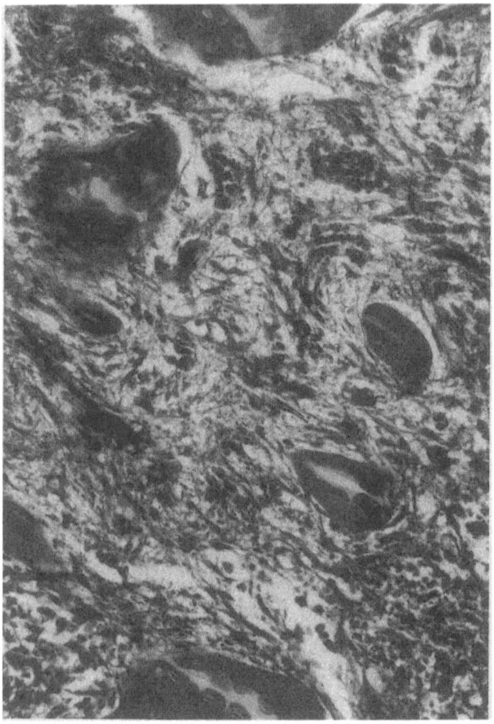

Fig. 10. Vascularized allograft stained for fibrin (phosphotungstic acid hematoxylin)

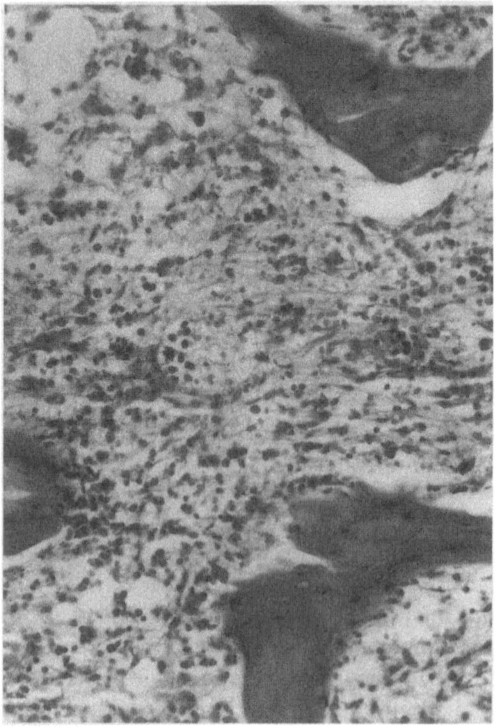

Fig. 11. Vascularized allograft stained for fibrin (hematoxylin and eosin)

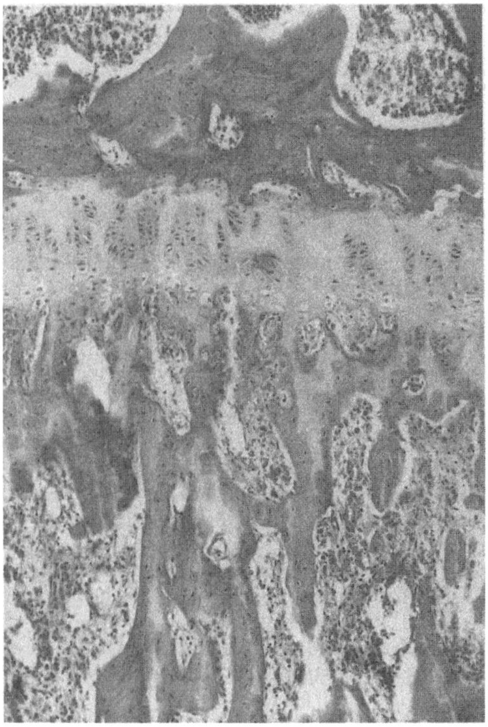

Fig. 12. Vascularized allograft stained for fibrin (hematoxylin and eosin)

suggest that ischemic damage secondary to immune-related vascular compromise is a significant factor in graft loss. New bone growth and host vascularization of these grafts had occurred by 12 weeks.

Conclusions

An approach to the study of the fate of vascularized bone grafts employing histology, fluorescent microscopy, microangiography, microradiography, and biomechanical testing has been presented in an effort to better understand their biological behavior. While a complete understanding of vascularized bone grafts is far from accomplished, an objective approach has been defined. Further investigation is prerequisite to define the potential value and role of free vascularized bone grafts clinically.

References

1. Albee FH (1972) Transplantation of a portion of the tibia into the spine for Pott's disease. Clin Orthop 87:5–8
2. Allgöwer M, Blocker TG Jr, Engley BWD (1952) Some immunological aspects of auto- and homolografts in rabbits tested in vivo and in vivo techniques. Plast Reconstr Surg 9:1–21

3. Alm A, Stromberg B (1974) Vascular anatomy of the patellar and cruciate ligaments: a microangiographic and histologic investigation in the dog. Acta Chir Scand [Suppl] 445:25
4. American Replantation Mission to China (1973) Replantation surgery in China. Plast Reconstr Surg 52:176
5. Andersson GBJ, Gaechter A, Galante JO, Rostoker W (1978) Segmental replacement of long bones in baboons using a fiber titanium implant. J Bone Joint Surg [Am] 60-A:31–40
6. Androsov PI (1956) New methods of surgical treatment of blood vessel lesions. Arch Surg 73:902
7. Ariyan S, Finseth FJ (1978) The anterior chest approach for obtaining free osteocutaneous rib grafts. Plast Reconstr Surg 62(5):676–685
8. Barth H (1895) Histologische Untersuchungen über Knochentransplantation. Beitr Path Anat Allg Pathol 17:65–142
9. Baschkerzeu NJ, Petrow NN (1912) Beiträge zur freien Knochenüberpflanzung. Dtsch Z Chir 113:490–531
10. Berggren A et al. (1981) The effect of different storage media and perfusion on osteoblast and osteocyte survival in free composite bone grafts revascularized by microvascular anastomoses. J Microsurg 2:273
11. Berggren A, Weiland AJ, Dorfman H (1982) The effect of prolonged ischemia time on osteocyte and osteoblast survival in composite bone grafts revascularized by microvascular anastomosis. Plast Reconstr Surg 69:290
12. Berggren A, Weiland AJ, Dorfman H (1982) Free vascularized bone grafts: factors affecting their survival and ability to heal to recipient bone defects. Plast Reconstr Surg 69(1):19–29
13. Berggren A, et al. (1982) Microvascular free bone transfer with revascularization of the medullary and periosteal circulation or the periosteal circulation alone: a comparative experimental study. J Bone Joint Surg [Am] 64A:73
14. Berggren A, Weiland AJ, Ostrup L (1982) Bone scintigraphy in evaluating the viability of composite bone grafts revascularized by microvascular anastomoses, conventional autogenous grafts, and free nonrevascularized periosteal grafts. J Bone Joint Surg [Am] 64A:799
15. Bergstedt HF, Korlof B, Lind MG, Wersall J (1978) Scintigraphy of human autologous rib transplants to a partially resected mandible. Scand J Plast Reconstr Surg 12:151–156
16. Boyd H (1943) The treatment of difficult and unusual non-unions. J Bone Joint Surg [Am] 25:535–552
17. Bright RW, Nelson FR, Stevenson JS, Strash AM (1973) Polyphosphate ^{99m}Tc scans: a quantitative method for evaluating clinical bone formation rates. Surg Forum 2:475
18. Brookes M (1971) The blood supply of bone. Butterworth, London
19. Brookes M, Elkin AC, Harrison RG, Heald CB (1961) A new concept of capillary circulation in bone cortex. Lancet i:1078–1081
20. Brookes M, Richards DJ, Singh M (1970) Vascular sequelae of experimental osteotomy. Angiography 21:355
21. Buncke HJ, Furnas DW, Gordon L, Achauer B (1977) Free osteocutaneous flap from a rib to the tibia. Plast Reconstr Surg 59:799–805
22. Buncke HJ, Schulz WP (1965) Experimental digital amputation and reimplantation. Plast Reconstr Surg 36:62
23. Buncke HJ, Schulz WP (1965) Total ear re-implantation in the rabbit utilizing microminiature vascular anastomoses. Br J Plast Surg 19:15
24. Burwell RG (1964) Biological mechanisms in foreign bone transplantation. Butterworths, Washington DC, (Modern trends in orthopaedics, vol. 4)
25. Burwell RG (1961) Studies in the transplantation of bone. VII. The fresh composite homograft-autograft of cancellous bone: an analysis of factors lending to osteogenesis in marrow transplants in marrow-containing bone. J Bone Joint Surg [Br] 46B:110–111

26. Campbell WC (1919) Transference of the fibula as an adjunct free bone graft in tibial deficiency. J Orthop Surg 7:625–631
27. Carrell A (1912) The preservation of tissues and its applications in surgery. J Am Med Assoc 59:523–527
28. Carrell A (1908) Results of the transplantation of blood vessels, organs, and limbs. J Am Med Assoc 51:1662–1667
29. Clark K (1959) A case of replacement of the upper end of the humerus by a fibular graft: reviewed after 29 years. J Bone Joint Surg [Br] 41B:365–368
30. Cobbett JR (1967) Microvascular surgery. Surg Clin North Am 47:521–542
31. Collins GM, Bravo-Shurgarman M, Terasaki PI (1969) Kidney preservation for transplantation. Lancet ii(632):1219–1222
32. Curtiss PH Jr, Powell AE, Herndon CH (1959) Immunological factors in homogenous bone transplantation: III. The inability of homogenous rabbit bone to induce circulatory antibodies in rabbits. J Bone Joint Surg [Am] 41A:1482–1488
33. Daniel RK, Taylor GI (1973) Distant transfer of an island flap by microvascular anastomoses. Plast Reconstr Surg 52:111–117
34. D'Aubigne RM, Meary R, Thomine JM (1966) La resection dans le traitement des tumeurs des os. Rev Chir Orthop 52:305–324
35. DeBruyn P, Kabish W (1955) Bone formation by fresh and frozen autogenous and homogenous transplants of bone, bone marrow, and periosteum. Am J Anat 96:375–417
36. Doi K, Tominaga S, Shabata T (1977) Bone grafts with microvascular anastomoses of vascular pedicles. J Bone Joint Surg [Am] 59A:809–815
37. Eadie DGA, DeTakats G (1966) The early fate of autogenous grafts in the canine femoral vein. J Cardiovasc Surg (Torino) 7:148
38. Enneking WF, Burchardt H, Puhl JJ, Piotrowski G (1975) Physical and biological aspects of repair in dog cortical bone transplants. J Bone Joint Surg [Am]57A:237–251
39. Gilbert A (1979) Vascularized transfer of the fibular shaft. Int J Microsurg 1(2):100–102
40. Goldhaber P (1979) The effect of hyperoxia in bone resorption in tissue culture. Arch Pathol 66:635
41. Gothman L (1960) The normal arterial pattern of the rabbit's tibia: a microangiographic study. Acta Chir Scand 120:201–210
42. Haas SL (1923) A study of the viability of bone after removal from the body. Arch Surg 7:213–226
43. Harashina T, Buncke HJ (1975) Study of Washout solutions for microvascular replantation and transplantation. Plast Reconstr Surg 56:542
44. Harashina T, Nakajima H, Imai T (1978) Reconstruction of mandibular defects with revascularized free rib grafts. Plast Reconstr Surg 62(4):514–522
45. Harmon PH (1945) A simplified surgical approach to the posterior tibia for bone grafting and fibular transference. J Bone Joint Surg [Am] 27:496–498
46. Haw CS, O'Brien BMC, Kurate T (1978) The microsurgical revascularization of resected segments of the tibia in the dog. J Bone Joint Surg [Br] 60B:266–269
47. Heiple K, Chase S, Herndon C (1963) A comparative study of the healing process following different types of bone transplantation. J Bone Joint Surg [Am] 45A:1593–1616
48. Herndon CH, Chase SW (1952) Experimental studies in the transplantation of whole joints. J Bone Joint Surg [Am] 34A:156–164
49. Herndon CH, Chase SW (1954) The fate of massive autogenous and homogenous bone grafts including articular surfaces. Surg Gynecol Obstet 98:273–290
50. Holt GP, Lewis FT (1905) A new technique for end-to-end anastomosis for small arteries. Surg Forum 11:242
51. Huntington TW (1905) Case of bone transference. Ann Surg 41:249–256
52. Hutchinson J (1952) The fate of experimental bone autografts and homografts. Br J Surg [Am] 39:552–561

53. Jacobson JH, Suarez EL (1960) Microsurgery in anastomoses of small vessels. Surg Forum 11:243
54. Johnson RW (1927) A physiological study of the blood supply of the diaphysis. J Bone Joint Surg 25:153–184
55. Kelly JF, Cagle JD, Stevenson JS, Adler GJ (1975) Technetium-99m radionuclide bone imaging for evaluating mandibular osseous allografts. J Oral Surg 33:11–17
56. Ketchum L, Masters F, Robinson P (1974) Mandibular reconstruction using a composite island rib flap: a case report. Plast Reconstr Surg 53:471–476
57. Lacroix P (1945) Recent investigation on the growth of bone. Nature 156:576
58. Levander G (1938) A study of bone regeneration. Surg Gynecol Obstet 67:704–714
59. Lexer E (1915) Blutige Vereinigung von Knochenbrüchen. Dtsch Z Chir 133:1970
60. Lexer E (1903) Die Entstehung entzündlicher Knochenherde und ihre Beziehung zu den Arterienverzweigungen der Knochen. Arch Klin Chir 81:1
61. Lexer E (1908) Substitution of whole or half joints from freshly amputated extremities by free plastic operation. Surg Gynecol Obstet 6:601–607
62. Lexer E, Kuliga, Turk (1904) Untersuchungen über Knochenarterien. Hirschwold, Berlin
63. Little JH, Cooper P, Sarwat A, Waisman J, Fonkalsrud EW (1973) Factors influencing endothelial injury and vascular thrombosis after perfusion. J Surg Res 14:221–227
64. Maatz R, Lentz W, Graf R (1954) Spongiosa test of bone grafts for transplantation. J Bone Joint Surg [Am] 36A:721–731
65. Mankin HJ, Fogelson FS, Thrasher AZ, Jaffer F (1976) Massive resection and allograft transplantation in the treatment of malignant bone tumors. N Engl J Med 194:1247–1255
66. Manktelow RT, McKee NH (1978) Free muscle transplantation to provide active finger flexion. J Hand Surg [Am] 3(5):416–426
67. Marchand (1900) Zur Kenntnis der Knochentransplantation. Verh Dtsch Pathol Ges 2:368–375
68. Matsui H (1968) Studies on replacement of the cervical and upper thoracic or intestinal segment. Arch Jpn Chir 37:817–834
69. Nakayama K, Tamiya T, Yamamoto K, Akimoto S (1962) A simple new apparatus for small vessel anastomoses (free autograft for sigmoid included). Surgery 52:918–931
70. Nettelblad H, Randolph MA, Weiland AJ (1984) Free microvascular epiphyseal plate transplantation: an experimental study. J Bone Joint Surg [Am] 66A:1421–1430
71. Nettelblad H, Randolph MA, Weiland AJ (1986) Heterotopic microvascular growth plate transplantation of the proximal fibula: an experimental canine model. Plast Reconst Surg 77(5):814
72. Nettelblad H, Randolph MA, Weiland AJ (1984) Physiologic isolation of the canine proximal fibular epiphysis on a vascular pedicle. Microsurgery 5(2):98–101
73. Nettelblad H, Randolph MA, Weiland AJ (1985) Short-term response of a skeletal growth plate to heterotopic microvascular transfer. J Reconstr Microsurg 1(3):177–183
74. O'Brien BM (1977) Microvascular free bone and joint transfer. In: Microvascular reconstructive surgery. Churchill Livingstone, New York, pp 267–289
75. Ottolenghi C (1972) Massive osteo and osteo-articular bone grafts: technical results of 62 cases. Clin Orthop 87:156–164
76. Parrish FF (1973) Allograft replacement of all or part of the end of a long bone following excision of a tumor: report of twenty-one cases. J Bone Joint Surg [Am] 48A:7–22
77. Parrish FF (1966) Treatment of bone tumors by total excision and replacement with massive autologous and homologous grafts. J Bone Joint Surg [Am] 48A:968–990
78. Phemister DB (1914) The fate of transplanted bone and regenerative power of various constituents. Surg Gynecol Obstet 19:303–333
79. Puranen J (1966) Reorganization of fresh and preserved bone transplants. Acta Orthop Scand [Suppl] 92

80. Ray RD, Degge J, Gloyd P, Mooney G (1952) Bone regeneration. J Bone Joint Surg [Am] 34A:638–647
81. Rhinelander FW (1973) Effects of medullary nailing on the normal blood supply of diaphyseal cortex. Instr Course Lect (AAOS) 22:161–187
82. Rhinelander FW (1968) The normal microcirculation of diaphyseal cortex and its response to fracture. J Bone Joint Surg [Am] 50A:784–800
83. Rhinelander FW, Baragry RA (1962) Microangiography in bone healing. I. Undisplaced closed fractures. J Bone Joint Surg [Am] 44A:1273–1298
84. Rhinelander FW, Phillips RS, Steel WM, Beer JC (1968) Microangiography in bone healing. II. Displaced closed fractures. J Bone Joint Surg [Am] 50A:643–662
85. Riordin DC (1945) Congenital absence of the radius. J Bone Joint Surg [Am] 27A:1129–1140
86. Rohlich K (1941) Bildung neuer Knochensubstanz in abgetöteten Knochentransplantation. A Mikrosk Anat Forsch 50:132–145
87. Rohlich K (1942) Über die Transplantation periost- und markloser Knochenstücke. A Mikrosk Anat Forsch 51:636–653
88. Salmon PA, Assimocopoulos CA (1964) A pneumatic needle holder suitable for microsurgical procedures. Surgery 55:446
89. Serafin D, Villarreal-Rios A, Georgiade N (1977) A rib-containing free flap to reconstruct mandibular defects. Br J Plast Surg 30:263–266
90. Shaw JL, Bassett CAL (1967) The effects of varying oxygen concentrations on osteogenesis and embryonic cartilage in vitro. J Bone Joint Surg [Am] 40A:73
91. Starr DE (1945) Congenital absence of the radius. J Bone Joint Surg [Am] 27:572–577
92. Stevenson JS, Bright RW, Dunson GL, Nelson FR (1974) Technetium-99m phosphate bone imaging: a method for assessing bone graft healing. Radiology 110:391–394
93. Tamai S, Komatsu S, Sakamoto K, Sano S, Sasauchi N, Hori Y, Tatsumi Y, Okuda H (1970) Free muscle transplants in dogs with microsurgical neurovascular anastomoses. Plast Reconstr Surg 46:219–225
94. Taylor GI (1977) Microvascular free bone transfer. Orthop Clin North Am 8:425–447
95. Taylor GI, Miller GDH, Ham FJ (1975) The free vascularized bone graft. Plast Reconstr Surg 55:533–544
96. Taylor GI, Townsend P, Corlett R (1979) Superiority of the deep circumflex iliac vessels as the supply for free groin flaps: clinical study. Plast Reconstr Surg 64(6):745–759
97. Taylor GI, Townsend P, Corlett R (1979) Superiority of the deep circumflex iliac vessels as the supply for free groin flaps: experimental study. Plast Reconstr Surg 64(5):595–605
98. Taylor GI, Watson N (1978) One-stage repair of compound leg defects with free revascularized flaps of groin, skin, and iliac bone. Plast Reconstr Surg 61:494–506
99. Trias A, Fery A (1979) Cortical circulation of long bones. J Bone Joint Surg [Am] 61A:1052–1059
100. Triplett RG, Kelly JF, Mendenshall KG, Vieras F (1979) Quantitative radionuclide imaging for early determination of fate of mandibular bone grafts. J Nucl Med 20(4):297–302
101. Trueta J, Caladias AX (1964) A study of the blood supply of the long bones. Surg Gynecol Obstet 118:485–498
102. Urdaneta LF, Gilsdorf RB, Leonard AS (1968) An evaluation of pedicle infiltration, organ perfusion, and prevention of vascular collapse during canine kidney procurement for transplantation. J Surg Res 8:314–319
103. Urist MR, McLean FC (1952) Osteogenetic potency and new bone formation by induction in transplants to the anterior chamber of the eye. J Bone Joint Surg [Am] 34A:443–470
104. Volkov M (1970) Allotransplantation of joints. J Bone Joint Surg [Br] 52B:49–53

105. Weiland AJ, Daniel RK (1979) Microvascular anastomoses for bone grafts in the treatment of massive defects in bone. J Bone Joint Surg [Am] 61A(1):98–104
106. Weiland AJ, Daniel RK, Riley LH Jr (1977) Application of the free vascularized bone graft in the treatment of malignant or aggressive bone tumors. Johns Hopkins Med J 140:85–96
107. Weiland AJ, Kleinert HE, Kutz JE, Daniel RK (1979) Free vascularized bone grafts in surgery of the upper extremity. J Hand Surg [Am] 4(2):129–144
108. Weiland AJ, Kleinert HE, Kutz JE, Daniel RK (1978) Vascularized bone grafts in the upper extremity. In: Serafin D, Buncke HJ Jr (eds) Microsurgical composite tissue transplantation, chap 41. Mosby, St Louis, pp 605–625
109. Weiland AJ, Phillips TW, Randolph MA (1984) Bone grafts: a radiologic, histologic, and biomechanical model comparing autografts, allografts, and free vascularized bone grafts. Plast Reconstr Surg 74(3):368–379

Biology of Osteoarticular Allografts *

V. M. Goldberg[1], C. H. Herndon[1], and E. Lance[2]

[1] Department of Orthopaedics, Case Western Reserve University, Cleveland, Ohio, USA
[2] Department of Orthopaedics, University of Honolulu, Honolulu, Hawaii, USA

Experimental and clinical investigations of whole joint transplantation have identified major problems that may compromise the biologic outcome of complex osteochondral grafts [1, 3–6, 10–12, 14, 16, 18–21, 24–26, 29, 30]. The problems that have led to failure include delayed and incomplete revascularization, inadequate new bone formation, and difficulty in preserving and maintaining the articular cartilage and soft tissue support. Although there is no doubt that the host responds to donor antigens with an immune reaction directed to osteochondral elements, the role of this response in the success or failure of a graft remains controversial [3, 7, 8, 20, 25, 26]. It would seem, then, that autogenous bone is the best solution for the clinical requirements of bone grafting. However, advances in the management of musculoskeletal tumors, the increasing requirement for reconstruction after trauma, and failed joint arthroplasties have resulted in an increasing demand for massive osteochondral grafts. Autogenous tissue is clearly not available in these circumstances, so that further exploration of the appropriate biological factors which may improve the acceptance of allogeneic tissue is critical to improve the clinical result. This chapter reviews the biological fate of both vascularized and nonvascularized osteoarticular (whole joint) allografts.

Nonvascularized Whole Joint Transplants

Early studies of nonvascularized whole joint transplants were concerned with mechanical factors such as internal fixation and soft tissue supports. Judet [15], Lexer [18], and others [1, 4, 12, 17, 22] demonstrated that although the articular surface of both autografts and allografts appears to survive for prolonged periods of time, the subchondral bone ultimately failed, and the entire construct collapsed. It appeared, therefore, that the major biological determinant of the transplant was the subchondral bone of the graft. Imamaliyev [14], Volkov [29], and more recently Seligman [26] in an attempt to modify the failure of the bone have studied the role of freezing in whole joint transplantation. Although there appeared to be some improvement in the overall survival of the transplant, only fresh autografts appeared to survive for a prolonged period of time and to function satisfactorily. Additionally, when the host was immunosuppressed with azathioprine, there appeared to be some prolongation of the allograft's survival and improvement in the overall function. Ultimately, subchondral bone necrosis ensued, and the resulting loss of mechanical integrity caused the transplant to fail.

* Research supported in part by NIH grant AM 22166.

Bone Transplantation
Eds.: M. Aebi, P. Regazzoni

There was no evidence that an immunological response, although present, determined the outcome of the graft.

Other investigators have evaluated the role of osteochondral shell grafts in an attempt to deduce the major determining component in the success or failure of whole joint transplants [22]. Although data suggested that fresh cartilagenous autografts survived and functioned for a prolonged period of time, any freezing appeared to be detrimental to the biological functioning of articular cartilage. Although shell grafts appeared to function somewhat better, ultimately either technical problems ensued, such as loss of fixation, or the entire bony construct collapsed. It is apparent, therefore, that with the increasing demand of large osteochondral grafts for clinical problems, further experimental studies are necessary to define biological factors which may improve the use of these grafts.

A detailed histological evaluation has been performed in our laboratory from 1 day to 2 years after transplantation of whole canine autogenous and allogeneic knee transplants in an attempt to define the biological fate of massive articular transplants [10, 13]. Three groups of grafts were studied; fresh autografts, fresh allografts, and frozen allografts. The allografts were frozen at −20 °C for 2 weeks and then transplanted to unrelated animals. The graft included the entire knee joint, including the cruciate and collateral ligaments and the meniscus but excluding the capsule and synovial membrane. Femoral and tibial osteotomies were fixed by utilizing wire fixation or self-compressing DCP plates. Animals were killed from 1 day to 2 years after surgery, and the entire transplant was removed. The graft was fixed in a buffered 10% formalin fixative, and specimens were decalcified in a 1 : 1 mixture of 50% formic acid and 20% sodium citrate. Longitudinal sections at 25 μ were stained with hematoxylin and eosin and evaluated.

The graft-host junction of the femoral and tibial osteotomies generally healed by 3 months after transplantation without any significant differences between autografts and allografts. The autografts demonstrated early necrosis of both cancellous and cortical bone. The osteocytes contained pyknotic nuclei, and empty lacunae were seen by 2 weeks after transplantation. However, there very rapidly appeared to be an early revascularization of the haversian system. Sequential resorption of necrotic spongiosa and cortical bone was seen by 3 weeks after transplantation, and appositional new bone followed quickly. Gradual reorganization proceeded in an orderly fashion and appeared almost complete by 12 months after surgery. The meniscus of the autogenous transplants generally showed a normal appearance during the first few months after surgery. However, by 4 months there appeared to be focal areas of necrosis and gradual ingrowth of fibroconnective tissue with replacement by new fibrocartilage. The articular cartilage demonstrated a normal histologic appearance during the 1st month after surgery. Focal cartilage necrosis occurred gradually and later progressed. Granulation tissue invading the articular surface was seen early, progressing from the periphery and migrating over the entire articular surface, which later became fibrocartilagenous in character. The bone marrow in these grafts rapidly became necrotic and was replaced by avascular connective tissue. Normal marrow replaced this tissue in a sequential manner and was present throughout the graft by 1 year. In general, the fresh autogenous grafts maintained their overall configuration and functioned clinically satisfactorily during the 24-month observation

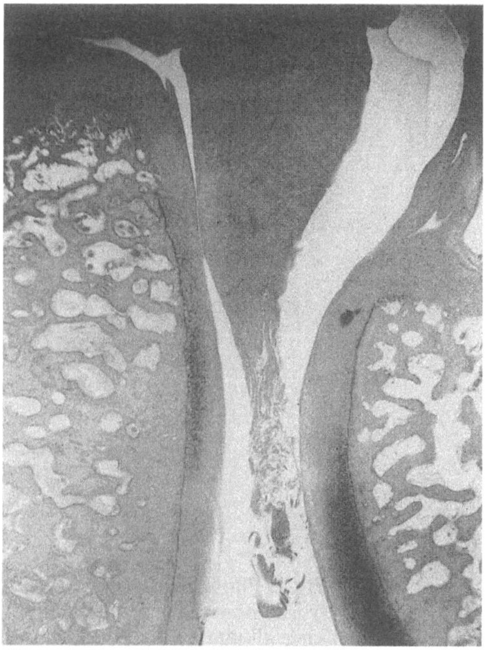

Fig. 1. Photomicrograph of a fresh nonvascularized canine knee autograft showing some viable cartilage and bone 24 months after transplantation. (hematoxylin and eosin, ×16)

period. However, a gradual deterioration of the articular surface was seen in all grafts (Fig. 1).

The fresh allografts demonstrated rapid widespread osseous necrosis which was present within the first 2 weeks after grafting. Cortical resorption occurred rapidly, and only sporatic appositional new bone was seen. Even at 2 years, the surviving allografts demonstrated widespread necrosis of bone and marked disorganization. Little cortical reorganization was seen at 2 years. The meniscus demonstrated early necrosis, and there was only a sparse attempt to replace it with new fibrocartilage during the 2nd year. Early widespread necrosis of the articular cartilage occurred during the first few weeks and a pannuslike ingrowth of granulation tissue developed over the entire surface. The bone marrow was invaded early by an active inflammatory process with cells suggestive of an immunological response. There was only an aborted attempt in focal areas to replace this inflammatory tissue with normal marrow.

The frozen allografts demonstrated changes similar to those in the fresh grafts, with rapid subchondral collapse, marked cortical resorption, and lack of reorganization occurring in most grafts. However, some maintenance of joint integrity was noted, and no active inflammation was present. After 2 years there was some attempt to replacement of the necrotic bone with appositional new bone. The meniscus was replaced with fibrous tissue, and only focal areas of fibrocartilage remained throughout the period of observation. The articular cartilage rapidly deteriorated during the first few months after grafting and was replaced by a fibroconnective tissue. The marrow was never transformed to active adult tissue and generally remained fibrotic (Fig. 2).

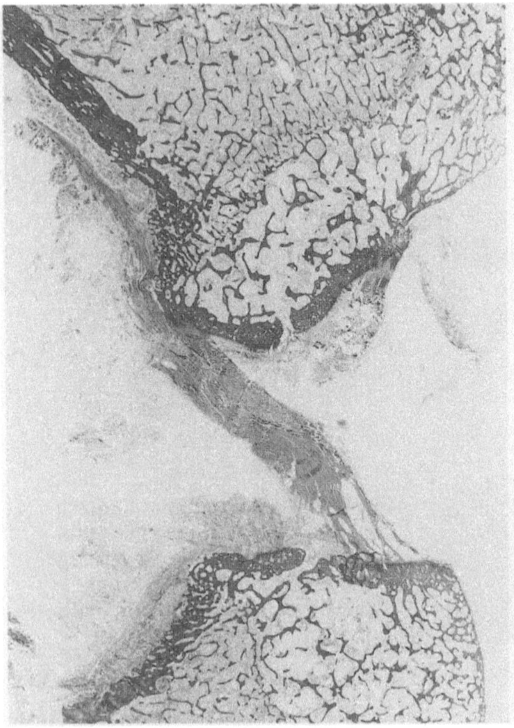

Fig. 2. Photomicrograph of a frozen nonvascuralized canine knee allograft illustrating widespread bony and cartilage necrosis 12 months after surgery. (hematoxylin and eosin, ×4)

The results of these studies indicate that the major cause of failure of whole joint transplants was delayed and incomplete revascularization of the bony components with inadequate new mineralization. This led to subchondral bone collapse and the disorganization of the entire joint.

Vascularized Whole Joint Transplants

Because of the problems seen with nonvascularized osteoarticular grafts, recent studies have been directed toward immediately vascularized transplants and modifications of the immune response of the recipient in order to improve the biological fate of the transplant. Early work by Buncke [2] and Slome and Reeves [23, 27] suggested that immediate revascularization improved the overall outcome and delayed the usual degenerative processes that have been described for nonvascularized joints. Autografts appeared to survive for a prolonged period of time with excellent function, while fresh vascularized allografts appeared to be rejected rapidly. Their data indicated that prolonged survival resulted when vascularized canine knee joints were transplanted to recipients immunosuppressed with azathioprine. We have also investigated whole knee joint transplantation in dogs in order to develop a model to study the role of immediate revascularization and intensive immunosuppression on allograft survival [9]. This model is described elsewhere in this volume, but, briefly, the canine knee joint can be isolated with a vascular pedicle while preserving the blood supply to the distal part of the extremity. The transplant includes the entire joint with its surrounding soft tissue. The femoral and tibial osteotomies are repaired by osteosynthesis. Microvascular techniques are used to repair the popliteal vein and artery, with the average ischemia time less then 2 h. The remaining periarticular soft tissue structures are repaired using standard surgical techniques. Blood volume is maintained and antibiotics administered prophylactically. Three groups of animals were studied; autografts, allografts immunosuppressed with azathioprine and prednisolone alone, and allografts immunosuppressed additionally with antilymphocyte serum. Animals were evaluated clinically and radiographically. Sequential angiograms were performed at 2-week intervals, and only animals with patent vascular pedicles were followed. At the time of sacrifice, from 1 week through 18 months, the entire joint was removed and fixed in 10% formalin and decalcified using a formic acid-sodium citrate technique. Serial sagittal sections were cut at 10 μm and stained with hematoxylin and eosin for evaluation.

There were 26 dogs in the autograft series that survived longer then 1 week with patent anastomoses. These dogs were followed for as long as 18 months after implantation. Radiographic evaluation demonstrated general maintenance of the overall joint configuration and healing of the osteotomies by the 4th month after surgery. The joints of animals which demonstrated failed vascular anastomoses deteriorated rapidly, as was seen previously in the nonvascularized series of dogs. Widespread necrosis was present, although there appeared to be some areas of replacement with new appositional bone. The articular surface and meniscus were replaced by a pannus ingrowth of fibrous tissue. An additional finding was necrosis in the anterior compartment of the leg, which resulted in loss of the soft tissue supports and frequent dislocations of the joint.

Long-term survivors whose anastomoses remained patent during the entire study functioned normally after transfer to an animal farm. All animals were fully weight-bearing and active. Radiographic appearance of the articular surface as long as 18 months after transplantation appeared normal, with only minimal joint narrowing. At the time of sacrifice the articular cartilage, meniscus, and ligaments were intact and appeared normal. There was little scarring of the periarticular muscles. Histologic evaluation demonstrated normal articular cartilage with only small focal areas of necrosis (Fig. 3). The subchondral bone was viable and the cortical bone demonstrated mostly living osteocytes. There was no evidence of disorganization of the joint or osteochondral fragmentation. There appeared to be an increase in the collateral circulation of the joint, with only mild narrowing of the popliteal artery at the site of the anastomosis.

By contrast, the allografts which were treated with azathioprine and prednisolone alone demonstrated failure of the vascular repair usually by 1 month after surgery. The rapid deterioration of the joint followed with necrosis of the periarticular soft tissue and joint dislocation. The vascular repair of 14 of the 24 allografts treated with azathioprine, prednisolone, and antilymphocyte serum also failed within the 1st month. Although the joint deteriorated rapidly, there was no evidence of an immune rejection at sacrifice. However, a marked destruction of the articular cartilage secondary to subchondral bone collapse was seen. Five of the animals in this group that survived with patent vessels longer than 1 month were lost because of systemic infection due to the intense level of immunosup-

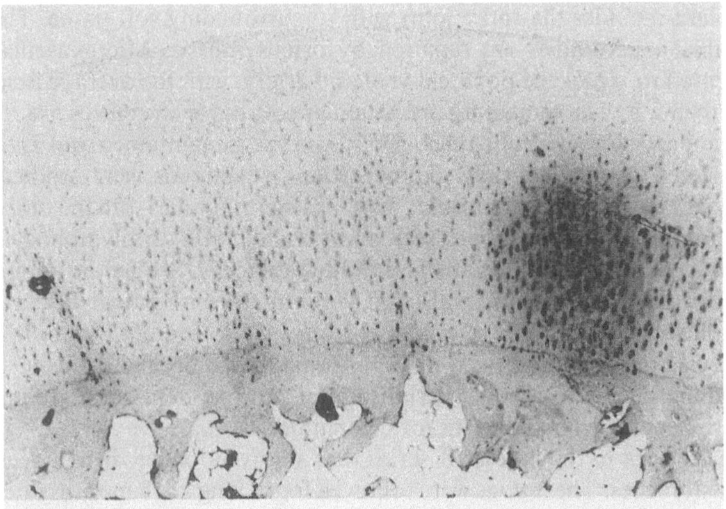

Fig. 3. Photomicrograph of a successfully vascularized canine whole knee autograft showing a normal articular surface 18 months after transplantation. (hematoxylin and eosin, ×16)

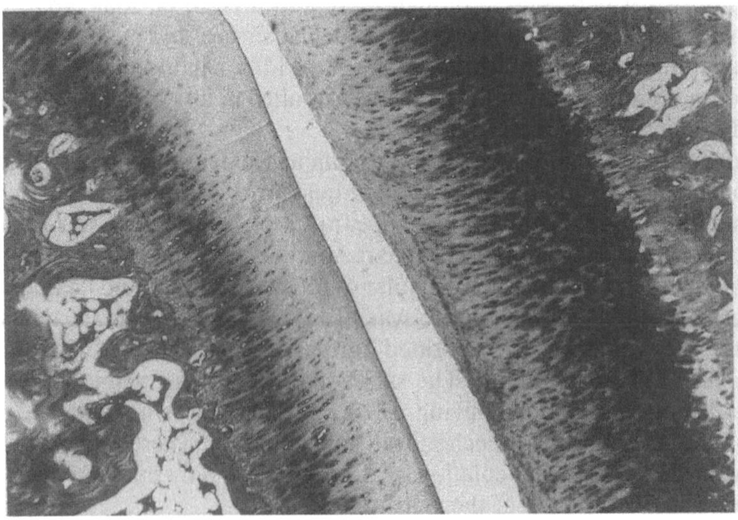

Fig. 4. Photomicrograph of a vascularized canine whole knee allograft demonstrating viable bone and cartilage 12 months after transplantation. (hematoxylin and eosin, ×16)

pression. The remaining five dogs functioned well on an open animal farm for 1 year after surgery, and although the transplanted knees functioned satisfactorily, the dogs demonstrated a restricted range of motion and muscular atrophy of the extremity. Two of the osteotomies did not heal, but all joints remained stable throughout the study. The joints demonstrated minimal narrowing of the articular cartilage on radiographs. Arteriograms demonstrated some narrowing at the repair site and an increased collateral circulation to the knee similar to that seen in the autografts. At the time of sacrifice, 12–18 months after transplantation, the entire joint surface was intact although there were focal areas of cartilage degeneration. The soft tissues generally demonstrated mild scarring, and there was a restricted range of joint motion. The articular cartilage and subchondral bone maintained a well-preserved histologic appearance. There were focal areas of cartilage loss. There were some areas of subchondral collapse seen in these dogs but without loss of the joint integrity. There was no evidence in these allograft survivors of an inflammatory response in the bone marrow. The soft tissues did not show the presence of any lymphocytes or plasma cells. Small portions of the meniscus were replaced by fibrous connective tissue pannus, but without any inflammation. Only minor necrotic areas were seen in the muscles of the anterior compartment. There was no evidence of any disorganization within the graft suggestive of a neuropathic process (Fig. 4).

Conclusion

Because of the increasing incidence of failures of total joint arthroplasties, biological alternatives still remain a viable alternative. But before wider application of this approach can be used, the factors which determine the outcome of joint transplantation must be further delineated. The present experimental data indicate that frozen allografts appear to do poorly. However, recent reports by Mankin et al. suggest that despite any immune response, allogeneic material is well tolerated, nontoxic, incorporated by host bone, and functions rather satisfactory for a prolonged period of time [19, 20]. There is no question that there is a definite "race" between revascularization, bony apposition, and mechanical failure of the transplant. If the data from our studies of vascularized osteoarticular grafts are to be used, further experimental studies are necessary. The problems which must be addressed are issues of tissue preservation and immune rejection. Advances in transplantation biology have demonstrated the value of tissue typing for transplantation antigens to improve clinical acceptance of allogeneic tissue. The use of cyclosporin-A and other newer less toxic immunosuppressive agents have been helpful in circumventing the immune response seen in other vascularized tissue [28]. The application of these methods and continued exploration of preservation techniques could result in the future successful transplantation of complex vascularized musculoskeletal allografts for clinical problems.

References

1. Aichroth P, Burwell RG, Laurence M (1972) Transplantation of synovial joint surfaces: an experimental study. J Bone Joint Surg [Br] 54B:747
2. Buncke HF Jr, Daniller AI, Schultz WP, Chase RA (1967) The fate of autogenous whole joints transplanted by microvascular anastomoses. Plast Reconstr Surg 5(39):333
3. Burwell RG (1974) Transplantation of cartilage and bone, biology and mechanical problems of osteoarticular allografting. The Knee Joint. International Congress Series no 324, Amsterdam, p 174
4. Campbell CJ, Ishida H, Takashashi J, Kelly F (1963) The transplantation of articular cartilage. An experimental study in dogs. J Bone Joint Surg [Am] 45A:1579

5. Cannon WD, Salama R, Burwell RG (1972) Massive Osteoarticular femoral grafts in sheep. J Bone Joint Surg [Am] 54A:1133
6. DePalma AF, Tsaltas TT, Mauler GG (1963) Viability of osteochondral grafts as determined by uptake of S-35. J Bone Joint Surg [Am] 45A:2565
7. Elves MW (1976) Newer knowledge of the immunology of bone and cartilage. Clin Orthop 120:232
8. Elves MW, Ford CH (1971) The development of humeral cytotoxic antibodies after the allografting of articular surfaces at the knee joint in sheep. J Bone Joint Surg 53B:554
9. Goldberg V, Porter B, Lance E (1980) Transplantation of the canine knee joint on vascular pedicles. J Bone Joint Surg [Am] 62A:414
10. Goldberg VM, Heiple KG (1983) Experimental hemijoint and whole-joint transplantation. Clin Orthop 174:43–53
11. Gross AE, Silverstein EA, Falk J, Falk R, Langer F (1975) The allotransplantation of partial joints in the treatment of osteoarthritis of the knee. Clin Orthop 108:7
12. Hamilton JA, Barnes R, Gibson T (1969) Experimental homografting of articular cartilage. J Bone Joint Surg [Br] 51B:566
13. Herndon CH, Chase SW (1952) Experimental studies in the transplantation of whole joints. J Bone Joint Surg [Am] 34A:564
14. Imamaliyev AE (1969) The preparation, preservation and transplantation of articular bone end. In: Apley AG (ed) Recent advances in orthopaedics. Churchill Livingstone, London, p 209
15. Judet H (1908) Essai sur la greffe des tissus articulaires. Comptes rendus de l'Association Française pour l'Avancement des Sciences. 146:600
16. Judet H, Padovani JP (1968) Transplantation d'articulation complète avec rétablissement circulatoire immediate par anastomoses arterielles et veineuses. Mem Acad Chir 94:520
17. Lane JM, Brighton CT, Otten HR, Lipton M (1977) Joint resurfacing in the rabbit using an autologous osteochondral graft. J Bone Joint Surg [Am] 59A:218
18. Lexer E (1908) Substitution of whole or half joints from freshly amputated extremities by free plastic operation. Surg Gynecol Obstet 6:601
19. Mankin HJ, Fogelson FS, Thrasher AS, Jaffer F (1976) Massive resection and allograft-transplantation in the treatment of malignant bone tumors. N Engl J Med 294:1247
20. Mankin HJ, Gebhardt MC, Tomford WW (1987) The use of frozen cadaveric allografts in the management of patients with bone tumors of the extremities. Orthop Clin North Am 18(2):275
21. Pap K, Krompecher S (1961) Arthroplasty of the knee: experimental and clinical experiences. J Bone Joint Surg [Am] 43A:523
22. Porter BB, Lance EM (1974) Limb and joint transplantation. Clin Orthop 104:249
23. Reeves B (1968) Studies of vascularized homotransplants of the knee joint. J Bone Joint Surg [Br] 50B:226
24. Schachar NS, Fuller TC, Wadsworth PL, Henry WB, Mankin HJ (1978) A feline model for the study of frozen osteochondral allografts. II. Development of lymphocytotoxic antibodies in allografts recipients. Trans Orthop Res Soc 3:131
25. Schachar NS, Henry WB, Wadsworth PL, Castronovo FP Jr, Mankin HJ (1978) A feline model for the study of frozen osteoarticular allografts. I. Quantitative assessment of cartilage viability and bone healing. Trans Orthop Res Soc 3:130
26. Seligman GM, George E, Yablon I, Vutik G, Cruess RL (1972) Transplantation of whole knee joints in the dog. Clin Orthop 87:332
27. Slome D, Reeves B (1966) Experimental homotransplantation of the knee joint. Lancet ii:205
28. Tutschka PJ (1982) Cyclosporin-A as a tool for experimental and clinical transplantation. Biomedicine 36:321–344
29. Volkov M (1970) Allotransplantation of joint. J Bone Joint Surg [Br] 52B:49
30. Yablon IG, Brandt KD, DeLellis R, Covall D (1977) Destruction of joint homografts. Arthritis Rheum 20:1526

Experimental Models for Bone Allografting

Y. Gotfried, T. Blum-Hareuveni, and D. G. Mendes

Research Center for Implant Surgery, Haifa Medical Center (Rothschild), Haifa, Israel

Chase and Herndon [16], in their excellent historical review on the fate of bone autografts and allogenous grafts, reported that the first scientific work on osteogenesis was done by Duhamel in 1739. However, Axhausen in 1907 was given credit for a major contribution to the basic principles of transplantation of osteogenic tissue in auto-, allo- and xenograft experimental animal models. Since then much knowledge has been accumulated and clinical experience gained on this complicated subject. The understanding of organ transplantation immunology significantly contributed to elucidating the close dynamic relationship between graft and recipient. This applied to vascularized and non-vascularized bone grafting. Accordingly, a schematic representation could be compiled (Fig. 1), outlining the reciprocal events between graft and recipient. Furthermore, different points of intervention altering one or more of the immunological factors were also defined in this scheme. Each point of intervention represents a clinical stage which directly influences the outcome of transplantation. Experimental models were developped adressing specifically these stages. Graft biology represents two main immunological aspects: genetically inherent antigenicity and the different cell and intercellular structures which are targets to the recipient immune response. Graft antigenicity can be reduced when graft and recipient are genetically matched. Using different physical agents results also in alteration of graft antigenicity. Recipient immune response can be altered using immunosuppression.

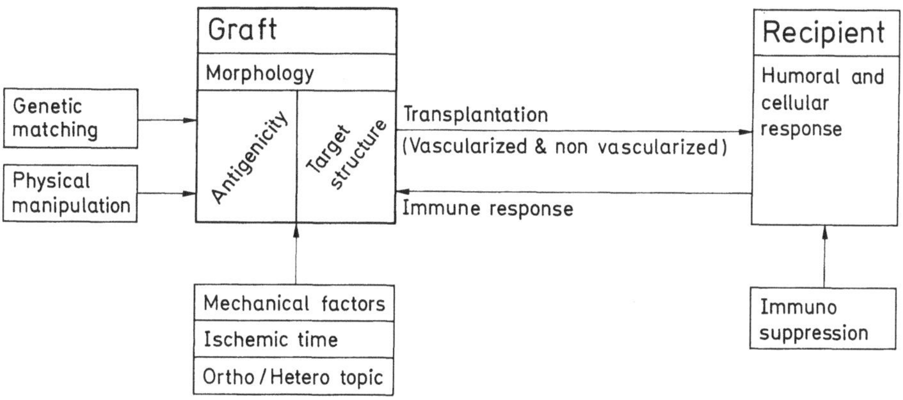

Fig. 1. Factors affecting bone graft transplantation

Bone Transplantation
Eds.: M. Aebi, P. Regazzoni

Different mechanical factors, such as ischemic time, heterotopic and orth(topic transplantation may directly influence the graft's target structures. Th topic, however, is not addressed in this paper.

Graft Physical Manipulation

Direct physical manipulation of the antigenic characteristics of bone grafts pre: ents the most widely used method of altering the quality of bone as immunoger Freezing [3, 4, 11, 14, 23, 46, 47, 49, 53] and freeze-drying [9–11, 14, 15, 23, 3! were the most common physical vectors used; graft boiling [11], removal of bor marrow [40] and irradiation [54] were also used. In addition, combinations of di ferent methods of physical manipulation were evaluated, including freezing an irradiation [42, 47], freezing and histocompatibility matching [5, 6, 21, 22, 31, 3‹ 50, 51], freezing and immunosuppression [47] and the effect of internal fixatio in the freeze-dried graft [39] (Table 1).

Various criteria are useful in the evaluation of the outcome of the transplar tation. The qualities of the graft-recipient interface (also referred to as graft fra(ture site) were evaluated histologically [3–6, 9, 12, 39, 47], radiologically [5, 9, 2: 39, 47] and biomechanically [9, 22, 34, 42]; revascularization [14], graft new bon formation [11, 15] and metabolic turnover [21] were evaluated as well. On th other hand, substantial information was gained when recording the host immun response in the form of histological evidence of inflammatory reaction [3, 4, 15 serum antibodies [5, 6, 10, 23, 31, 40, 50, 51] and lymphocyte-mediated cytoto› icity [5, 6, 23, 40, 50]. Second-set skin reaction were also used as an immunologicε parameter for qualifying bone graft antigenicity [6, 10, 11, 15].

Experimental models of physically manipulated bone allografts showed tha freezing [5] and freeze-drying [15] provoked less immune response. Concernin graft incorporation and fracture healing, the combination of freezing and irrad ation gave better results than freezing and immunosuppression, which in turn wa better than freezing alone [47]. Although freeze-drying was not found to protec cortical allograft from rejection [9], an increased revascularization was reporte in frozen and freeze-dried allografts [14]. The importance of rigid internal fixatio in the freeze-dried grafts was demonstrated when compared with cast immobil zation [39]. In addition to freezing and freeze-drying, when immunologicε

Table 1. Physical manipulation of grafts

Frozen
Irradiation
Histocompatibility matching
Immunosuppression
Freeze-dried
Different internal fixation
Boiled
Removal of bone marrow
Irradiation

matching was carried out, it was demonstrated that the greater the histocompatibility barrier, the less are the healing and remodelling [5]. No differences in incorporation of frozen syngeneic and major and minor histocompatibility allografts was reported [6]. These findings were confirmed biomechanically. The strength and compliance of frozen syngeneic and disparate allografts was equal [22]. However, metabolic turnover studies showed that calcium replacement appears to be more effective in frozen syngeneic than in frozen allografts [21].

Conflicting results were reported on recipient immune response. While some authors found no antibody immune response following frozen [5, 31] and freeze-dried [23] allografting, as well as no lymphocyte-mediated cytotoxicity [5], others found measurable host immune response [6, 23] and generated specific cytotoxic lymphocytes [6, 23]. Second-set skin reaction was found useful in assessing the effect of different methods used to alter bone antigenicity. Freeze-dried bone allografts were shown to prolong skin survival [10, 11, 15]. On the other hand, frozen, major histocompatibility different allografts were found to accelerate skin rejection [6], while other researchers reported no acceleration following boiled and frozen allografting [11]. It was noted, however, that alterations in immunological response to various preservation techniques was not accompanied by an advantageous graft incorporation as measured by torsion testing up to 16 weeks [42]. Bone in toto was found to evoke stronger humoral and cellular immune response than bone subject to physical removal of marrow. It was therefore concluded that major histocompatibility antigens are present in the bone itself [40].

Genetic Matching

Non-vascularized [5, 6, 21, 22, 30, 31, 34, 40, 48, 50, 51] and vascularized [28, 29, 37, 41, 46, 52, 55] models are commonly used. Canine models are mostly matched on the basis of correlation between serological types [5]. In these animals, segmental ulna [5], fibula [48] and proximal radius [50, 51] were applied. Major and minor histocompatibility matching is used in the rat models in which iliac crest [6], femor [21, 22, 34, 40], knee joint [28, 29, 41, 52, 55], tibia [40] and whole limb [37] are preferable grafts. Mice with major histocompatibility differences at H-2 and H-Y and syngeneic models were useful in evaluating tibia grafting [30, 31].

The advantage of genetic matching between donor and recipient was well demonstrated in various models of bone grafting. Syngeneic transplanted rat limb showed normal function with regard to growth. Bone scan and radiological examination were also normal [37]. Preserved vascularization of the grafts was demonstrated in major histocompatibly matched dogs [48]. The rejection phenomena were found to be quite different in vascularized major and minor histocompatible rat allografts [29]. Rejection time and target cells were directly altered by genetic matching. Bone marrow and osteoblasts at the primary spongiosa were the most sensitive target cells in both, while articular and growth plate cartilage was rejected in the major but not in the minor difference grafts. Osteocytes were primarily assaulted by the host immune response in the major, however ischemia was the cause of cell death in the minor difference group [29]. No beneficial effect of matching on frozen cartilage survival was reported by other authors [51].

Frozen bone allograft had a reduced rate of union in strong histocompatibility barriers [5, 30] and no difference in weak barriers and autografts [5]. Similarly, more effective calcium replacement was found in frozen syngeneic than in allogenic grafts [21]. On the other hand, other observers found no difference in the fate of fracture healing and incorporation regardless of histocompatibility [6]. No difference in compliance and loads to failure were observed between frozen syngeneic and disparate allografts [22, 34].

Upon evaluating the recipient immune response, allogeneic grafts with two allelic differences gave a stronger reaction than semi-allogeneic grafts with one allelic difference; this indicated a gene-dose effect [40]. Accelerated skin graft rejection following major histocompatibility difference bone grafting [6, 41] and a hypersensitivity type of humoral immune response in rats regrafted with allogeneic or semi-allogeneic bone [40] suggested that the type of immune response is dependent on the graft's relative immunogenicity. Freezing and tissue-antigen matching significantly reduced synovial anti-donor DLA antibodies [51].

Immunosuppression

Immunosuppression presents a most effective way of altering recipient immune response, both humoral and cellular. Amongst the different agents used are: azathioprine [7, 8, 47], cyclosporin A [1], imuran [44], and the combinations of azathioprine and anti-lymphocytic serum (ALS) [43], ALS and prednisolone [27], ALS and cyclosporin A, [52] and double-dose cyclosphosphamide [45].

Graft survival following immunosuppression was followed for 6 months [8], 1 year [7] and 18 months [44] up to sacrifice. This included non-vascularized [7, 8] as well as vascularized allografts [1, 43, 44]. Results indicated that in the non-vascularized allografts the effect of short-term azathioprine immunosuppression (3 weeks) is as effective as long-term treatment regarding graft incorporation [7]. The beneficial effect of ALS in combination with prednisolone on the healing of vascularized allografts [27] as well as the superior results of bone viability and remodelling following cyclosporin A immunosuppression [1] were extensively elaborated and documented.

Assessing the effect of recipient immunosuppression combined with graft physical manipulation rendered valuable information on the importance of each of these manipulative methods. Comparing quality of graft incorporation following freezing and irradiation against freezing and azathioprine regimen demonstrated the superiority of the freezing irradiation method. However, the combination of azathioprine and freezing was superior to freezing alone [47]. In an analogous fashion the effect of cyclosporin A and ALS was evaluated. Both delayed rejection and allowed growth to continue. ALS alone delayed rejection only in weak histocompatibility differences while cyclosporin A was also effective in delaying rejection in strong histocompatibility barriers [52].

A major disadvantage of immunosuppression is the generalized effect of the agents. These depend on the quality, quantity and duration of the usage. Incomplete immunosuppression results in knee graft survival, however massive invasion of fibrous tissue was observed [44]. Using double-dose cyclophosphamide, no significant inhibition of antibody production was noted while increased leukopenia and animal mortality was recorded [45].

Morphology

Osteocartilagenous grafts present a composite mesenchymal tissue, including bone, cartilage, bone marrow elements, vessels and nerve tissue. Each of these elements presents an entire spectrum of cell maturation as well as differences depending on anatomical locations (such as cartilage at the growth plate and articular surface). A wide variety of tissue responses is therefore expected following transplantation. Furthermore, different physical manipulations and immunosuppressive agents may alter the immunological characteristics of different cells in different ways. It is therefore important to observe the various models of bone allografts from the point of view of morphology.

Articular Cartilage. The articular cartilage used was taken from the knee joint [2, 13, 14, 28, 29, 44], distal or proximal radius [13, 50, 51, 53], femural head [20, 17] or proximal humerus [46]. The mechanical factor of internal fixation plays a significant role in the success of these models. In a sheep model of shell osteoarticular allografts, most of the grafts underwent mechanical derangement 10 weeks following surgery [2]. However, improvement could be achieved once the technique was changed to dowel shell allografts with snug fitting to the recipient site [2]. In addition, it was found that the graft must be sufficiently thick to prevent fracture [2] and facilitate rigid internal fixation [2, 53].

Using ^{35}S autoradiography in evaluating distal femoral articular cartilage, the superficial two-thirds of the cartilage in fresh grafts remained viable, while frozen and freeze-dried grafts displayed cell death [14]. Other investigators reported degenerative changes in fresh cartilage with viable foci and cartilage disintegration when subjected to weight bearing [13]. Similarly, fresh allografts had areas of cell destruction while plasma-stored allografts survived 30 days of storage [20]. On the other hand, deep-frozen cryopreserved articular cartilage displayed metabolic activities approaching normal values, steadily increasing up to 12 months [46], and no erosion was reported in most of the cases [17].

Using a vascularized model of different histocompatibility barriers, significant differences in rejection were observed. Articular cartilage at a strong histocompatibility difference was subjected to a vigorous rejection while those at the weak histocompatibility difference were not rejected. Similar findings were made at the growth plate cartilage, indicating the observation that articular cartilage does possess antigenic characteristics [29].

Joint and Hemijoint. Experimental models for hemijoint transplantation were reported on the distal femur [12, 14, 33] and the proximal and distal radius [12, 50, 51, 53]. Hemijoint transplantation revealed information on the fate of massive bone allografting. Replacement by creeping substitution of the cancellous bone was found to be rapid, however degeneration of articular cartilage did occur and was slow [12]. Graft revascularization could be improved when frozen or freeze-dried grafts were used instead of fresh ones [14]. The amount of subchondral bone in hemijoint transplantation may be of significant importance, as grafts with a larger amount were rapidly rejected [26]. Frozen allografts with a smaller amount of subchondral bone usually maintained the overall joint configuration and in time eventually degenerated [26]. Complications of massive bone allografts could be demonstrated in animal models, including diaphyseal fractures and collapse of the distal femoral condyles [14].

Massive bone graft transplantation, including whole joint transplants, were used to evaluate graft incorporation, behaviour of articular cartilage and host immune response. The knee joint was primarily used [27–29, 43, 44, 47, 54, 55], but limb transplantation was also reported [37, 38]. Most of these models used vascularized transplants [28, 29, 43, 54]. Non-vascularized knee, frozen, frozen irradiated and azathioprine-immunosuppressed grafts were reported as well [47]. The effects of immunosuppression on vascularized whole joint transplantation were evaluated by other researchers [27, 44, 54]. The fate of articular cartilage in these models as well as graft incorporation and healing are discussed elsewhere in this paper.

Vascularized Bone Allografts

The introduction of microsurgical techniques in orthopaedic surgery has been a major contribution to successful replantation of severed digits and limbs as well as to autotransplantation. Technical barriers no longer exist for bone graft allotransplantation, and laboratory models were developed for this purpose [1, 27–29, 37, 38, 41, 43, 44, 48, 52, 54, 55]. The effect of immunosuppression [1], the fate of graft target structures [29], vascular anastomoses [41, 43, 54] and the quality of graft incorporation and viability with and without recipient immunosuppression were extensively evaluated. Whole joints and segmental bone grafts [1, 48, 52] were studied.

Vascularized bone allografts depend entirely on the patency of the anastomoses, which may be subjected to mechanical and to immunological injuries. Vascularized knee transplants were used to study this problem [41, 43, 54]. Long pedicles with anastomoses in the thigh were reported to be more successful than long- and short-pedicle popliteal grafts [43]. Using strong histocompatibility barriers it was found that an anastomosed vessel remained patent long after the bone graft was rejected; the vessels, however, ultimately clotted [29].

Bone grafts are transplanted as organs when immediately anastomosed, securing blood supply. The effect of recipient immunosuppression was evaluated on these models [27, 44, 52, 54]. Prolonged graft survival could be demonstrated [44, 52], however concomitant side effects encouraged further improvements in the searching for better immunosuppressive agents. Segmental bone grafts [1, 52] were used to assess the effect of cyclosporin A on graft viability, which was found to be significantly improved. Genetically matched vascularized rat models were evaluated for cell viability following treatment with ALS and cyclosporin A immunosuppression. The results indicate that prolonged survival of fully allogenic grafts could be achieved with both. Genetic matching alone in vascularized transplanted fibular grafts resulted in preserving regional blood flow and repair [48]. Vascularized limb models in rats [37, 38] were useful in assessing the clinical function of the transplanted knee joint as well as bone viability, healing, limb growth and donor-specific antibody production.

References

1. Aebi M, Regazzoni P, Perren SM, Schwarzenbach C (1985) Free vascularized allografts of bone segments with immunosuppression by cyclosporin. Trans Orthop Res Soc 10:288
2. Aichroth PM, Burwell RG, Laurence M (1972) Transplantation of synovial joint surfaces. Bone Joint Surg [Br] 54B(4):747
3. Bonfiglio M, Jeter WS (1972) Immunological responses to bone. Clin Orthop 87:19–27
4. Bonfiglio M, Jeter WS, Smith CL (1955) The immune concept: its relation to bone transplantation. Ann NY Acad Sci 59:417–432
5. Bos GD, Goldberg VM, Powell AE, Heiple KG, Zika JM (1983) The effect of histocompatibility matching on canine frozen bone allografts. J Bone Joint Surg [Am] 65A(1):89–96
6. Bos GD, Goldberg VM, Zika JM, Heiple KG, Powell AE (1983) Immune responses of rats to frozen bone allografts. J Bone Joint Surg [Am] 65A(2):239–246
7. Burchardt H, Glowczewskie FP, Enneking WF (1981) Short-term immunosuppression with fresh segmental fibular allografts in dogs. J Bone Joint Surg [Am] 63A(3):411–415
8. Burchardt H, Glowczewskie FP, Enneking WF (1977) Allogeneic segmental fibular transplants in azathioprine – immunosuppressed dogs. J Bone Joint Surg [Am] 59A(7):881–894
9. Burchardt H, Jones H, Glowczewskie F, Rudner C, Enneking WF (1978) Freeze-dried allogeneic segmental cortical-bone grafts in dogs. J Bone Joint Surg [Am] 60A(8):1082–1090
10. Burwell RG (1976) The fate of freeze-dried bone allografts. Transplant Proc VIII(2) [Suppl 1]:95–111
11. Burwell RG (1963) Studies in the transplantation of bone. V. The capacity of fresh and treated homografts of bone to evoke transplantation immunity. J Bone Joint Surg [Br] 45B(2):386–403
12. Campbell CJ (1972) Homotransplantation of a half or whole joint. Clin Orthop 87:146–155
13. Campbell CJ, Ishida H, Takahashi H, Kelly F (1963) The transplantation of articular cartilage. J Bone Joint Surg [Am] 45A(8):1579–1592
14. Cannon WD, Salama R, Burwell RG (1972) Massive osteoarticular femoral grafts, in sheep. J Bone Joint Surg [Am] 54A(5):1133
15. Chalmers J (1959) Transplantation immunity in bone homografting. J Bone Joint Surg [Br] 41B(1):160–179
16. Chase SW, Herndon CH (1955) The fate of autogenous and homogenous bone grafts. A historical review. J Bone Joint Surg [Am] 37A(4):809–841
17. Chesterman PJ (1968) Cartilage as a homograft. J Bone Joint Surg [Br] 50B(4):878
18. Chesterman PJ, Smith AU (1968) Homotransplantation of articular cartilage and isolated chondrocytes. J Bone Joint Surg [Br] 50B(1):184–197
19. Curtiss PH, Powell AE, Herndon CH (1959) Immunological factors in homogenous-bone transplantation. J Bone Joint Surg [Am] 41A(8):1482–1487
20. Depalma AF, Tsaltas TT, Mavler GG (1963) Viability of osteochondral grafts, as determined by uptake of S-35. J Bone Joint Surg [Am] 45A(8):1565–1578
21. Dollinger B, Klein L, Goldberg V, Powell A, Zika J (1984) Metabolic fate of frozen osteochondral allografts, in genetically imbred rats. Trans Orthop Res Soc 9:267
22. Dollinger B, Verdin P, Davy D, Goldberg V (1984) Strength and compliance of frozen osteochondral allografts, in genetically inbred rats. Trans Orthop Res Soc 9:268
23. Friedlander GE, Strong DM, Sell KW (1976) Studies on the antigenicity of Bone. J Bone Joint Surg [Am] 58A(6):854–858

24. Friedlander GE, Prasod V, McKay J (1984) Effects of law-dose irradiation on bone allograft immunogenicity. Trans Orthop Res Soc 9:264
25. Goldberg VM, Lance EM (1972) Quantitative studies of bone transplantation: the role of the allograft barrier. J Bone Joint Surg [Am] 54A(5):1133
26. Goldberg VM, Heiple KG (1983) Experimental hemijoint and whole joint transplantation. Clin Orthop 174:43–53
27. Goldberg V, Porter BB, Lance EM (1973) Transplantation of the canine knee joint on vascular-pedicles. J Bone Joint Surg [Am] 55A(6):1314
28. Gotfried Y, Yaremchuk MJ, Randolph MA, Weiland AJ (1985) Vascularized bone allografts: characteristics of minor histocompatibility differences. Trans Orthop Res Soc 10:286
29. Gotfried Y, Yaremchuk MJ, Randolph MA, Weiland AJ (1987) Histological characteristics of acute rejection in vascularized bone allografts. J Bone Joint Surg [Am] 69:410–425
30. Halloran PF, Ziv I, Lee EH, Langer F, Pritzker KPH, Gross AE (1979) Orthotopic bone transplantation in mice. Transplantation 27(6):414–419
31. Halloran PF, Lee EH, Ziv I, Langer F, Gross AE (1979) Orthotopic bone transplantation in mice. Transplantation 27(6):420–426
32. Harris WR, Martin R, Tile M (1965) Transplantation of epiphyseal plates. J Bone Joint Surg [Am] 47A(5):897–914
33. Henry WB, Schachar NS, Wadsworth PL, Castronovo FP, Mankin HJ (1985) Feline model for the study of frozen osteoarticular hemijoint transplantation: qualitative and quantitative assessment of bone healing. Am J Vet Res 46(8):1714–1720
34. Kraay MJ, Davy DT, Goldberg VM, Klein L, Powell A, Gordon N (1986) Mechanical behavior of frozen osteochondral allografts in rats with known histocompatibility barriers. Trans Orthop Res Soc 11:273
35. Langer F, Czitrom A, Pritzker KP, Gross AE (1975) The immunogenicity of fresh and frozen allogenic bone. J Bone Joint Surg [Am] 57A(2):216–220
36. Laurence M, Smith A (1968) Experiments in chondrocyte homografting in the rabbit. J Bone Joint Surg [Br] 50B(1):226
37. Lipson RA, Kawano H, Halloran PF, McKee NH, Pritzker KPH, Langer F (1983) Vascularized limb transplantation in the rat. Transplantation 35(4):293–299
38. Lipson RA, Kawano H, Halloran PF, McKee NH, Pritzker KPH, Langer F (1983) Vascularized limb transplantation in the rat. Transplantation 35(4):300–304
39. Malinin TI, Mnaymneh W, Wanger JL, Borja F (1985) Healing of internally fixed intercalary canine allografts of freeze-dried bone. Trans Orthop Res Soc 10:289
40. Muscolo DL, Kawai S, Ray RD (1976) Cellular and humoral immune response analysis of bone allografted rats. J Bone Joint Surg [Am] 58A(6):826–832
41. Nettelblad H, Yaremchuk MJ, Randolf MA, Weiland AJ (1984) The effect of genetic disparity on vascularized bone allograft survival in the rat. Trans Orthop Res Soc 9:244
42. Pelker RR, McKay J, Panjabi MM, Friedlaender GE (1986) Biomechanical evaluation of allograft incorporation. Trans Orthop Res Soc 11:272
43. Reeves B (1969) Orthotopic transplantation of vacularised whole knee joint in dogs. Lancet i:500–502
44. Reeves B (1968) Studies of vascularised homotransplants of the knee joint. J Bone Joint Surg [Br] 50B(1):226
45. Rodrigo JJ, Gray JM, Thompson EC (1984) Temporary suppression of humoral cytotoxic antibodies with double dose cyclophosphamide treatment in rats receiving distal femur allografts. Trans Orthop Res Soc 9:265
46. Schachar N, Lam S, MacDonald D, Heard J (1984) Articular cartilage survival after transplantation of deep-frozen cryopreserved osteoarticular allografts. Trans Orthop Res Soc 9:216
47. Seligman GM, George E, Yablon I, Nutik G, Cruess RL (1972) Transplantation of whole knee joints in the dog. Clin Orthop 87:332–344
48. Shaffer JM, Field GA, Goldberg VM (1984) Regional blood flow and repair following successful vascularized fibula allografts. Trans Orthop Res Soc 9:243

49. Sondenaa K, Alho A, Nielsen R (1985) Cryopreservation of osteo-chondral grafts in rabbits. Acta Orthop Scand 56:218–222
50. Stevenson S, Templeton JW (1985) The immune response to fresh and frozen, DLA matched and misimatched osteochondral allografts. Trans Orthop Res Soc 10:287
51. Stevenson S, Dannucci G, Sharkeg N (1986) Fresh and cryopreserved, DAL-matched and mismatched massive osteochondral allografts. Trans Orthop Res Soc 11:274
52. Steward JA, Langer F, Halloran P, Gross AE (1984) Vascularized bone and joint transplantation in the rat. The effect of antilymphocyte serum and cyclosporin immunosuppression. Trans Orthop Res Soc 9:266
53. Tomford WW, Henry WB, Trahan CA, Mankin HJ (1984) The fate of allograft articular cartilage: fresh and frozen. Trans Orthop Res Soc 9:217
54. Yaremchuk MJ, Sedacca TN, Schiller AL, May JW (1983) Vascular knee allograft transplantation in a rabbit model. Plast Reconstr Surg 71(4):461–471
55. Yaremchuk MJ, Nettelblad H, Randolph MA, Weiland AJ (1985) Vascularized bone allograft transplantation in a genetically defined rat model. Plastic Reconstr Surg 75(3):355–362

Experimental Models for Joint Allografting *

V. M. Goldberg

Department of Orthopaedics, Case Western Reserve University,
Cleveland, Ohio 44106, USA

Advances in the management of musculoskeletal tumors have enabled surgeons to perform limb-sparing procedures. Salvage procedures for periarticular trauma, congenital abnormalities, and degenerative processes also require large osteochondral bone grafts [11, 14, 18–20, 29]. Resurfacing osteochondral surfaces with allografts for degenerative joint disease has also been performed with varying success [11]. As a result, there has been an increased need for osteochondral grafts. Judet in 1908 first reported experimental transplantation of hemijoints and whole joints with a preservation of joint surface geometry, but with gradual cartilage deterioration and bony collapse [15]. Subsequently, many reports have confirmed these results with both autografts and allografts and have identified the major problems leading to failure [14, 18–20, 29]. These include technical difficulties with fixation and joint fit and biological causes such as delayed and incomplete revascularization and inadequate mineralization. When allografts have been used, an immune response directed toward donor antigens may be responsible for graft failure, but no studies to date have correlated the clinical outcome with this event. These problems are still unsolved, and additional experimental studies are necessary to delineate the role of these factors in determining the success or failure of osteoarticular grafts. This chapter reviews some of the experimental models that have been utilized to study hemijoint and whole joint transplantation.

Hemijoint Transplantation

Transplantation of a partial joint with a minimum amount of subchondral bone constructed as a "shell" graft is an attractive model, considering that a major portion of the immunogenicity of osteochondral grafts appear to reside in the subchondral bone [3, 7, 8]. Osteoarticular shell grafts have been studied in dog and sheep [1, 3, 5, 6, 12, 21, 22]. Three methods of fixation were evaluated: adhesive, cement, and internal fixation pins. In addition, studies have used thin and thick osseous portions of the allograft. Techniques of fixation and joint fit determined to a great extent the outcome. The important features of success included: grafts of adequate thickness rigidly fixed to the underlying bone and congruous fit between the graft and its host. These studies concluded that the major cause of graft deterioration and failure was inadequate fixation or poorly fitting grafts rather than immune rejection.

---

* Supported in part by NIH grant AM 22166.

Bone Transplantation
Eds.: M. Aebi, P. Regazzoni

Studies by Lane et al. using a rabbit autogenous osteochondral shell graft followed for up to 12 months, confirmed that in technically successful grafts the articular cartilage remained viable and biochemically intact in terms of proteoglycan, collagen, and cell content when compared with normal control animals [17]. They demonstrated that the subchondral bone was replaced in less than 6 weeks by a process that continued to maintain the integrity of the articular surface.

Other investigations of this type of osteochondral shell allografts have been directed toward delineation of the immune response to allografts. Elves and Ford identified cytotoxic antibodies in sheep 3 weeks after fresh shell and massive osteochondral allografts [7, 8]. The response, however, was not diminished by minimizing the subchondral bone. Frozen allografts evoked a similar response while freeze-dried grafts produced variable results. Yablon et al. have studied immune response of dogs after shell osteochondral hemijoint allografting [30]. They demonstrated specific cellular and humoral responses to link protein and proteoglycan fractions of the cartilage matrix of these allografts. An immune response was noted histologically in the host synovium at 6 weeks after grafting. When technical problems such as fixation were overcome, as reported by Hamilton et al. in a canine hip joint model, fresh allografts did survive and function well [12]. Ultimately, they deteriorated, and when animals were killed 2 years after transplantation, histological examination showed round cell infiltration and follicular hyperplasia of the regional lymph nodes, suggesting a chronic immune rejection. It thus appears at least experimentally that in most circumstances the immune system is an important determinant of the biological outcome of even shell allografts.

The concept of hemijoint shell grafts was extended by Porter and Lance to a whole joint model using the knee joint of dogs [22]. Although early sepsis followed 6 of 31 procedures, they were able to show that leaving a thicker bony shell of up to 7 mm had no detrimental affect on the allograft function. In addition, technically successful allografts generally showed no delay in bony union, and joint function was generally preserved. Again, internal fixation was an important technical consideration.

All of these studies indicate that if technical aspects of shell allografts can be overcome, biological problems may be surmountable, and long-term successful clinical applications may result. However, additional investigations should be directed toward cartilage and bone preservation for appropriate storage to enable osteoarticular shell grafts to be clinically useful.

Large "block" osteochondral allografts have been studied for many years. Pap and Krompecher initially reported that technical factors, including graft fixation and congruity of the articular surface, influenced the ultimate outcome [21]. Graft survival also depended upon the thickness of the subchondral bone since grafts with more than 5 mm of bone demonstrated bony necrosis and usually failed. Both autografts and allografts were followed for as long as 2.5 years after transplantation. Histological data suggested that articular cartilage appeared relatively viable in many instances, however the subchondral bone was gradually resorbed. Bony union did occur, but slowly. These early results in small block allografts were confirmed by Campbell et al., who demonstrated that during the first 6 months there were no differences histologically between fresh autogenous and allogeneic grafts [4]. Bony union was seen by 1 year. All of the allografts demonstrated degenerative changes of the articular cartilage and gradual disorganization of the grafts. The results for frozen allografts was in contrast to those previously reported by Pap and Krompecher. Burwell has also reported gradual deterioration of fresh allografts in a similar dog model, with gradual cartilage degeneration and subchondral bone necrosis [3]. Major obstacles blocking the successful outcome of these block allografts appear to be appropriate fixation, surface congruity, and an immune response.

Experimental models of "massive" hemijoint allografts have centered primarily on the study of frozen or freeze-dried material because of the studies of Elves and Ford showing the marked immunogenicity of fresh bone allografts [7, 8]. However, although antibody responses to donor transplantation antigens have been demonstrated with both fresh and frozen massive hemijoint allografts, there was no correlation of the immune response with graft survival or with creeping substitution of the donor bone by host tissue [24, 25]. Imamaliyev has attempted to modify the results seen in fresh massive canine osteoarticular grafts by using frozen allografts [14]. Satisfactory incorporation of these massive hemijoint transplants resulted when the donor tissue was frozen at −70 °C for 30 days. However, Cannon et al. undertook similar investigations in a sheep model and were unable to demonstrate satisfactory results in hemijoint transplants of knees [5]. Osteoarticular fractures of the femoral condyles resulted, and resorption of the distal osteoarticular portion took place. Recently Schachar et al., has studied a feline and a rabbit model of osteoarticular transplantation [24, 25]. They preserved the grafts with 10% dimethylsulfoxide and freezing to −80 °C for at least 1 week prior to transplantation and reported preservation of overall graft integrity. The osteosynthesis site of the allografts healed although somewhat slower than in autograft controls. The host bone seemed to replace donor tissue slowly and predictably, and although an immune response was detected, no correlation to graft survival or bone replacement was seen.

Stevenson studied a similar model in dogs utilizing the proximal radius and was able to show similar results but extended these studies to genetic typing [28]. This study indicated that the immune system was important in the ultimate acceptance and function of massive osteoarticular grafts. DLA-matched transplants appeared to function better and demonstrated improved articular cartilage characteristics and subchondral bone preservation.

In summary, these experimental models have demonstrated that not only are there technical considerations in the ultimate success or failure of osteoarticular hemijoint allografts but biological considerations are important. These considerations are the host immune response to donor antigens and revascularization and creeping substitution of the bony components. Futher studies are indicated to delineate the importance of each factor and to define better methodologies for preservation of cartilage and bone.

Whole Joint Transplantation

Models of whole joint transplantation have included both vascular and nonvascularized joint transplants. The early experimental studies in nonvascularized joint transplantation were initiated by Judet [15] and Lexer [18] in the early part of this century. They demonstrated a slow deterioration of fresh whole joint autografts or allografts, although the overall joint surfaces were maintained for a prolonged time and functioned acceptably until the bony support collapsed. Because of the failure of bone, other investigators have utilized models which transplanted whole canine knee joints after freezing the grafts to −80 °C for at least 30 days prior to transfer [14, 26, 29]. These grafts demonstrated satisfactory articular surfaces, and the bony components appeared to be replaced by new tissue. However, when fresh allografts were used, the joint rapidly degenerated. Other investigators have utilized frozen irradiated allografts stored for periods of 1–4 weeks as well as frozen allografts supplemented by immunosuppression of the host with azathioprine [26]. These grafts were compared to fresh autografts and frozen allografts preserved at −20 °C for 1–4 weeks prior to grafting. Autografts uniformly gave the best results while the irradiated frozen allografts demonstrated the best incorporation of the allograft group. The articular cartilage did not survive the freezing and the transplant procedure. Immunosuppression with azathioprine had some effect, but these grafts ultimately failed. The cause of these failures was attributed to bony collapse because of inadequate mineral accretion and poor revascularization.

Herndon and Chase, in the present author's laboratory, investigated canine whole knee transplants using a detailed histological examination to study the biological outcome [13]. The entire joint, excluding the capsule and synovial membrane, was transplanted, and both fresh and frozen autogenous and allogeneic transplants were studied over a 2-year period. Fresh autografts maintained their overall structure during the observation period and demonstrated sequential and orderly revascularization, resorption, and replacement of bony tissue. The articular cartilage was initially normal, but gradually cartilage necrosis ensued and was followed by a fibrous pannus formation which appeared to replace the surfaces with a new fibrocartilage (Fig. 1). By contrast, both fresh and frozen allografts demonstrated rapid bony necrosis with only a sporadic attempt at replacement with new bone. These grafts usually deteriorated. These investigations of nonvascularized whole joint transplants indicated again that the major causes of failure of both autografts and allografts were delayed and incomplete revascularization of the subchondral bone and the lack of adequate new bony replacement.

Recent studies have utilized immediately vascularized transplants and modifications of the immune response of the recipient to improve the results of whole joint transplantation. Buncke et al. reimplanted small whole joints in monkeys with immediate revascularization and reported that the usual degenerative process that was described for nonvascularized joints did not occur [2]. The grafts appeared to function normally for a long period of time. Slome and Reeves demonstrated in preliminary work using a vascularized canine knee replaced heterotopically in the neck or orthotopically that autografts survived for a prolonged period of time [23, 27]. Fresh allografts, in contrast, were rejected almost immediately, while when the recipients were treated with azathioprine, some of the allotransplants survived for 18 months. Further studies using azathioprine and antilymphocyte serum appeared to improve survival of allogeneic transplants. Judet and

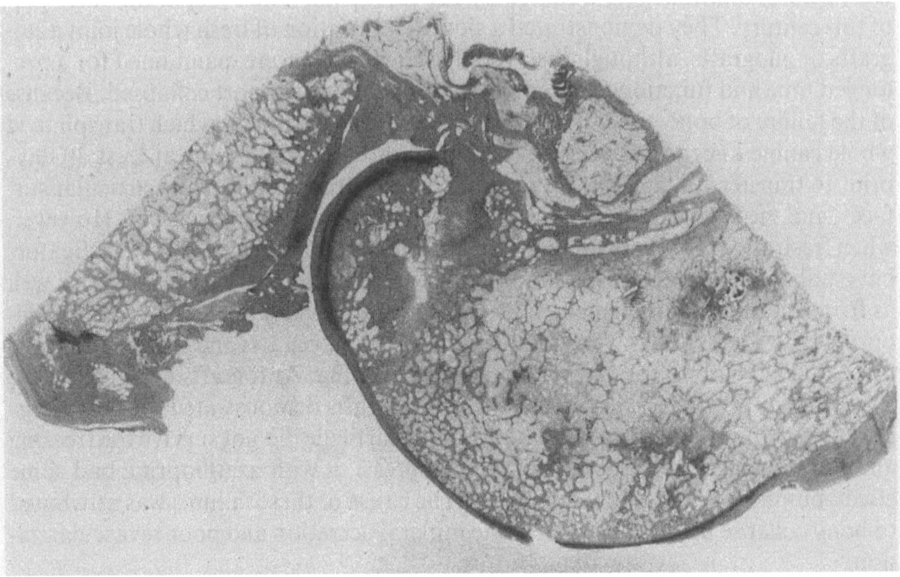

Fig. 1. Photomicrograph of fresh whole joint autograft 18 months after surgery, showing viable subchondral and cortical bone and a well-maintained articular surface (hematoxylin and eosin ×4)

Padovani reported similar results in autografts but without any prolonged allografts survivals [16].

We have investigated a similar model of vascularized canine knee joint transplants in beagles and greyhounds [9, 10]. This model is based on the concept that the vascular supply to the canine knee joint can be isolated while maintaining perfusion to the distal limb by the medial saphenous artery. The popliteal artery and vein are isolated and the periarticular muscle sectioned 4 cm from the bony attempts. The femur and tibia are osteotomized transversely approximately 5 cm from the joint. At this point the artery and vein are transsected between two vascular clamps and the joint perfused with low molecular weight dextran 40, containing heparin and 2% procaine. Either reimplantation (autograft) or a simultaneous exchange (allograft) with an unrelated animal are performed by first repairing the osteotomy using 4.5-mm self-compressing DCP plates. The vein and artery are repaired using standard microvascular technique. The remaining periarticular structures are repaired using standard technique. The major complication seen with this model is failure of the vascular anastomosis. Whenever this occurred, rapid necrosis of the soft tissue occurred, and the joint failed. When the vascular anastomoses were successful, autografts were observed for as long as 18 months and demonstrated normal function with excellent articular cartilage and subchondral bone (Fig. 2). Allografts exchanged between unrelated pairs of animals treated with azathioprine and prednisolone were uniformly unsuccessful, however when these immunosuppressive drugs were used in combination with antilymphocyte serum, long-term successful grafts were seen. However, function

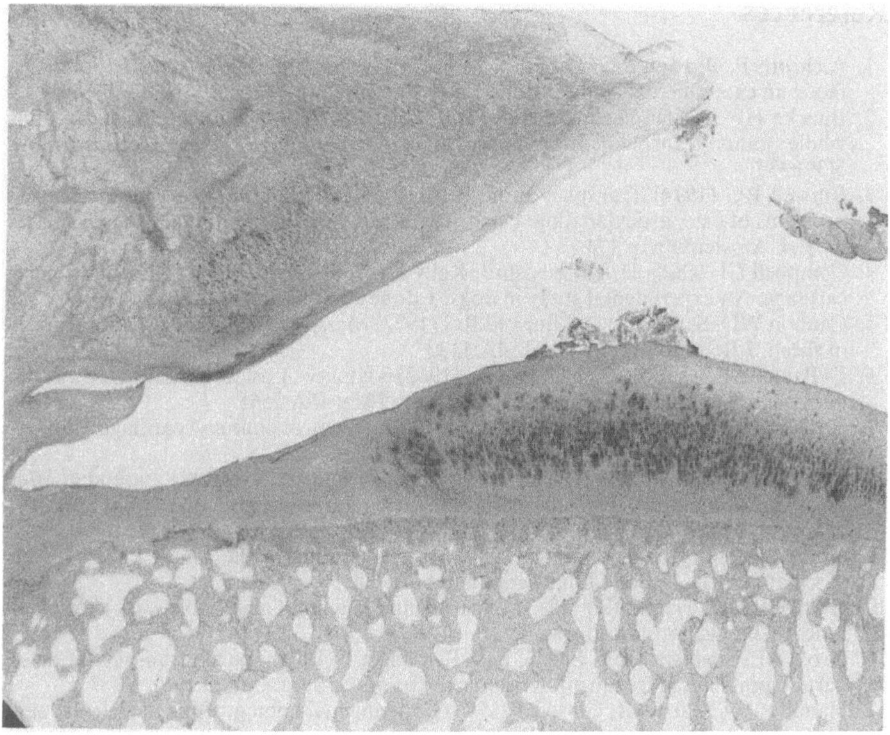

Fig. 2. Photomicrograph of a fresh vascularized autograft 12 months after surgery, demonstrating viable bone and articular cartilage. (hematoxylin and eosin ×16)

was fair when compared to the contralateral knee, and although the overall configuration of the joint was maintained, there was gradual deterioration of the articular cartilage and meniscus as well as a moderate amount of bony necrosis.

Conclusion

The studies of both hemijoint and whole joint transplantation have demonstrated the feasibility of using these models of osteochondral grafting with and without vascular pedicles. These models are useful for further study of the biological implication of immediate vascular supply in transplanting massive osteochondral grafts as well as to define the role of the immune system in the success or failure of allogeneic grafts. Further studies developing appropriate techniques for the preservation of musculoskeletal and vascular tissue must be carried out so that clinical use of these large osteochondral grafts will be based on sound scientific data.

References

1. Aichroth P, Burwell RG, Laurence M (1972) Transplantation of synovial joint surfaces: an experimental study. J Bone Joint Surg [Br] 54B:747
2. Buncke HF Jr, Daniller AI, Schultz WP, Chase RA (1967) The fate of autogenous whole joints transplanted by microvascular anastomoses. Plast Reconstr Surg 5(39):333
3. Burwell RG (1974) Transplantation of cartilage and bone, biology and mechanical problems of osteoarticular allografting. The Knee Joint. International Congress Series no 324, Amsterdam, p 174
4. Campbell CJ, Ishida H, Takashashi J, Kelly F (1963) The transplantation of articular cartilage. An experimental study in dogs. J Bone Joint Surg [Am] 45A:1579
5. Cannon WD, Salama R, and Burwell RG (1972) Massive osteoarticular femoral grafts in sheep. J Bone Joint Surg [Am] 54A:1133
6. DePalma AF, Tsaltas TT, Mauler GG (1963) Viability of osteochondral grafts as determined by uptake of S-35. J Bone Joint Surg [Am] 45A:2565
7. Elves MW (1976) Newer knowledge of the immunology of bone and cartilage. Clin Orthop 120:232
8. Elves MW, Ford CH (1971) The development of humeral cytotoxic antibodies after the allografting of articular surfaces at the knee joint in sheep. J Bone Joint Surg [Br] 53B:554
9. Goldberg V, Porter B, Lance E (1980) Transplantation of the canine knee joint on vascular pedicles. J Bone Joint Surg [Am] 62A:414
10. Goldberg VM, Heiple KG (1983) Experimental hemijoint and whole-joint transplantation. Clin Orthop 174:43–53
11. Gross AE, Silverstein EA, Falk J, Falk R, Langer F (1975) The allotransplantation of partial joints in the treatment of osteoarthritis of the knee. Clin Orthop 108:7
12. Hamilton JA, Barnes R, Gibson T (1969) Experimental homografting of articular cartilage. J Bone Joint Surg [Br] 51B:566
13. Herndon CH, Chase SW (1952) Experimental studies in the transplantation of whole joints. J Bone Joint Surg [Am] 34A:564
14. Imamaliyev AE (1969) The preparation, preservation and transplantation of articular bone end. In: Apley AG (ed) Recent advances in orthopaedics. Churchill Livingstone, London, p 209
15. Judet H (1968) Essai sur la greffe des tissus articulaires. Comptes rendus de l'Association Francaise pour l'Avancement des Sciences. 146:600
16. Judet H, Padovani JP (1968) Transplantation d'articulation complète avec rétablissement circulatoire immédiate par anastomoses arterioelles et veineuses. Mem Acad Chir 94:520
17. Lane JM, Brighton CT, Otten HR, Lipton M (1977) Joint resurfacing in the rabbit using an autologous osteochondral graft. J Bone Joint Surg [Am] 59A:218
18. Lexer E (1908) Substitution of whole or half joints from freshly amputated extremities by free plastic operation. Surg Gynecol Obstet 6:601
19. Mankin HJ, Fogelson FS, Thrasher AS, Jaffer F (1976) Massive resection and allograft transplantation in the treatment of malignant bone tumors. N Engl J Med 294:1247
20. Mankin HJ, Gebhardt MC, Tomford WW (1987) The use of frozen cadaveric allografts in the management of patients with bone tumors of the extremities. Orthop Clin North Am 18(2):275
21. Pap K, Krompecher S (1961) Arthroplasty of the knee: experimental and clinical experiences. J Bone Joint Surg [Am] 43A:523
22. Porter BB, Lance EM (1974) Limb and joint transplantation. Clin Orthop 104:249
23. Reeves B (1968) Studies of vascularized homotransplants of the knee joint. J Bone Joint Surg [Br] 50B:226
24. Schachar NS, Fuller TC, Wadsworth PL, Henry WB, Mankin HJ (1978) A feline model for the study of frozen osteochondral allografts. II. Development of lymphocytotoxic antibodies in allografts recipients. Trans Orthop Res Soc 3:131

25. Schachar NS, Henry WB, Wadsworth PL, Castronovo FP Jr, Mankin HJ (1978) A feline model for the study of frozen osteoarticular allografts. I. Quantitative assessment of cartilage viability and bone healing. Trans Orthop Res Soc 3:130
26. Seligman GM, George E, Yablon I, Vutik G, Cruess RL (1972) Transplantation of whole knee joints in the dog. Clin Orthop 87:332
27. Slome D, Reeves B (1966) Experimental homotransplantation of the knee joint. Lancet ii:205
28. Stevenson S (1987) The immune response to osteochondral allografts in dogs. J Bone Joint Surg [Am] 69A:573–582
29. Volkov M (1970) Allotransplantation of joint. J Bone Joint Surg [Br] 52B:49
30. Yablon IG, Brandt KD, DeLellis R, Covall D (1977) Destruction of joint homografts. Arthritis Rheum 20:1526

The Incorporation and Function of DLA-Matched and -Mismatched, Fresh and Cryopreserved Massive Allografts in Dogs

S. Stevenson [1], N. Sharkey [2], G. Dannucci [2], and R. Martin [2],

[1] Department of Orthopaedics, Case Western Reserve University, Cleveland, Ohio, USA
[2] Orthopaedic Research Laboratory, University of California, Davis, California, USA

Postoperative problems after the implantation of massive osteochondral allografts include degenerative joint disease and inadequate bony incorporation of the graft and result in significant morbidity. An understanding of the long-term effects of the immune response to the grafts would be helpful in preventing and treating these complications.

Dog leukocyte antigen (DLA) matched and mismatched, fresh and cryopreserved (10% DMSO, −80 °C) allografts of the proximal radius were implanted in beagles which were followed for 11 months after the surgery. Specimen radiographs and histologic sections of the articular cartilage were graded, and the cartilage was analyzed biochemically. The host-graft interface was tested in uniaxial tension, and graft incorporation was evaluated by histology and quantitated by histomorphometry. Interactive analyses of variance were used to analyze the data.

Clinically, all dogs did well, and there were no noticable differences in the appearance of allografts and autografts on in vivo radiographs. Specimen, high-detail radiographs revealed poorer incorporation of allografts than of autografts and of frozen grafts than of fresh grafts ($p < 0.05$), typified by cortical resorption, loss of trabecular detail, and subchondral bone cysts.

The synovial membrane of all operated joints underwent mild fibrosis and synovial hyperplasia. Only those of allografts, particularly fresh DLA-mismatched, showed severe fibrosis, hyperplasia, and an inflammatory response. The gross appearance of the cartilage of autografted and sham-operated joints was normal. Thinning, dullness, and roughening were noted in all allografts. Invasive pannus was present in fresh grafts and erosion to subchondral bone was sometimes present in fresh, DLA-mismatched grafts. Cartilage of grafts which had been frozen appeared to be consistently thinner than cartilage transplanted fresh. The histological and biochemical analysis of transplanted cartilage correlated well. Frozen grafts received significantly worse histologic scores, and had significantly less GAG and a lower Gal : Glu ($p < 0.001$).

There were no differences in the stiffness of the host-graft interface. Histologically, all grafted bone was necrotic and covered to a greater or lesser extent by new host bone. Incorporation of cortical bone was initiated by resorption, and there was a significant correlation between porosity and live bone. The apposition rate and number of remodeling osteons was significantly greater in the cortex of grafted segments than in the cortex of sham-operated segments ($p < 0.01$), but no statistically significant differences were noted between groups. The cortical bone

Bone Transplantation
Eds.: M. Aebi, P. Regazzoni

of autografts had more live bone than that of allografts, but the difference was only occasionally statistically significant ($p < 0.05$). New bone formation and normal marrow contents were noted in the metaphyseal cancellous bone of autografts and DLA-matched allografts. Little new bone formation and extremely fibrotic bone marrow were present in DLA-mismatched allografts, particularly fresh ones.

Segmental Vascularized and Non-vascularized Bone Allografts

O. Schwarzenbach, P. Regazzoni, and M. Aebi

Department of Orthopedic Surgery, University of Bern, and Department of Surgery, University of Basel, Switzerland

Segmental defects in diaphyseal bone resulting from congenital deformity, trauma, or tumor resection remain a challenging therapeutic problem. To bridge such defects, cancellous grafts, vascularized and nonvascularized cortical autografts, and nonvascularized segmental allografts have been used. The data available until now suggest that the optimal conditions for bone grafting include good viability of the graft, internal fixation, and orthotopic transplantation. Vascularized autografts therefore have several advantages as compared with avascular grafts. Autograft harvesting, however, creates an additional lesion in the patient, and the procedure has its own morbidity. Especially considering the availability of these grafts even in the context of hemijoint and whole joint replacements, bone allografting therefore seems a promising alternative in the treatment of large segmental bone defects. But fresh allogeneic bone is highly immunogenic, and for this reason immunosuppression of the host might be beneficial for the outcome of bone allografts.

The objectives of our study were to investigate the bone healing pattern of large segmental bone allografts in a technically standardized model and to analyze possible benefits of microsurgical revascularization and short- or long-term immunosuppression on the viability and remodeling of the graft.

A total of 47 mature, immunologically unmatched mongrel dogs were analyzed. In all, eight different groups were operated on: the autologous control groups, the allogeneic groups without immunosuppression, with short-term (4-week) immunosuppression, and with long-term (20-week) immunosuppression with cyclosporine A (daily dosage 15 mg/kg). The surgical procedure consisted of transplanting an 8-cm long trapezoid midshaft segment of the donor tibia. For microsurgical revascularization the nutrient vessels were used and anastomosed to the anterior tibial vessels. The periosteum of the graft was totally stripped. Therefore, if primary revascularization occurred, it was due to the anastomosed vessels. Internal fixation was performed using 12 whole 3.5-dynamic ASIF compression plates. The smallest possible number of screws to achieve the necessary stability for immediate weight bearing was implanted in order to avoid interference with vascularization of the graft. During the postoperative survival of 20 weeks the animal bone was labeled with fluorochromes. At sacrifice date all animals were injected intravenously with disulfine blue. Standardized X rays were done after removing the whole tibia, and the bones were then worked up histologically.

Radiological evaluation of the graft-host interface healing showed optimal results in the autografts and long-term immunosuppressed allografts, but with sta-

Bone Transplantation
Eds.: M. Aebi, P. Regazzoni

tistical significance only in the revascularized allografts without immunosuppression. The radiological quality of the grafted bone showed statistical significance between the best group, the autografts, and all the allografts without immunosuppression and with only short-term immunosuppression, but comparable results with the long-term immunosuppressed allografts. The radiological findings could be confirmed by fluorescent mircoscopy.

Disulfine blue perfusion tells us about the actual vascularity of the graft at sacrifice date. Beside the autografts, only the long-term immunosuppressed allografts have a negligible amount of unperfused bone. Unperfused bone areas are mainly found in the vascularized allografts without immunosuppression, in a lesser amount in the nonvascularized allografts without immunosuppression, and in the short-term immunosuppressed groups (Fig. 1).

One parameter of the viability of the graft is the remodeling of the grafted bone. We were able to show two different remodeling patterns. Mainly in nonvascularized grafts we found a creeping substitution starting from periosteal sites moving towards the endosteal surface. In contrast, we found predominantly in revascularized grafts a haversian type of remodeling along the intracortical vascular system, preserving the architecture of the cortex. A quantitative evaluation of the number of living, labeled osteons per mm^2 in different areas of interest of the

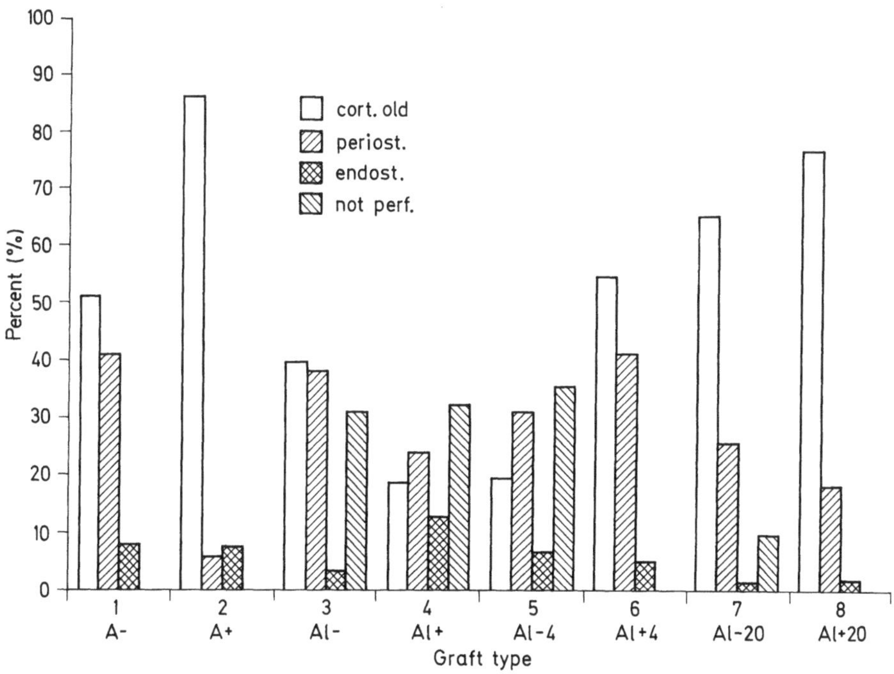

Fig. 1. Percentage of perfusion in different areas of autografts and allografts. *A−/A+*, nonvascularized/vascularized autografts; *Al−/Al+*, nonvascularized/vascularized allografts without immunosuppression; *Al−4/Al+4*, nonvascularized/vascularized allografts with 4-week immunosuppression; *Al−20/Al+20*, nonvascularized/vascularized allografts with 20-week immunosuppression

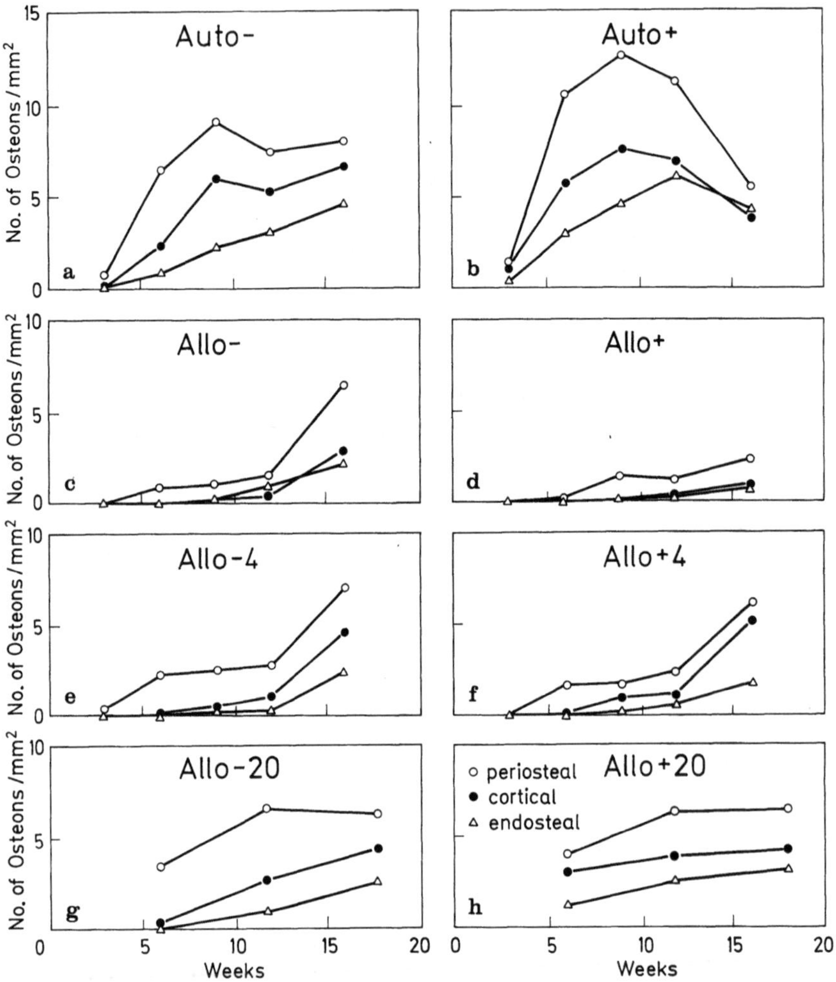

Fig. 2. Rates of remodeling of periosteal, cortical, and endosteal bone in different graft types. **a** Nonvascularized autograft. **b** Vascularized autograft. **c** Nonvascularized allograft without immunosuppression. **d** Vascularized allograft without immunosuppression. **e** Nonvascularized allograft with 4-week immunosuppression. **f** Vascularized allograft with 4-week immunosuppression. **g** Nonvascularized allograft with 20-week immunosuppression. **h** Vascularized allograft with 20-week immunosuppression

midgraft cortical bone showed a high level of early labeled osteons in all three cortical areas (periosteal, midcortical, endosteal) in both autograft groups. The long-term immunosuppressed groups remodel to a lesser, but still significantly high, amount. Compared to the short-term immunosuppressed grafts the remodeling starts earlier and on a clearly higher level (Fig. 2). Revascularization in the short-term immunosuppressed group does not change the remodeling pattern of the graft, and there is no significant difference between the short-term immunosuppressed groups and the nonvascularized allografts without immunosuppression. The remodeling in these three groups starts late in the second half of the experimental period. The vascularized allografts without immunosuppression do not show remodeling activity throughout the cortex, except for a mild periosteal creeping substitution starting at the end of the experiment. Either these allografts consist of dead bone, or a large part of the cortex has been resorbed and replaced by soft tissue.

In conclusion, this study indicates that histoincompatibility is the limiting factor for bone graft survival. Primary stable internal fixation allows rapid bone healing at the graft-host interface, if important bone resorption – due to graft rejection – does not cause a secondary instability. Short-term immunosuppression improves graft survival, but long-term immunosuppression is necessary to obtain the full benefit of primary microvascular anastomoses and to induce the allograft to be incorporated in a way very much like that of analogous autografts.

Research on the Biology of Microvascular Bone Grafts

G. Stefani, P. Guizzi, B. Battiston, and G. Brunelli

Orthopedic Department, Brescia University Medical School, Italy

More and more often the orthopedic surgeon must treat large bone defects due to bone tumors, resections, osteomyelitis, congenital pseudarthrosis, and post-traumatic bone defects that require large bone grafts. In these cases, conventional autogenous corticocancellous bone grafts can hardly solve the problem. Using vascularized bone grafts, which do not undergo creeping substitution, which heal swiftly, and which are not parasitic of surrounding tissues, yields better, safer and quicker results [2, 4]. To better understand the recovery of vascularized grafts as compared to conventional ones, research on rabbits has been done comparing the biological features of repair by means of scintigraphic, radiographic, and histologic methods [1, 3].

We used adult white rabbits weighting 3.0–3.5 kg. We chose the radius as the best bone for the study because of its good vascularization and because the animals do not disturb the bone fixation after the operation since their weight is supported mainly by the ulna. In all, 24 animals were operated on: 12 by means of vascularized grafts and 12 by means of nonvascularized ones. The graft was obtained by a double transversal osteotomy, preserving the vessels in 12 rabbits and cutting them, thus completely isolating the graft, in the other 12. Then the graft was synthetized, fixing it by means ot two transversal Kirschner wires securing the radius to the ulna. Postoperatively eight animals (four vascular and four nonvascular) were injected with ^{99}Tc methylene diphosphonate at 7 days. After 3 h a scintigraphic evaluation by gamma camera with high resolution was made. In six cases the operated radius was examined by means of a Geiger counter after killing the animal. In eight animals (four vascular and four nonvascular) the operated radius was withdrawn at 20 and 40 days and fixed in formalin. These were then decalcified, placed in paraffin, and stained by the Cajal-Gallego method. Eight more animals (four vascular and four nonvascular) were studied by means of tetracycline labeling, injecting rolitetracycline for 2 days postoperatively and again for 4 days after an interval of 12 days. The specimens were withdrawn 20 and 40 days after the operation, fixed in methylmethacrylate, cut, and observed by fluorescent microscopy.

The scintigraphic evaluation showed a better uptake, both at osteotomies and at diaphyseal level, in the vascularized grafts. More reliable data were obtained by the Geiger counter: the microvascular grafts always showed a superior activity of the radioisotope. The histology (decalcified specimens) revealed in the conventional grafts that the central channel of the osteons had an altered edge, and that the central vessel was degenerated (Fig. 1). The cells were picnotic, and several lacunae were empty. Vascular grafts, on the other hand, showed normal lacunae

Bone Transplantation
Eds.: M. Aebi, P. Regazzoni

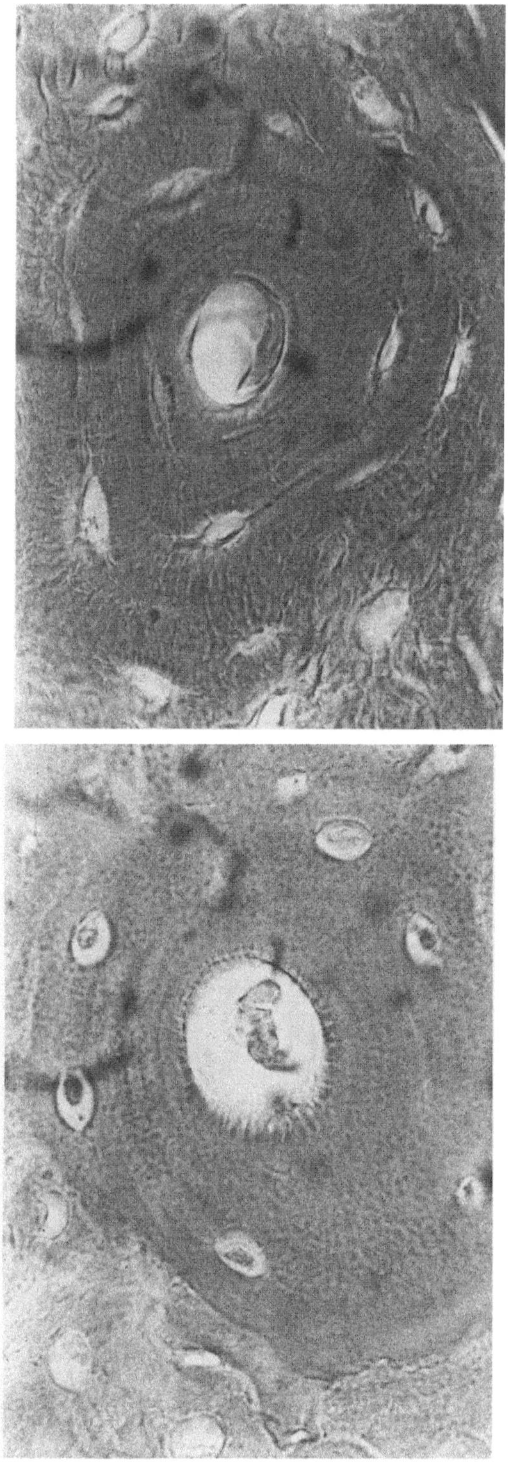

Fig. 1. a Necrosis of osteocytes and central vessel in avascular grafts. **b** Viability of osteocytes with normal lacunae and normal central vessel in vascular grafts. Decalcified specimens ($\times 100$)

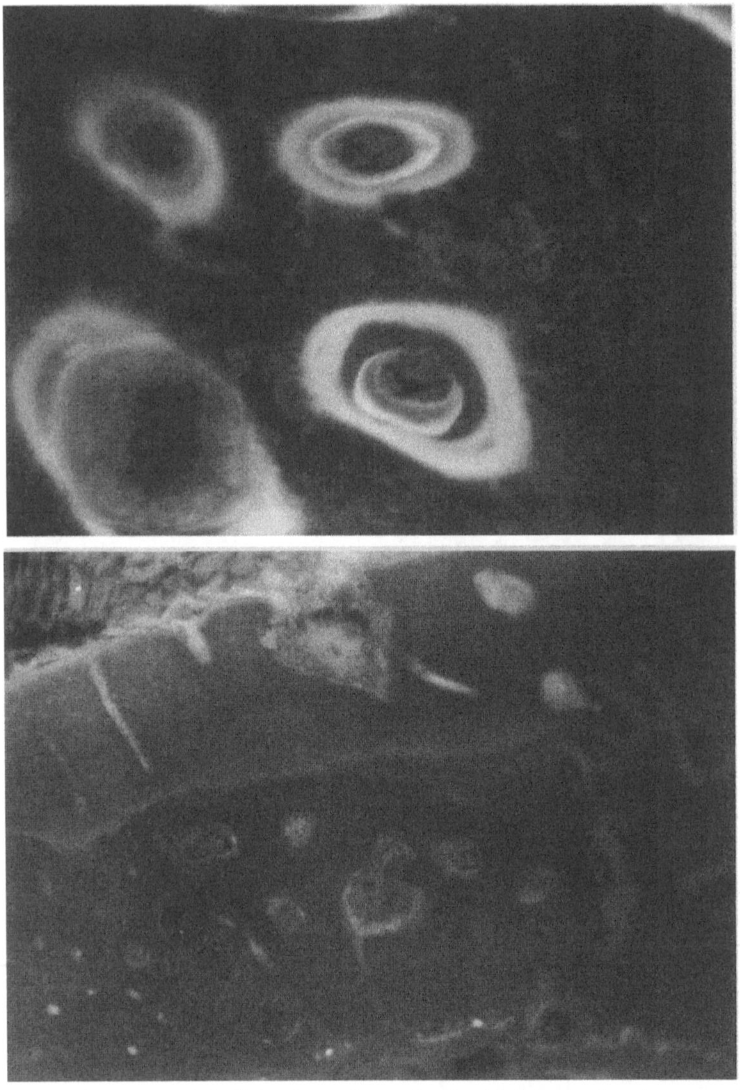

Fig. 2. a Osteogenesis in living bone shown by double labeling in microvascular grafts. Nondecalcified specimen at fluorescence microscopy (× 100). **b** No sign of living bone remodeling in avascular grafts. Nondecalcified specimen at fluorescence microscopy (× 25)

filled by normal osteocytes and good central vessel. The fluorescent histology showed that tetracycline uptake was high in the vascular grafts, with double labeling present both in the periosteal area and in the central osteons. The double labeling is a clear index of living bone remodeling (Fig. 2). However, in the conventional grafts either there was no fluorescence, or, if present, it consisted of single labels just in the periosteal area. Finally, the radiographic examination demonstrated (at 20 and 40 days) a better and much earlier callus formation in the vascularized bone.

This experimental research demonstrated the viability and superiority of vascularized grafts and the poor survival of nonvascularized grafts. This confirms clinical results and the indications for the use of microvascular bone grafts, especially in those cases in which a large loss of substance and bad local conditions render healing by conventional grafts very difficult.

References

1. Allieu Y, Teissier J, Bonnel F (1983) Etude expérimentale du comportement biologique d'une greffe osseuse cortical vascularisée et problèmes mécaniques. SOFCOT [Suppl 2]:69
2. Brunelli G (1980) Utilizzazione di innesti ossei microvascolari nella chirurgia dell'arto superiore. Riv Chir Mano 17(2):285
3. Shaffer et al. (1984) A vascularized fibula model to study vascularized canine bone grafts. Microsurgery 5:185
4. Weiland J (1979) Free vascularized bone grafts in surgery of the upper extremity. J Hand Surg [Am] 4:129

A Comparison of Vascularized and Conventional Bone Grafts for Large Defects in Weight-Bearing Bones

J. F. Welter and K. L. B. Brown

Montreal Children's Hospital, Montreal, Quebec, Canada

The increasing use of limb-sparing surgery for major tumor excisions has created a demand for a reliable method of bridging large bony gaps. Conventional grafts require long periods of immobilization and often fail, especially when very large defects are bridged or the recipient bed is poorly vascularized. Microsurgery can be used to reestablish the blood supply to bone autografts, thus circumventing much of the repair process. Clinically, vascularized grafts heal faster, hypertrophy more, and are more reliable in poorly vascularized beds. Recent animal experiments have not duplicated the excellent results claimed in clinical studies, particularly with regard to hypertrophy. These experimental models use non-weight-bearing grafts or grafts shielded by plates. The ability to hypertrophy rapidly is a key advantage for a bone graft since it reduces the immobilization period and lessens complications.

To resolve this controversy, we used a model which more closely resembles the clinical situation. A total of 38 adult dogs were operated. In one forelimb, 7-cm segments of both radius and ulna were removed. A 9-cm vascularized fibula was harvested from one hindlimb. A conventional 9-cm fibular graft was obtained subperiosteally from the other leg. The dogs were divided into two groups. In group 1, the radial gap was bridged by the vascularized graft while the ulnar defect was bridged by the conventional graft. In group 2, the positions were reversed. An external fixator was used to stabilize the forelimb. Grafts placed in the radius were subjected to much greater weight-bearing loads than those placed in the ulna. X rays were taken biweekly to determine union time and to assess hypertrophy. Graft hypertrophy was measured from the radiographs using a Bioquant image analyzer. The dogs were sacrified at 2, 3, 4, 6, and 12 months, after receiving two doses of tetracycline to label new bone formation. The grafts were twisted to failure using an Instron materials-testing machine. The applied torque and resulting angular deformation were recorded. Undecalcified sections were obtained from four sites of the grafts. Bone formation and resorption rates were quantified from these sections.

All conventional grafts were revascularized within 2 months. Union time of the conventional and vascularized grafts was the same. In group 1, vascularized transplants doubled in size within 12 weeks; conventional grafts hypertrophied more slowly and did not reach the size of the vascularized transplants until after 6 months. In group 2, the vascularized transplants also hypertrophied faster than the conventional grafts in the first 6 months, but the differences were considerably smaller. In group 1, vascularized grafts were significantly stronger than conventional grafts at 4 and 6 months. This corresponds to the maximum difference in

Bone Transplantation
Eds.: M. Aebi, P. Regazzoni

size between the two types of graft. Histologically, the vascularized transplants showed marked peripheral bone formation and little activity in the center of the graft, leaving the original bone intact for about 6 months and then gradually remodeling. Conventional grafts became highly porous while bone deposition was minimal at first and gradually increased.

In this study, vascularized transplants hypertrophied faster and became stronger than conventional grafts. The pattern of repair was different in the two types of graft. The amount of stress placed on the grafts appeared to be important, as the vascularized grafts hypertrophied much more when placed in the radius. In dogs, the radius is reported to be the main weight-bearing bone of the forelimb. This seems to indicate that combined weight-bearing stress and microsurgical revascularization allow bone grafts to perform most reliably in large reconstructive procedures.

Experimental Vascularized Bone Allograft Transplantation *

M. J. Yaremchuk, A. J. Weiland, M. A. Randolph, H. Nettelblad, Y. Gotfried, S. Kesmarky, P. C. Innis, J. P. Paskert, L. W. Clow, J. F. Burdick, W. P. A. Lee, and Y. C. Pan

Department of Orthopaedic Surgery, Division of Plastic Surgery, Division of Transplantation Surgery, Johns Hopkins University School of Medicine, Baltimore, Maryland, USA

The immediate vascularization of bone allografts by microsurgical anastomosis of donor and host vessels is a theoretically appealing way to avoid problems related to graft nonviability inherent in nonvascularized bone allografts. However, these grafts are subjected to immunologic rejection similar to organ allografts. To determine the immunologic and morphologic consequences of the transplantation of vascularized bone allografts, a series of experiments using a genetically defined rat model was performed. The specific aims were (a) to develop a reliable model for heterotopic and orthotopic vascularized bone allograft transplantation; (b) to determine the role of genetic disparity on allograft survival; (c) to define histologic criteria for rejection; (d) to assess the cellular and humoral arms of the immune response to vascularized bone allografts; (e) to determine the role of nonspecific (cyclosporine) and specific (tolerance, enhancement) immunosuppression on graft survival; and (f) to assess the healing properties of vascularized bone allografts.

Heterotopic and orthotopic models for vascularized bone grafting were developed using inbred Lewis rats. The heterotopic model consisted of the complete knee joint of the rat, which included the distal 1 cm of the femur, the proximal 1 cm of the tibia, and a minimal muscle cuff. The vascular supply was based on the femoral vessels dividing into the genicular and popliteal branches. These transplants were placed subcutaneously on the abdominal wall in the inguinal region with microvascular anastomoses between the graft pedicle and the host femoral vessels. Similarly, the orthotopic model consisted of the distal 1 cm of femur with muscle cuff and vascular pedicle. The graft was fixed in an orthotopic site with an intramedullary Kirschner wire and a metal suture around the knee joint. Nonvascular controls were performed in the same manner without muscle and vascular pedicle. Lewis grafts (major histocompatibility locus designated $RT1^{l}$) were transplanted across weak and strong histocompatibility barriers to Fischer-344 ($RT1^{lv}$) and Brown Norway ($RT1^{n}$) recipients respectively. More than 600 transplants were performed and serially analyzed with standard histologic, histochemical, and bone fluorochrome labeling procedures. The humoral immune response by the host was assessed using a complement-dependent ^{51}Cr cytotoxic antibody assay. The cell-mediated response was evaluated using host splenocytes in mixed lymphocyte cultures. After 6 days in culture, these cells were used in a

* Supported by NIH grant AM 25791.

Bone Transplantation
Eds.: M. Aebi, P. Regazzoni

^{51}Cr cell-mediated lymphocytotoxicity assay against donor lymphocytes. Nonspecific immunosuppression was achieved by the administration of cyclosporine (10 mg/kg per day subcutaneously) to graft recipients. Specific immunosuppression was induced by administering donor-specific blood (DSB), UV-irradiated DSB, DSB with a short course of cyclosporine, and third-party blood transfusions. All studies were 12 weeks in duration.

Results were as follows: (a) Viable isograft transplantation proved the reliability of both models. (b) Vascularized bone allografts transplanted across a strong histocompatibility barrier were victims of an acute rejection response at 7–10 days, leading to total graft necrosis and never regaining the potential to form new bone. However, transplants across a weak barrier showed a less pronounced, prolonged rejection reaction, with new bone formation apparent in the grafts by 12 weeks. (c) Histologically, rejection was characterized by marrow disruption, with fibrin deposition and osteoblast damage in the primary spongiosa below the growth plate. (d) Unlike nonvascularized corticocancellous allografts, both of which elicit only an early cellular response, vascularized bone allografts provoked both early cellular and humoral responses, evident as early as 5 days posttransplantation. (e) Only continuous cyclosporine prevented rejection and allowed healing in transplants across a strong genetic barrier. DSB regimens demonstrated enhanced rejection over nontreated control allografts, indicating a sensitized response to the transplants. (f) Short-term cyclosporine prevents rejection for a sufficient period to allow healing in weak-barrier transplants. However, chronic rejection results in collapse of these grafts when placed in an orthotopic position.

Vascularized bone allografts are as susceptible to rejection as are other primarily vascularized organ allografts, and genetic disparity is a primary determinant of the timing and nature of the rejection process. The cellular and humoral responses to vascularized bone allografts are different from nonvascularized grafts in timing and intensity, suggesting a different mechanism of rejection. Therefore, data available from nonvascularized transplantation may not be applicable to vascularized transplantation. Short-term cyclosporine immunosuppression in weak histocompatibility barrier transplantation allowed bone healing but did not avoid chronic rejection of the graft. Successful orthotopic transplantation required continuous cyclosporine in transplantation across a strong histocompatibility barrier. Thus, clinical vascularized bone allograft transplantation may require both genetic matching and immunologic manipulation of host and/or graft.

Implants of Frozen and Decalcified Allogeneic Bone in Rats

P. Yde[1], G. S. E. Dowd[1], G. Bentley[1], F. Handelberg[2], P. P. Casteleyn[2] and P. Opdecam[2]

[1] Institute of Orthopaedics, R. N. O. H., Stanmore, UK
[2] Department of Orthopaedics and Traumatology, Academic Hospital, Free University Brussels, Belgium

A standardized non-healing bone defect, described by Siegel et al. (1972), was performed on rat femora. The defect consisting of the midsection of the femur was immobilized by internal fixation, using an omega-shaped intramedullary distraction pin. The gaps were filled by two types of allogeneic bone: (a) frozen cancellous bone (−70 °C) and (b) decalcified cortical bone (0.6 N HCl). In a control group, autologous bone grafts were used. The animals were sacrificed at 6 and 12 weeks. The samples were analysed by X rays and in histological preparations.

Results were as follows: (a) Autologous bone was, compared to frozen and decalcified bone, the best material for bone grafting. (b) The frozen bone grafts were well surrounded by new bone formation near the callus of the femur; further away from this site, the frozen grafts were necrotic, with no new bone formation. (c) The decalcified bone grafts gave good results, comparable to those of the frozen grafts, near the callus site; further away from the callus formation, the decalcified grafts still were surrounded by new bone, although not in continuity with the callus. In poorly vascularized areas, cartilage was formed.

In this experiment autologous bone proved to be the best grafting material. The results of the frozen and decalcified bone grafts were comparable to each other. Decalcified bone grafts have an osteogenetic capacity.

Bone Transplantation
Eds.: M. Aebi, P. Regazzoni

Immunology

Introduction to Transplantation Immunology

P. C. Hiestand

Preclinical Research, Sandoz Ltd. 4002 Basel, Switzerland

Introduction

This is not intended to be an exhaustive account of all the facts and findings which have been shown to contribute to graft rejection, but rather a short introduction to the mechanisms leading to rejection.

Transplant rejection is a multistep process initiated by the recognition of foreign antigens on the grafted tissue by the recipient's immune cells. This recognition leads in turn to the activation of various T lymphocyte subsets, B lymphocytes and accessory cells. All these activated cells contribute to rejection process by being directly cytotoxic to the graft [cytotoxic T lymphocytes (CTL), cytolytic macrophages], by supplying help in the form of lymphokines required for lymphocyte activation, clonal expansion and differentiation, or by producing antibodies which in turn bind to alloantigens, thereby enhancing antibody-mediated cytotoxicity. Antibodies, however, play only a minor role in acute or chronic graft rejection.

Antigen Recognition

Recognition of alloantigens by the immune system was known even before T and B lymphocytes were defined. Since the discovery of T and B lymphocytes in 1968, it has been clear that graft rejection is mediated mainly by T lymphocytes. However, it is also clear that the formation of alloantibody is detrimental to the transplanted tissue and that pre-existing alloantibodies cause hyperacute rejection, probably by activation of the complement cascade.

The antigens which are recognized on the graft are the major histocompatibility complex [MHC; also called human lymphocyte antigen (HLA)] products expressed on the cell surface. These MHC or HLA products are divided into two distinct classes, class I and class II antigens.

Class I antigens, which are expressed on the surface of all nucleated cells, are composed of two noncovalently associated, glycosylated polypeptides: a heavy chain of M_r 44000 and β_2-microglobulin, M_r 12000. While the light chain (β_2-microglobulin) is identical in all class I antigens, the heavy chain exhibits extensive polymorphism and is coded for by the K, D and L genes of the mouse H-2 complex and the A, B and C genes of the human HLA complex. Class I antigens are recognized in the killing of virus-infected cells by CTL and are the target antigens recognized by CTL during graft rejection. The CTL carry the CD8 (T8) products as phenotypic surface markers.

Bone Transplantation
Eds.: M. Aebi, P. Regazzoni

Class II antigens are expressed constitutively on B lymphocytes and other accessory cells (e.g., dendritic cells) and can be induced on other cell types like macrophages, epithelium and vascular endothelium. They are composed of two non-covalently associated glycosylated polypeptides: α chain, M_r 32000, and β chain, M_r 28000. Class II antigens include murine I-A and I-E and human HLA-DR, -DQ and -DP antigens. Class II antigens are recognized by T helper (T_H) cells. T_H cells carry the CD4 (T4) antigen which can be used as a phenotypic surface marker.

Recognition and binding of either soluble antigens or MHC (HLA) from grafted tissue is to the T cell receptor. While the MHC molecules bind directly to the receptor, soluble antigens need to be processed by antigen presenting cells (APC) and expressed on the surface of the APC in context with the APC's own MHC antigens.

The T cell receptor consists of the T_i α/β heterodimer, which carries the clonal specificity through its variable regions and has apparently coevolved to interact with another gene family, the proteins of the MHC. The function of another heterodimer, γ/δ, expressed on about 5% of T cells, is unknown. Furthermore, as T cells mature they undergo stringent selection, allowing only a small percentage of precursor cells to develop. T cells bearing receptors that recognize the host's own molecules are deleted, a process known as tolerance induction, and the remaining cells are probably also selected positively for the ability to interact with self-MHC molecules (= MHC restriction).

Three other molecules, termed CD3, are physically associated with the T cell receptor heterodimer on the cell surface and serve as signal transducing elements.

Additional structures on T cells stabilize the binding of the foreign antigen to the T cell receptor. These structures are in the case of the CTL, the CD8 molecule, in the case of the T_H lymphocyte, the CD4 molecule. They play no role in the specificity of binding but rather enhance the avidity of these cell-cell interactions by binding to monomorphic determinants of the appropriate MHC molecule on the target cell.

Cell Activation

Since all grafts express class I antigens (especially vascular endothelial cells are rich in class I expression), CTL are among the first cells to be activated. Subsequently, or concomitantly, T_H cells are activated either by passenger leukocytes bearing class II antigens or by graft antigens generated during cell death of at least part of the grafted tissue and then processed by and presented on the cell surface of accessory cells in conjunction with self-MHC, or by a combination of the two processes.

Interaction of the alloantigen-MHC complex with the T cell receptor results in a series of intracellular events eventually leading to the expression of interleukin-2 (IL-2) receptor molecules on the T cell surface. Upon receiving a signal from activated APC, in the form of IL-1, the lymphocytes respond by producing IL-2 which binds to the IL-2 receptors on their own cell membrane and on cells in the near vicinity. IL-1 is not only a required signal for the T_H cells but is probably important for the activation of unprimed CTL. Additional lymphokines, like γ-interferon, are also formed upon T cell activation. While most of the IL-2 is produced by T_H cells, a certain amount is also formed by CTL. Binding of IL-2 to the surface receptor results in proliferation of both T_H lymphocytes and CTL (called clonal expansion) and maturation of CTL to effector cells. The fully activated CTL is now ready to lyse the target cell to which it binds via the T cell receptor.

Augmentation

Release of γ-interferon from activated T cells will have the following two major consequences. γ-Interferon serves as an activating lymphokine for monocytes, causing them to release mediators (chemotactic factors) which attract more leukocytes to the grafted tissue and may therefore potentiate an inflammatory response. γ-Interferon is also known to be a potent inducer for both MHC class I and class II antigen expression. Enhanced expression, especially of class II antigen, on the grafted tissue makes the graft more vulnerable to effector mechanisms. Other factors with adverse effects on graft survival are the complement and the coagulation system. Chemotactic activity of activated complement induces and sustains inflammatory processes and vascular leakage. Microthrombus formation and coagulation processes also contribute to graft rejection.

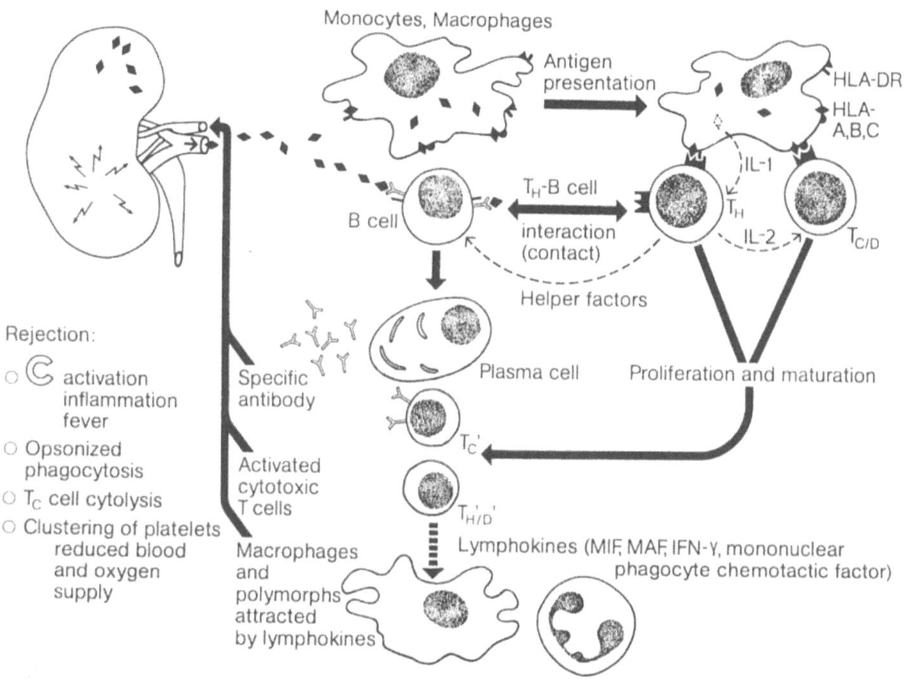

Fig. 1. Mechanism of transplant rejection. T_H, T helper; T_C, T cytotoxic; T_D, T de layed type hypersensitivity; prime (') indicates activated. IL-1, IL-2, interleukin-1, -2; *MIF*, macrophage-inhibiting factor; MAF, macrophage-activating factor; *IFN*-γ, γ-interferon. ◆, antigen; C, complement

Graft Destruction

Occupation of the T_i-CD3 complex of the CTL causes calcium influx which acts as a signal for the so-called lethal hit phase, during which specific toxic proteins are released by the CTL onto target cells which then undergo lysis. These proteins include the pore-forming protein perforin (cytolysin), proteolytic enzymes and tumor necrosis factor (TNF). Perforin produces transmembrane lesions after binding to and insertion into a biological membrane. Pores formed by perforin are large enough to permit ion exchange, which ultimately leads to cell death. Pore formation by perforin is in many aspects similar to the channel formation induced by the ninth component of complement or bacterial and amebal toxins. The involvement of proteolytic enzymes and of TNF-β (formerly called lymphotoxin) in the process of target cell destruction is still controversial.

Conclusion

Due to the complexity of the subject only an overview of the mechanisms involved in graft rejection could be presented. Many of them still require further investigation to be completely understood. A list of relevant references has been added for the interested reader.

Acknowledgement. I would like to thank Dr. P. Geiser, Sandoz Ltd., for the illustration.

Further Reading

General

Roitt I (1980) Essential immunology. Blackwell, Oxford
Stites DP,, Stobo JD, Wells JV (1987) Basic and clinical immunology. Appelton & Lange, Norwalk, Connecticut
Bier OG, da Silva WD, Götze D, Mota I (1986) Fundamentals of immunology. Springer, Berlin Heidelberg New York

Recognition

Moeller E (1987) Recognition and response to alloantigens. Transplant Proc 19:40–44

Structure and Function of T Cell Receptor and MHC (HLA) Molecules

Thorsby E (1987) Structure and function of HLA molecules. Transplant Proc 19:29–35
Capra JD, Hoover ML (1987) The immunoglobulin gene superfamily and human disease. Transplant Proc 19:25–28
Marrack P, Kappler J (1987) The T cell receptor. Science 238:1073–1079

Cell activation

Activation antigens and signal transduction in lymphocyte activation (1987) Immunol Rev 95
Smith KA (1988) Interleukin-2: inception, impact, and implications. Science 240:1169–1176

Regulation of Alloantigen Expression

Fabre JW, Milton AD, Spencer S, Settaf A, Houssin D (1987) Regulation of alloantigen expression in different tissues. Transplant Proc 19:45–49

Effector Mechanisms

Tschopp J, Jongeneel CV (1988) Cytotoxic T lymphocyte mediated cytolysis. Biochemistry 27:2641–2646
Hall BM (1987) Cellular infiltrates in allografts. Transplant Proc 19:50–56
Ascher NL (1987) Effector mechanisms in allograft rejection. Transplant Proc 19:57–60

General Aspects of Organ Transplantation Surgery

F. Harder and J. Landman

Department of Surgery, University of Basel, Basel, Switzerland

Of the notable events in renal transplantation now a routine clinical treatment option, the following are of particular significance: definition of the major histocompatibility complex in man, with consequent typing and matching of donor-recipient pairs, of value especially in the highly sensitized recipient; the advent of azathioprine, prednisolone and, later, anti-lymphocyte globulin and cyclosporin A to control rejection reactions; and organ preservation of up to 48 h in kidney transplantation, which has made organ distribution by way of large exchange organizations possible, so realizing optimal matching. Preservation extended over 48 h as a routine procedure allowing antigen-specific recipient conditioning has not as yet been possible. In renal transplantation surgical techniques are well standardized, bringing surgical complications down to a very low level. Effective immunosuppression tailored to the needs of the individual has replaced past policies of saving the graft at all costs, often in the face of life-threatening infections. However, long-term immunosuppression still presents serious risks, e.g., induction or facilitation of cancer and infection. When weighing risks against benefits, one must distinguish between organ transplantations that are necessary to support life and these "only" to improve the quality of life. In the latter case the long-term risks taken must be restricted.

This paper refers only to renal transplantation, where all the basic principles of clinical transplantation which have emerged over two decades of world-wide experience are demonstrated. Striking progress has been made, to a large extent on the basis of clinical trial-and-error, resulting in an increase in animal experiments attempting to confirm or clarify clinical experience. With regard to osteochondral joint transplantation with primary vascular anastomosis, the graft is initially certainly to be regarded as any other clinically transplanted organ. Animal experiments in this area should respect all clinical criteria, such as immediate perfusion, rigid fixation, immediate mobility and controlled stress. Currently used immunosuppression protocols can then be applied in these models. Limited nonspecific or antigen-specific immunosuppression by way of conditioning of the host or by modification of the immunogenecity of the graft must remain a future objective.

If we look at the long-term results in human renal transplantation, the first fact to remember is that genetic disparity determines long-term graft survival. After the initial post-operative phase of 3–6 months, a constant attrition is observed, where the slope on a semi-logarithmic plot follows a straight line. This slope reflects the degree of disparity in large samples of donor-recipient pairs – in terms of progressively steepening slope: identical twins, HLA-identical siblings,

Bone Transplantation
Eds.: M. Aebi, P. Regazzoni

parent-to-child, and cadaver donor organ transplantation. It is an interesting observation that improved immunosuppression does not modify this, i.e. the curve expressing graft loss between the 2nd and 10th post-operative years does not flatten out but continues with the slope unchanged. In other words, the 1-year graft survival is being constantly improved. The important events as a consequence of donor-recipient disparity occur mostly in the first 3–6 months, and these are more successfully controlled with today's immunosuppression. The later fate of the graft under optimal treatment is determined by chronic rejection, recurrent disease, infection, technical complications, and disease or side effects consequent to long-term immunosuppression affecting the host rather than the graft itself.

Following the firm establishment of azathioprine and prednisone and the later introduction of anti-lymphocyte or anti-thymocyte globulin, subsequent minor modifications in immunosuppressive therapy have only marginally improved kidney graft survival. Two distinct milestones have markedly improved the efficiency of immunosuppressive therapy in renal transplantation and initiated an impressive boost in the field of transplantation of other organs in man.

Until about the mid 1970s it was virtual dogma that even marked anaemia in uraemic patients on chronic haemodialysis should not be treated with liberal blood transfusions, as these were likely to sensitize the future recipient, induce lymphocytotoxic antibody formation and promote graft rejection, as shown in numerous animal experiments. Skin grafts, transplantation of allogeneic tumours, injection of splenic tissue or lymph node cells etc. were all thought to accelerate rejection of any solid graft with the same genetic background as the sensitizing tissue. Then, however, it was found that larger mammals receiving third-party blood transfusions prior to grafting with a primarily vascularized solid organ such as a kidney and treated with low-dose immunosuppression, had an improved survival rate compared to those with low-dose immunosuppression alone. Experimental bone grafting and osteochondral transplants in animals led to the conventional belief that these tissues behave unlike all others. In fact, it is becoming increasingly evident that bone reacts just like any other solid organ when used in physiological fashion, i.e. primarily perfused, fixed in a stable fashion and exposed to stress. A distinction should be made among such experiments between (a) those that aim at perfecting the incorporation of a compound graft in order to replace large segments or the more important articulations and (b) those studying immunological events, the phenomenon of rejection, graft conditioning and so on, where only partial aspects are studied. Care must be taken not to translate partial aspects directly into the clinical situation, as had been the case in the erroneous belief that blood transfusions promote accelerated rejection.

Since 1977 we have not transplanted cadaveric kidneys into untransfused recipients [2]. Analysis of our results in 1977 showed that nontransfused patients had a 1-year graft survival expectation of less than 50%, whereas all groups of patients receiving either 1–5, 6–10 or over 10 transfusions had a graft survival of about 70% at 1 year. The first retrospective analysis of Opelz et al. [3] showed that only 30% of a large group of nontransfused patients retained their graft, but following pre-operative transfusions graft survival reached 40%–65%. These figures were confirmed by several centres between 1976 and 1978. Since then, about 90% of all cadaver renal graft recipients have received planned pre-transplant blood transfusions.

The second event with an impact on clinical transplantation was the discovery of cyclosporin A by Borel. In animal experiments it proved to be strongly immunosuppressive without conjunctive treatment. The first clinical series, published by Calne et al. [4], confirmed the experimental findings, but besides a superiority to conventional treatment they revealed a remarkable nephro- and hepatoxicity amongst other side effects in the high doses originally used. The European multicentre trial [5] involving seven centres besides our own, tested the new compound as the sole immunosuppressive treatment against the conventional immunosuppression regimen of their own centre. Steroids were allowed only to treat rejection episodes. Each of the eight centres using the new compound found an improvement in 1-year graft survival, which increased from an average of 52% to one of 72%. In order to reduce the side effects of cyclosporin, dose reductions and combination with other drugs such as cortisone, azathioprine and anti-thymocyte globulin were introduced, and results further improved. Cyclosporin as part of a treatment programme has replaced conventional immunosuppression in most places. In Basel we have attained a 1-year graft survival of 90% in a cadaver renal transplant programme, a figure that one would not dare to have imagined even 10 years ago [6]. Thus, multi-drug immunosuppression is establishing itself in organ transplantation in analogy to cancer polychemotherapy or antibiotic treatment of infection.

What about other forms of immunosuppression? Today's immunosuppression is nonspecific in regard to the identity of the foreign antigens introduced into the host. Although tolerance induction by pretreatment of the host is possible under certain conditions in animal experiments, it has not been so in the clinical situation in regard to cadaveric renal transplantation. It is unlikely that composite osteoarticular vascularized grafts will be clinically introduced on a large scale unless selectively specific immunosuppression is available. At present, the risks of long-term immunosuppression seem to be unacceptable for joint replacement or bone transplantation.

Modification of host-graft interactions have been tried using Rx irradiation: irradiation of blood flowing in close proximity to a radiation source by means of a device such as a Scribner shunt or by irradiation of the graft itself during rejection episodes. Both proved to be inefficient. However, total lymphoid irradiation, comparable to radiotherapy for Hodgkin's lymphomas, applied post-operatively with cortisone, tapered to doses below 10 mg/day have been used successfully in small clinical series. In the baboon, tolerance induction was demonstrated when at 1-year after renal allotransplantation using TLI, a third-party renal allograft was rejected in a first-set fashion, leaving the function of the first renal transplant undisturbed [7]. TLI causes sustained depression of the lymphokine-producing T helper cells whereas suppressor T cells recover very rapidly.

Monoclonal antibodies have been used diagnostically to identify various T-cell subsets, for instance, in the allograft. They have also been tested clinically as a means of treating acute steroid-resistant rejection of renal, hepatic and heart allografts. Although able to control rejection [8], monoclonal antibodies as long-term immunosuppression seem an unlikely choice.

Donor and organ conditioning in order to modify the antigenicity of the transplant has until now been relatively unsuccessful. The basic idea is to eliminate the so-called antigen-presenting cells, such as dendritic cells, macrophages and Kupffer cells, all of which are very immunogenic. In the experimental situation their elimination from the graft is associated with improved graft survival. In clinical renal transplantation their elimination has been attempted by treating beating-heart cadaveric donors with lethal doses of cytotoxic drugs, very high doses of steroids, anti-lymphocyte serum or Rx irradiation, as well as ex vivo perfusion of the kidney. No real success has been noted. However, graft modification (especially of osteochondral grafts) and prolongation of organ preservation both demand continuing investigation.

An interesting observation made by several authors, and retrospectively in our clinic [9], is that kidneys from polytransfused cadaveric donors have a better 1-year graft survival rate than those from nontransfused donors. In the rat, a favourable dose-dependent effect has been demonstrated after third-party blood transfusion to the donor in renal and heterotopic heart transplantation [10]. It is very likely that both the donor and the graft can in future be conditioned before transplantation in such a way that will somehow induce a weaker immune response by the recipient, which in turn will require decreased immunosuppression. This is certainly an absolute necessity if bone transplantation is ever to become a treatment modality on a large scale.

The risks of long-term immunosuppression are by no means negligible. They include the induction of cancer de novo or facilitation of micrometastases following resection of primary tumours as well as the risk of infections. Data from the international cancer registry for graft recipients in Cincinnati indicate an overall cancer risk for long-term immunosuppressed graft recipients of about three times that of the general population [11]. The cancers most often seen are skin cancers, for which the risk is between four and seven times the norm, and in areas with very strong sunlight is elevated by up to 20 times. Other characteristic cancers are non-Hodgkin's lymphomas, located preferentially in the central nervous system, and Kaposi's sarcoma, with intervals between start of immunosuppression and appearance of the tumour of 36 and 23 months, respectively. Among other cancers with a markedly higher incidence are cancer of the vulva and anus, hepatobiliary cancer and cervical cancer. Infections seen in immunosuppressed patients are viral infections in 50%, bacterial in 30%, fungal in 5% and polymicrobial and protozoal infections in about 15%.

The analysis of events which have marked the evolution of renal allotransplantation in man concern the tentative reduction of antigenic disparity between host and donor brought about by the discovery of the major histocompatibility complex, the discovery of the blood transfusion effect in conventionally immunosuppressed patients (azathioprine, prednisone +/− ALG), and the trend towards multi-drug immunosuppression following the introduction of cyclosporin A, which not only improved renal transplantation but induced a flurry of clinical organ transplantations besides those of the kidney. Long-term immunosuppression is known to induce cancer and facilitate infection. To further improve results and widen the scope of clinical transplantation extending it to other organs, including composite osteochondral grafts, the following points must be elucidated: donor/organ conditioning, organ preservation, selective immunosuppression aimed at precise events during induction of the immune response combined with refined monitoring, and finally an antigen-specific immunosuppression with the aim of inducing a tolerant state needing only limited multi-drug immunosuppression.

References

1. Takiff H, Mickey MR, Terasaki PT (1986) Factors important in 10-years kidney transplant survival. In: Terasaki PT (ed) Clinical transplant 1986. UCLA Tissue Typing Laboratory, Los Angeles, pp 157–164
2. Harder F, Jeannet M, Brunner F et al. (1977) Bluttransfusion und Nierentransplantation. Schweiz Med Wochenschr 107:694–698
3. Opelz G, Senger DPS, Mickey MR, Terasaki PT (1973) Effect of blood transfusion on subsequent kidney transplants. Transplant Proc 5:253–259
4. Calne RY, Rolles K, White DJG et al. (1979) Cyclosporin A initially as the only immunosuppressant in 34 reciepients of cadaveric organs: 32 kidneys, 2 pancreas and 2 livers. Lancet ii:1033–1036
5. European Multicenter Trial (1983) Cyclosporine in cadaver renal transplantation: 1-year follow-up of a multicenter trial. Lancet ii:986–989
6. Landmann J, Huser B, Thiel G, Harder F Nierentransplantation – 7 Jahre mit Cyclosporin. Langenbecks Arch Chir (in press)
7. Hyburgh JA, Smit JA (1985) Delineation, predictability and specificity of operational tolerance with total lymphoid irradiation in baboon kidney transplantation. Transplant Proc 17:1442–1445
8. Cosimi AB, Cho SI, Delmonico FL et al. (1987) A randomized clinical trial comparing OKT3 and steroids for treatment of hepatic allograft rejection. Transplantation 43:91–94
9. Harder F, Müller M, Landmann J et al. (1984) Effect of transfusions of cadaver donors on survival of first kidney graft in transfused recipients. Transplant Proc 16:1170–1171
10. de Bruin RWF, Marquet RL, Heinimann E, Jeekel J (1987) Attempts to ameliorate transfusion – induced sensitisation to heart grafts by additional multiple blood transfusions. Transplant Proc 19:1425–1426
11. Penn I (1986) Cancer is a complication of severe immunosuppression. Surg Gynecol Obstet 162:603–610

Bone Transplantation, Passenger Cells and the Major Histocompatibility Complex

A. A. Czitrom

Combined Orthopaedic Division, Toronto General Hospital and Mount Sinai Hospital, Departments of Surgery and Immunology, University of Toronto, Toronto, Ontario, Canada

Introduction

A point that may be obvious to many is the notion holding that host immunity controls the fate of transplanted bones. This implies that bone allografts are rejected while autografts or syngeneic transplants are not (Fig. 1). Yet, at meetings of bone transplanters, one often hears statements expressing doubt about "the importance of immunology" for the outcome of non-vascular bone allografts. Given that all agree that fresh autografts incorporate and heal more quickly than their allogeneic counterparts (a dogma based on ample experimental and clinical evidence), these doubts make very little sense. The only difference between a bone autograft and an allograft is that the former is a self and the latter is a non-self component of the organism. Immunology, by definition, is the science of self and non-self discrimination. One can conclude then, without doing a single immunological assay, that host immunity controls the fate of transplanted bones, just as it controls the outcome of any other organ transplant. Clearly, considerations with regard to fit and mechanical performance may become important when the graft rejection problem is under some sort of control.

This chapter reviews our knowledge on immunology related to bone transplantation and then examines an issue of current concern to transplantation scientists regarding passenger cells and their mysterious control by the major histocompatibility complex (MHC).

Immunology of Bone Transplantation

Scholars of bone transplantation have been busy for the past three decades investigating immune responses to transplanted bones. Humoral immunity has been demonstrated in many experimental studies [16, 19, 24, 33, 38, 41, 44] and also in patients receiving osteochondral grafts [20, 34, 42]. Cellular immunity to bone allografts was demonstrated in early work by second-set rejection of subsequent skin grafts or regional lymph node enlargement [8–10, 28]. In later studies, cell-mediated immune responses to allogeneic bone grafts were detected by in vitro assays [19, 33, 38]. Collectively, these findings indicate that bone allografts elicit both humoral and cellular immunity and thus are capable of sensitising recipients to donor cell surface alloantigens.

A brief digression is warranted to clarify the antigenic property of matrix components. Both proteoglycan subunits and collagen are antigenic and have been shown to induce humoral and cellular sensitivity in experimental animals result-

Bone Transplantation
Eds.: M. Aebi, P. Regazzoni

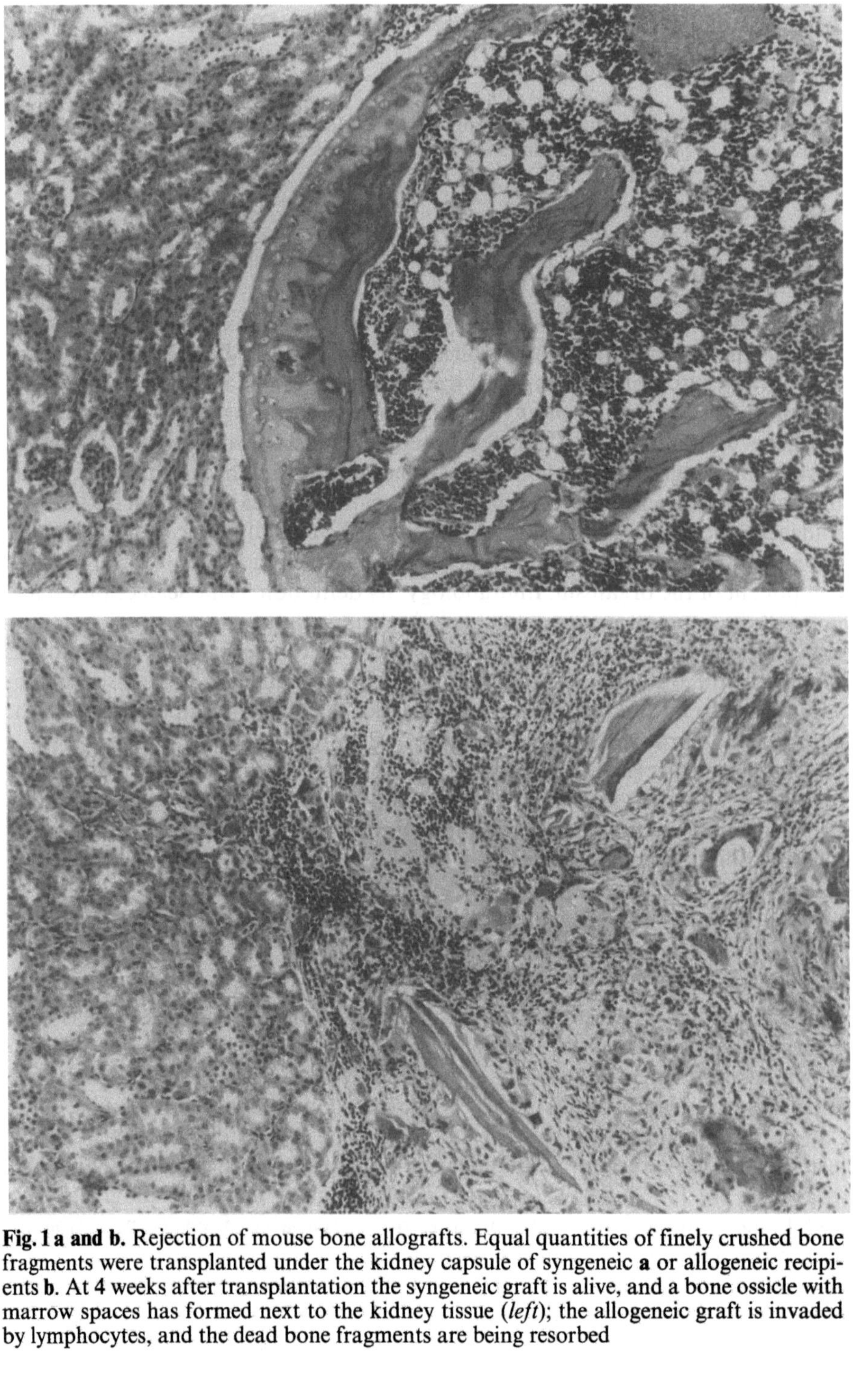

a

b

Fig. 1 a and b. Rejection of mouse bone allografts. Equal quantities of finely crushed bone fragments were transplanted under the kidney capsule of syngeneic **a** or allogeneic recipients **b**. At 4 weeks after transplantation the syngeneic graft is alive, and a bone ossicle with marrow spaces has formed next to the kidney tissue (*left*); the allogeneic graft is invaded by lymphocytes, and the dead bone fragments are being resorbed

ing in autoimmune arthritis [11, 12, 15, 21, 50, 51]. While this issue is of great relevance for autoimmunity, it is not likely to matter in alloreactivity because: (a) matrix components are not polymorphic within a species and (b) any possible sensitisation by self-matrix components of an allograft would be heavily overridden by the massive immune response directed at alloantigens on the cell surface. It seems reasonable, therefore, not to worry about the matrix in the context of bone transplantation experiments. Indeed, one only finds occasional reference to this in the literature [18, 52].

Returning to the subject of immune responses to cell surface alloantigens, it should be noted that humoral and cellular immunity has been demonstrated in many different animal models, and in most studies particular attention was paid to responses elicited by fresh versus frozen versus freeze-dried bone allografts. More recently, work in this field has concentrated on examining the effect of histocompatibility differences on immune responses and/or outcome of transplantation of both non-vascular and vascular bone allografts. This was done either by controlling genetic differences in inbred animals [5, 23, 29, 35] or by examining the effects of histocompatibility matching [37, 47, 48]. Finally, a large number of studies have investigated the effect of immunosuppression during transplantation of fresh or preserved, non-vascular or vascular bone allografts [1, 2, 7, 22, 25–27, 30, 36, 39, 43, 49, 53].

The knowledge gained from these numerous studies, many of which are somewhat repetitive, can be summarised as follows: (a) bone allografts induce humoral and cellular immunity to cell surface alloantigens; (b) fresh allografts are the most immunogenic, followed by frozen and then by freeze-dried bone; (c) MHC-compatible bone grafts (different at minor histocompatibility loci) fare better than MHC-incompatible grafts (different at major and minor loci); (d) histocompatibility matching seems to improve the outcome of bone transplantation; and (e) immunosuppression dampens humoral and cellular responses and improves allograft survival (best demonstrated with vascular bone allografts).

Even though this summary is an oversimplification of a great deal of solid work, it is representative of what is known in the field of immunology related to bone transplantation. The scholars of this discipline have, at best, duplicated for bone what was already known for other transplanted organs. They have failed to deliver novel approaches for solving the fundamental questions related to the mechanism of transplantation immunity and the specific abrogation of graft rejection. These questions are still unresolved even though recent developments in immunology and molecular genetics offer new approaches of investigation. It is to be hoped that the school of osteochondral transplantation will take part in these events by close collaboration with transplantation scientists and apply new technology to its specific field.

Passenger Cells and the MHC

The aim of this section is to explore certain new perspectives on transplantation immunity that are relevant for attempts to manipulate grafts in a specific way in order to avoid rejection. Efforts to apply some of these methods and knowledge to bone transplantation are currently in progress in my laboratory.

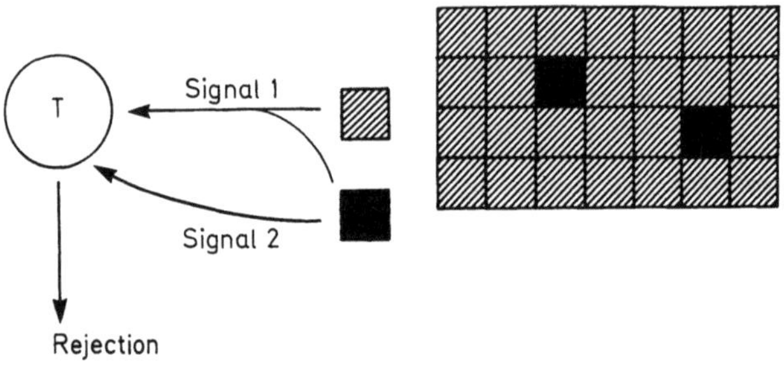

Fig. 2. Two signal model of alloreactivity. T-cell immunity and rejection are triggered by two signals: (**a**) alloantigen expressed on all parenchymal cells (*hatched squares*) and (**b**) a signal from specialised, bone marrow derived cells that reside in the graft (*full squares*)

The perspectives are based on two dogmas that, in my view, are supported by sufficient evidence to be accepted as such for future experimentation: (a) the two-signal model of alloreactivity and (b) MHC restriction of transplantation immunity.

The two-signal model of alloreactivity is based on a variety of experimental data showing that T cell immunity, and therefore rejection, is triggered by two signals: (a) alloantigen and (b) a signal from specialised, bone marrow derived cells that reside in the graft (Fig. 2) [32]. These specialised cells are antigen-presenting cells (APC), known by transplanters as "passenger leukocytes". We know today that passenger cells are heterogeneous. They have been studied in lymphoid tissues where they belong to the dendritic cell and macrophage categories and are uniquely powerful stimulators of T cell responses [14, 46]. Similar cells are Kupffer cells in liver, Langerhans' cells in skin, and oligodendrocytes in brain, to name just a few.

It is clear that any strategy designed to eliminate passenger cells from tissues must deal with the correct identification of these cells. Are there specific, bone marrow derived cells in bone allografts? Reconstitution experiments performed by Esses and Halloran have shown that immunogenic cells within bone are indeed bone marrow derived [17]. T. Axelrod in my laboratory recently investigated the nature of APC in bone marrow. He fractionated bone marrow cells by density gradients and separated various cell types by surface markers in order to test their allogeneic stimulator property in a standard cytotoxic T lymphocyte assay in vitro. He isolated a cell (to over 95% purity) that has the same physical properties as dendritic cells from spleen and is at least as powerful in stimulating allospecific T cells. The morphological features of this cell on both light and electron microscopy were not those of dendritic cells but rather those of an early myeloid cell of the granulocyte lineage [13]. This cell is the likely candidate passenger cell in bone grafts that one should eliminate for successful transplantation.

The concept of eliminating passenger cells is based on the two-signal model of alloreactivity: if APC are missing, there is no second signal to trigger rejection, as alloantigen per se is poorly immunogenic (Fig. 3) [4, 32]. There are a number of methods for removing passenger cells that have been successful experimentally. Freezing, as employed for bone, is not one of them; killing the tissue is a high price to pay for reducing immunogenicity! Culturing grafts in high oxygen tension or

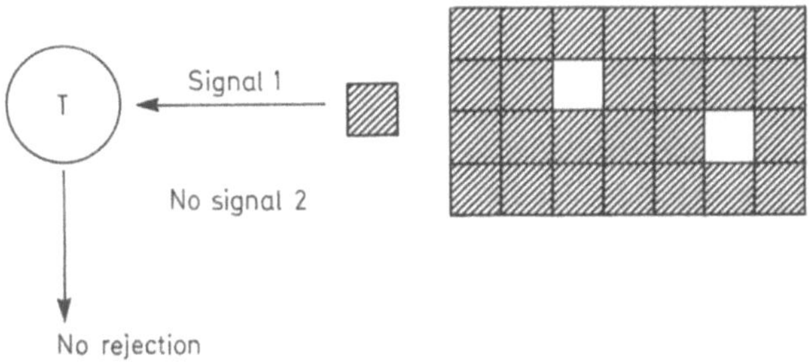

Fig. 3. Allotransplantation without "passenger" antigen-presenting cells (APC). If passenger APC are missing (*empty squares*), there is no second signal to trigger rejection as alloantigen per se (*hatched squares*) is poorly immunogenic

at low temperature has been shown to work for pancreatic islet cells [6, 31]. Deoxyguanosine effectively depletes passenger cells from allogeneic thymus grafts [40]. The most important clue from these experiments is that each tissue has different culture requirements. So, if we are to do this for bone, we must work out the method from the basics. O. Schwarzenbach has recently begun to do this in my laboratory. A small segment of rat diaphyseal bone was cultured under various conditions to remove passenger cells. Although the outcome of the transplantation experiment is not yet known, preliminary evidence indicates that the bone grafts remain viable under the culture conditions in vitro as shown by autoradiography with [^{3}H]cytidine.

MHC restriction of transplantation immunity is the second dogma that brings new perspectives to our possible ability to manipulate grafts. This topic is discussed here briefly with the special aim to show how the MHC, in a mysterious way, can help or negate manipulations of transplanted grafts.

MHC restriction is a property of T cells that "restricts" their receptors to react to antigen only when it is seen together with self-MHC glycoprotein on the surface of other cells [54]. Interesting recent evidence from Silvers' laboratory indicates that similar restriction operates in transplantation immunity [3, 45]. A small part of their data, that dealing with the survival of fresh and cultured endocrine tissues in mice and rats, is summarised in a simplified form in Table 1. The first two rows of the table show that fresh allografts, differing for multiple minor, non-

Table 1. The MHC mysteriously controls passenger cells in organ transplantation

Host		Graft		Graft type	Rejection
MHC	APC	MHC	APC		
A	A	B	B	Fresh	Yes
A	A	A	A	Fresh	Yes
A	A	B	–	Cultured	No
A	A	A	–	Cultured	Yes

A, MHC of host; B, MHC of graft. In each case host and graft also differ for multiple minor, non-MHC alloantigens.

MHC alloantigens are rejected, regardless of whether they are MHC-incompatible or -compatible with the host. In these cases, donor passsenger cells (APC) are present in the graft and can stimulate host immunity and rejection. The third and fourth rows show that cultured grafts (depleted of passenger cells) survive if they are MHC-incompatible but are rejected, like their fresh counterparts, if they are MHC-compatible with the host. Thus, in the absence of donor passenger cells, there is a need for MHC identity between host and graft for rejection to take place. This can be explained by a requirement for self-MHC restricted recognition by T cells of graft-derived transplantation antigens for effective transplantation immunity. The exact mechanism of this phenomenon is not clear. Without donor passenger cells, host APC must present donor alloantigens to host T cells. The question whether the observed MHC restriction operates at the level of APC and graft interaction or effector T cell and target recognition is amenable to experimental testing.

It is clear from such data that MHC compatibility may actually negate benefits that can be obtained from removing passenger cells from grafts. One would never suspect such subtle but important effects without controlling for genetic differences in transplantation experiments. It is known that MHC compatibility normally helps allograft survival. Curiously, then, the MHC has a mysterious control over passenger cells during transplantation immunity, either enhancing or negating graft survival, depending on manipulations imposed upon the graft. While it is important to elucidate the mechanism of this effect, its immediate relevance for clinical organ transplantation cannot be underestimated.

Acknowledgement. The author thanks Reginald Gorczynski and Douglas Carlow for discussing ideas contained in this paper and Georgina Parigoris for secretarial assistance.

References

1. Aebi M, Regazzoni P, Perren SM, Schwarzenbach O (1985) Free vascularized allografts of bone segments with immunosuppression by cyclosporin. Trans Orthop Res Soc 10:288
2. Aebi M, Schwarzenbach O, Regazzoni P (1987) Long-term versus short-term immunosuppression in experimental bone allotransplantation. Trans Orthop Res Soc 12:89
3. Bartlett ST, Naji A, Silvers WK, Barker CF (1983) Influence of culturing on the functioning of major histocompatibility complex-compatible and incompatible islet grafts in diabetic mice. Transplantation 36:687
4. Batchelor JR, Welsh KI, Burgos H (1978) Transplantation antigens per se are poor immunogens within a species. Nature 273:54
5. Bos GD, Goldberg VM, Powell AE, Heiple KG, Zika JM (1983) THe effect of histocompatibility matching on canine frozen bone allografts. J Bone Joint Surg [Am] 65A:89
6. Bowen KM, Lafferty KJ (1980) Reversal of diabetes by allogeneic islet transplantation without immunosuppression. Aust J Exp Biol Med Sci 58:441
7. Burchardt H, Glowczewskie FP, Enneking WF (1977) Allogeneic segmental fibular transplants in azathioprine-immunosuppressed dogs. J Bone Joint Surg [Am] 59A:881
8. Burwell RG (1963) Studies in the transplantation of bone. V. The capacity of fresh and treated homografts of bone to evoke transplantation immunity. J Bone Joint Surg [Br] 45B:386

9. Burwell RG, Gowland G (1962) Studies in the transplantation of bone. III. The immune responses of lymph nodes draining components of fresh homologous cancellous bone and homologous bone treated by different methods. J Bone Joint Surg [Br] 44B:131
10. Chalmers J (1959) Transplantation immunity in bone homografting. J Bone Joint Surg [Br] 41B:160
11. Champion BR, Poole AR (1981) Immunity to homologous cartilage proteoglycans in rabbits with chronic inflammatory arthritis. Coll Res 1:453
12. Champion BR, Sell S, Poole AR (1983) Immunity to homologous collagen and cartilage proteoglycans in rabbits. Immunology 48:605
13. Czitrom AA, Axelrod T, Fernandes B (1985) Antigen presenting cells and bone allotransplantation. Clin Orthop 197:27
14. Czitrom AA, Sunshine GH, Reme T, Ceredig R, Glasebrook AL, Kelso A, MacDonald HR (1983) Stimulator cell requirements for allospecific T cell subsets: specialized accessory cells are required to activate helper but not cytolytic T lymphocyte precursors. J Immunol 130:546
15. Eden van W, Holoshitz J, Nevo Z, Frenkel A, Klajman A, Cohen I (1985) Arthritis induced by a T-lymphocyte clone that responds to Mycobacterium tuberculosis and to cartilage proteoglycans. Proc Natl Acad Sci USA 82:5117
16. Elves NW (1974) Humoral immune response to allografts of bone. Int Arch Allergy Appl Immunol 47:708
17. Esses SI, Halloran PF (1983) Donor marrow-derived cells as immunogens and targets for the immune response to bone and skin allografts. Transplantation 35:169
18. Friedlaender GE, Mankin HJ (1981) Bone banking: current methods and suggested guidelines. In: Murray D (ed) AAOS Instructional Course Lectures, vol 30. Mosby, St. Louis, p 36
19. Friedlaender GE, Strong DM, Sell KW (1976) Studies on the antigenicity of bone. I. Freeze-dried and deep-frozen bone allografts in rabbits. J Bone Joint Surg [Am] 58A:854
20. Friedlaender GE, Strong DM, Sell KW (1977) Donor graft specific anti-HL-A antibodies following freeze-dried bone allografts. Trans Orthop Res Soc 2:87
21. Glant T, Hadas E, Nagy M (1979) Cell-mediated and humoral immune responses to cartilage antigenic components. Scand J Immunol 9:29
22. Goldberg VM, Bos G, Powell A, Zika J, Heiple KG (1982) The effect of immunosuppression on frozen bone allografts in histocompatibility mismatched dogs. Trans Orthop Res Soc 7:173
23. Gotfried Y, Yaremchuk MJ, Randolph MA, Weiland AJ (1985) Vascularized bone allografts: characteristics of minor histocompatibility differences. Trans Orthop Res Soc 10:286
24. Halloran PF, Lee EH, Ziv I, Langer F, Gross AE (1979) Orthotopic bone transplantation in mice. II. Studies of the alloantibody response. Transplantation 27:420
25. Innis PC, Randolph MA, Paskert JP, Burdick JF, Clow LW, Yaremchuk MJ, Weiland AJ (1987) Vascularized bone allografts: in vitro assessment of the cell-mediated and humoral responses. Trans Orthop Res Soc 12:116
26. Kesmarky S, Randolph MA, Yaremchuk MJ, Weiland AJ (1987) Vascularized bone allografting: the effect of cyclosporin in an orthotopic rat model. Trans Orthop Res Soc 12:118
27. Kliman M, Halloran PF, Esses S, Lee E (1981) Orthotopic bone transplantation in mice. III. Determinants of graft immunogenicity and effects of immunosuppression. Transplantation 31:34
28. Kossowska-Paul B (1966) Studies on the regional lymph node blastic reaction evoked by allogeneic grafts of fresh and preserved bone tissue. Bull Acad Polon Sci 14:651
29. Kraay MJ, Davy DT, Goldberg VM, Klein L, Powell A, Gordon N (1986) Mechanical behavior of frozen osteochondral allografts in rats with known histocompatibility barriers. Trans Orthop Res Soc 11:273
30. Kraay MJ, Davy DT, Goldberg VM, Shaffer JM, Klein L, Powell A (1986) Influence of cyclosporin-A treatment and sham surgery on mechanical properties in a canine fibular graft model. Trans Orthop Res Soc 11:275

31. Lacy PE, Davie JM, Finke EH (1979) Prolongation of islet allograft survival following in vitro culture (24 degrees C) and a single injection of ALS. Science 204:312
32. Lafferty KJ; Andrus L, Prowse SJ (1980) Role of lymphokine and antigen in the control of specific T cell responses. Immunol Rev 51:279
33. Langer F, Czitrom A, Pritzker KP, Gross AE (1975) The immunogenicity of fresh and frozen allogeneic bone. J Bone Joint Sürg [Am] 57A:216
34. Langer F, Gross AE, West M, Urovitz EP (1978) The immunogenicity of allograft knee joint transplants. Clin Orthop 132:155
35. Lee EH, Langer F, Halloran P, Gross AE, Ziv I (1979) The effect of major and minor histocompatibility differences on bone transplant healing in inbred mice. Trans Orthop Res Soc 4:60
36. Moore JR, Phillips TW, Weiland J, McDonald DF (1982) Influence of immunotherapy on allogenic transplants of bone revascularized by microvascular anastomoses. Trans Orthop Res Soc 7:175
37. Muscolo DL (1982) Histocompatibility matching in massive bone allografting. Trans Orthop Res Soc 7:172
38. Muscolo DL, Kawai S, Ray RD (1976) Cellular and humoral immune response analysis of bone allografted rats. J Bone Joint Surg [Am] 58A:826
39. Paskert JP, Yaremchuk MJ, Randolph MA, Weiland AJ (1986) Prolonging survival in vascularized bone allograft transplantation without chronic immunosuppression: developing specific immune unresponsiveness. Trans Orthop Res Soc 11:277
40. Ready AR, Jenkinson EJ, Kingston R, Owen JJT (1984) Successful transplantation across major histocompatibility barrier of deoxyguanosine-treated embryonic thymus expressing class II antigens. Nature 310:231
41. Rodrigo JJ (1977) Distal rat femur allografts: a surgical model for the induction of humoral cytotoxic antibodies. Trans Orthop Res Soc 2:265
42. Rodrigo JJ, Fuller TC, Mankin HJ (1976) Cytotoxic HL-A antibodies in patients with bone and cartilage allografts. Trans Orthop Res Soc 1:131
43. Rodrigo JJ, Thompson EC, Gray JM (1983) Inhibition of the antibody response with cyclosporin A after distal femur allografts in rats. Trans Orthop Res Soc 8:165
44. Schachar NS, Fuller TC, Wadsworth PL, Henry WB, Mankin HJ (1978) A feline model for the study of frozen osteoarticular allografts. II. Development of lymphocytotoxic antibodies in allograft recipients. Trans Orthop Res Soc 3:131
45. Silvers WK, Kimura H, Desquenne-Clark L, Miyamoto M (1987) Some new perspectives on transplantation immunity and tolerance. Immunology Today 8:117
46. Steinman RM, Gutchinov B, Witmer MD, Nussenzweig MC (1983) Dendritic cells are the principal stimulators of the primary mixed leukocyte reaction in mice. J Exp Med 157:613
47. Stevenson S, Dannuci G, Sharkey N (1986) Fresh and cryopreserved, DL-A matched and mismatched massive osteochondral allografts: the fate of articular cartilage. Trans Orthop Res Soc 11:274
48. Stevenson S, Templeton JW (1985) The immune response to fresh and frozen, DLA matched and mismatched osteochondral allografts. Trans Orthop Res Soc 10:287
49. Stewart J, Kiuchi T, Langer F, Halloran P, Gross AE (1983) The effect of immunosuppression on vascularized bone grafts. Orthop Trans 6:492
50. Terato K, Hasty KA, Cremer MA, Stuart JM, Townes AS, Kang AH (1985) Collagen induced arthritis in mice. Localization of an arthritogenic determinant to a fragment of type II collagen molecule. J Exp Med 162:637
51. Trentham DE, Tones AS, Kang AH, David JR (1978) Humoral and cellular sensitivity to collagen in type II collagen induced arthritis in rats. J Clin Invest 61:89
52. Yablon IG, Brandt KD, DeLellis RA (1977) The antigenic determinants of cartilage: their role in the homograft rejection. Trans Orthop Res Soc 2:90
53. Yaremchuk MJ, Sedacca T, May JW Jr (1982) Vascularized knee allograft transplantation in a rabbit model. Trans Orthop Res Soc 7:174
54. Zinkernagel RM, Doherty PC (1979) MHC-restricted cytotoxic T cells: studies on the biological role of polymorphic major transplantation antigens determining T cell restriction specificity, function and responsiveness. Adv Immunol 27:51

The Target Cells in Vascularized Bone Allografts

Y. Gotfried, J. Yaremchuk, M. A. Randolph, and A. J. Weiland

Johns Hopkins University School of Medicine, Department of Orthopaedic Surgery, Baltimore, Maryland, USA

Immediate vascularization of bone allografts by microsurgical anatomoses of donor and host arteries and veins is a theoretically appealing way to avoid problems of prolonged nonviability inherent in massive bone transplantation [1, 22, 24]. This includes nonunion, sepsis, and fatigue fracture [14–16, 18–20, 23, 25] until the grafts are revascularized by host vessels and repopulated by host osteocytes. In order to study the immunological consequences and sequelae of the primary vascularization of bone, transplanted as an organ, a genetically defined heterotopic rat model has been developed. The question was whether the immunologic events and target tissues are different in transplantation across strong and weak barriers, and whether transplantation across a weak genetic barrier would result in a less intense host response. To examine these, we carried out a histologic and histochemical analysis of the acute rejection process in vascularized bone allografts transplanted across both strong and weak histocompatibility barriers.

Materials and Methods

Animal Model. Vascularized knee from a genetically defined rat was transplanted to another genetically defined rat [26]. The knee was isolated on the popliteal vessels, including a small muscle cuff, which provide periosteal blood supply with endosteal communication. The femoral vessels were included as well. Transplantation was accomplished by anastomosing the graft artery and vein end-to-end to the host femoral artery and vein (Fig. 1). The graft was placed under the recipient abdominal skin. Lewis rates with the MHC, referred to as RTl^{l}, were used as graft donors in all instances. Fischer-344 rats vary slightly from the Lewis strain in the TLA region of the RTl locus and are designated RTl^{lv} (lv symbolizing Lewis variant). These differences reflect a relatively weak histocompatibility barrier for transplantation between these two strains. Brown-Norway rats are vastly disparate from Lewis rats at the RTl locus and are designated RTl^{n}. This disparity at the MHC provides a strong histocompatibility barrier for transplantation between these two strains. Lewis grafts were transplanted to Lewis recipients as isograft controls, to Brown-Norway rats as transplants across a strong histocompatibility barrier, and to Fischer-344 rats as transplants across a weak histocompatibility barrier. Intraperitoneal sodium pentobarbital, 50 mg/kg, ws used for general anesthesia. A total of 160 transplants were evaluated. Donor and recipient rats weighed 200 ± 20 g and were a minimum age of 10 weeks (range, 10–12 weeks) so as to assure maturity of their immune systems. One-half of the isografts and transplants across a strong histocompatibility barrier were nonvascularized.

Bone Transplantation
Eds.: M. Aebi, P. Regazzoni

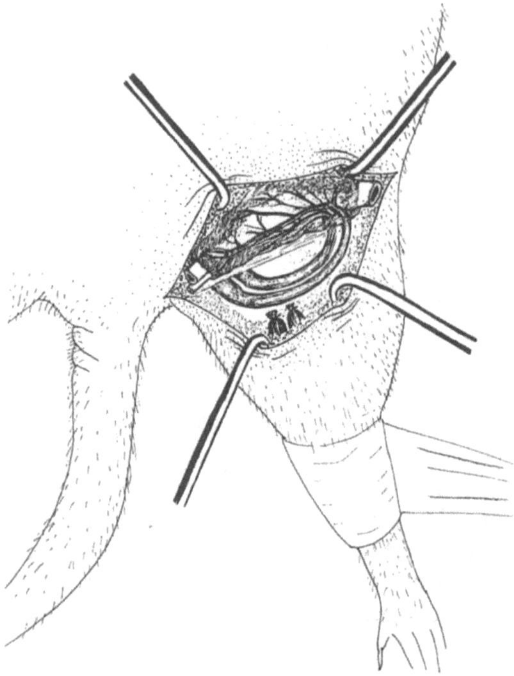

Fig. 1. The heterotopic vascularized knee allograft model. The graft is placed beneath the abdominal skin. Graft femoral vessels are microsurgically anastomosed end-to-end to the host femoral vessels

The nonvascularized grafts were harvested and transplanted in the same fashion as the vascularized counterparts with the exception that no revascularization was performed. Nonvascularized grafts were transplanted to define the histologic picture of the ischemic death of these grafts. Samples from isografts and strong histocompatibility barrier allografts were harvested at 3, 5, 7, 14, 42, and 84 days while specimens from weak histocompatibility barrier allografts were harvested at 7, 14, 42, and 84 days. Ten specimens were harvested at each time interval.

Histological and Histochemical Techniques. All animals received the fluorochrome labels: DCAF 1 day postoperatively and alizarin complexone 1 day prior to killing. The initial label was given to demonstrate successful microsurgical revascularization. Horseradish peroxidase was also used to evaluate the microcirculation [7]. Immediately prior to sacrifice, the vascular pedicle was identified and its patency determined by inspection of forceps patency test. At autopsy, both the graft and the unoperated contralateral host knee were harvested. The femoral component was fixed in 10% buffered formalin for histology. The tibia was divided longitudinally, one portion fixed in 2% glutaraldehyde for enzyme analysis and peroxidase localization, the remaining portion in absolute alcohol for fluorochrome verification [12].

The femoral component was demineralized in 90% formic acid and embedded in paraffin, stained with hematoxylin and eosin (H&E), safranin-O [21], Mallory's phosphotungstic acid hematoxylin (PTAH), and Verhoeff's van Gieson stain. The portions of the tibia placed in glutaraldehyde were lysosomal acid phosphatase labeled by a modified Gomori method [4, 6]. Lysosomal acid phosphatase appears as black crystals by this method. Their presence in cells was, therefore, interpreted as an indirect indicator of cell viability [2].

Cryostat sections of horseradish peroxidase were reacted with 3,3′-diaminobenzidene (DAB). With this assay, areas which had been perfused with the horseradish peroxidase stained brown [3, 4, 8].

To quantitate bone viability, an index was developed for counting the acid phosphatase-positive lysosomes in the cells [7].

Determination of the thickness of the growth cartilage in the heterotopic grafts and unoperated control knees of comparably aged Lewis donors was performed with an eyepiece [7].

Results

Vascularized Isografts. Vascularized isograft specimens remained viable but did show changes due to heterotopic transplantation. Fluorochrome bone labels were present in all portions of the grafts, demonstrating that the process of endochondral ossification continued throughout the experiment. Peroxidase could be localized in osteocyte lacunae and canaliculi. The marrow retained a normal appearance with erythrocytes confined to capillaries and sinusoids. The osteocytes in both the cortex and trabeculae as well as the osteoblasts in the primary spongiosa were identical to those of the contralateral unoperated host knee. A minor thickening of the growth cartilage occurred during the first 7 days after transplantation. Some specimens showed segmental areas of epiphyseal closure with bony bridges crossing the growth cartilage at 84 days.

Nonvascularized Grafts. No differences were noted between the nonvascularized bone allografts and nonvascularized bone isografts. By 3 days, ischemic changes were noted in all components of the graft. The nuclei of the chondrocytes in the growth plate became eosinophilic and lost their characteristic columnar orientation. No viable osteoblasts were discernible in the primary spongiosa, Osteocyte nuclei became pyknotic and a few empty lacunae were noted. Acid phosphatase labeling indicated that the cells had started to lyse.

By 7 days, many of the lacunae in the trabeculae and cortices were devoid of nuclei. The marrow demonstrated necrosis. Fibrin deposition could not be detected. Lysosomal acid phosphatase was almost undetectable, indicating lysis of the majority of cells. No fluorochrome labels were present.

By 14 days, the lacunae in the metaphysieal trabeculae were empty, while in the epiphyses some lacunae contained pyknotic nuclei. The articular cartilage appeared nonviable, without fibrin deposition.

Specimens at 6 and at 12 weeks showed similar changes without evidence of new bone formation or revascularization.

Strong Histocompatibility Barrier. Only minimal changes were noted in 3-day specimens. In the 5-day specimens macroscopic, histologic, and histochemical changes became obvious and were most pronounced in the 7-day specimens. At 5 days, the muscle cuff surrounding the bone graft was swollen and pale. In the

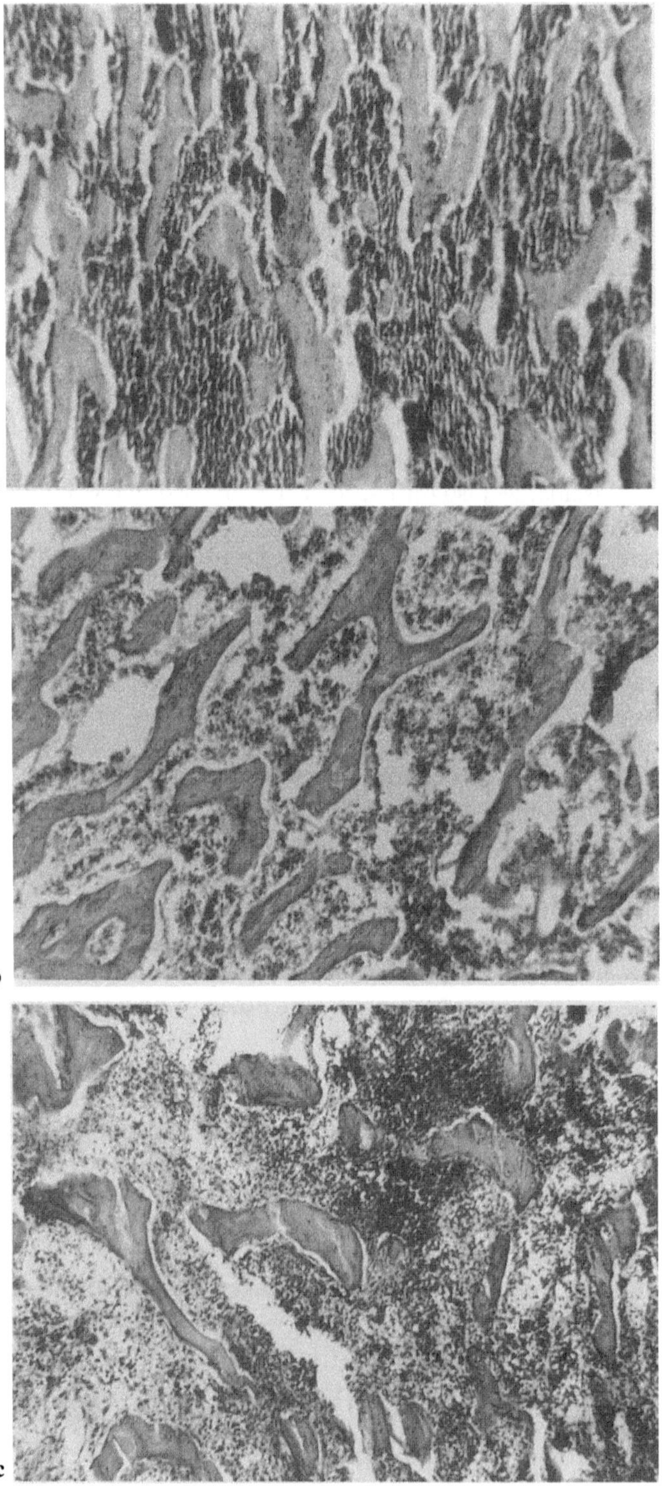

a

b

c

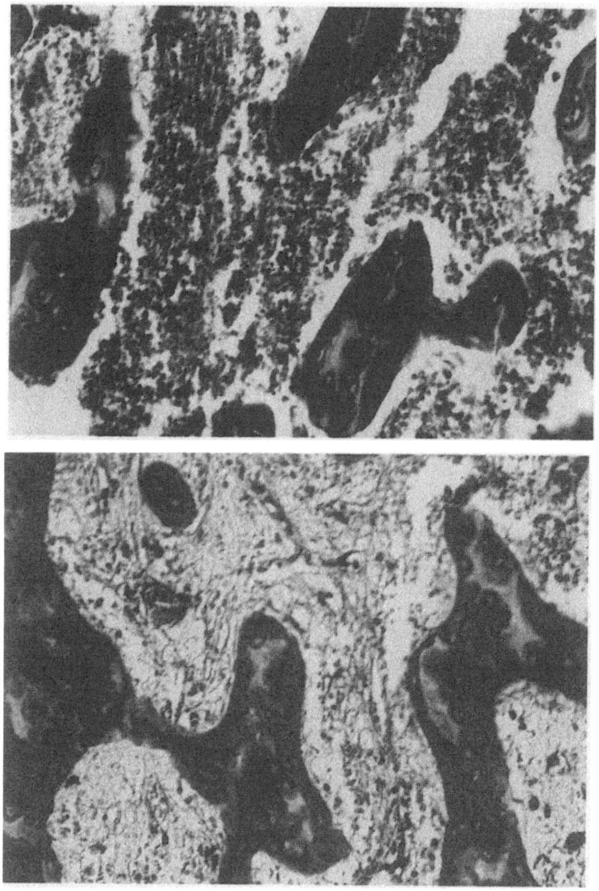

a

b

Fig. 3a and b. Nonvascularized and vascularized allograft across a strong histocompatibility barrier 7 days post transplantation (phosphotungstic acid hematoxylin, × 50). **a** Nonvascularized graft, no fibrin deposition. **b** Vascularized allograft, marked deposition of fibrin mesh within fibrotic bone marrow

Fig. 2 a–c. The fundamental difference between ischemic and rejected bone graft at the early stage. Sections of the metaphysis of nonvascularized or vascularized isograft and allograft that were transplanted across a strong histocompatibility barrier, 5 days after transplantation (H&E, × 20). **a** Vascularized isograft, bone and marrow appear normal. **b** Nonvascularized allograft, necrosis and fragmentation of the marrow as well as osteocyte damage have started by this time. **c** Vascularized allograft that was transplanted across a strong histocompatibility barrier: Capillary disruption resulting in massive extravasation. Round cell infiltration

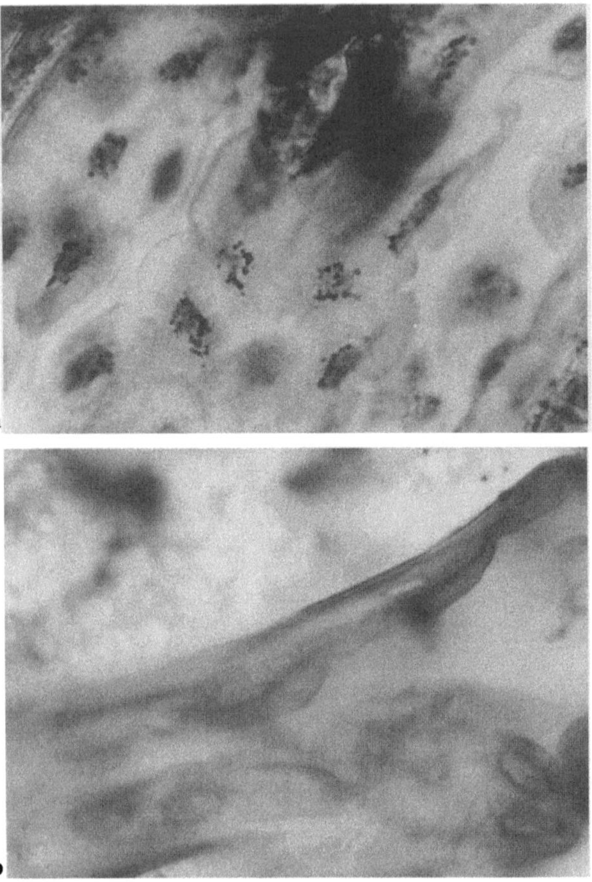

a

b

Fig. 4 a and b. Acid phosphatase activity at 7 days post transplantation across a strong histocompatibility barrier (lysosomal acid phosphatase, × 200). **a** Control knee, osteocyte lysosomes are positively acid phosphatase labelled, indicating high viability index. **b** Rejected graft, area of empty lacunae with no viable osteocytes

cartilaginous growth plate, chondrocytes showed decreased basophilic staining, and the matrix demonstrated decreased staining with safranin-0. The marrow began to lose its structural pattern, with the disruption of capillaries and sinusoids resulting in a massive red cell extravasation (Fig. 2). There was no obvious loss of bone marrow cells concomitant with fibrin deposition. Intact osteoblasts were no longer evident in the primary spongiosa. In this area, bone fluorochromes were not evident despite moderate labeling in all other portions of the graft. Throughout the graft, osteocyte viability as determined by the acid phosphatase assay was estimated at approximately 75% of control. Patency of the microcirculation to the osteocytes lacunae, as demonstrated by peroxidase staining, was only slightly decreased.

In 7-day specimens, only remnants of bone marrow cells and capillaries were observed, along with marked deposition of fibrin mesh (Fig. 3). Osteocyte damage progressed with an increased number of pyknotic, chromatin-dense nuclei;

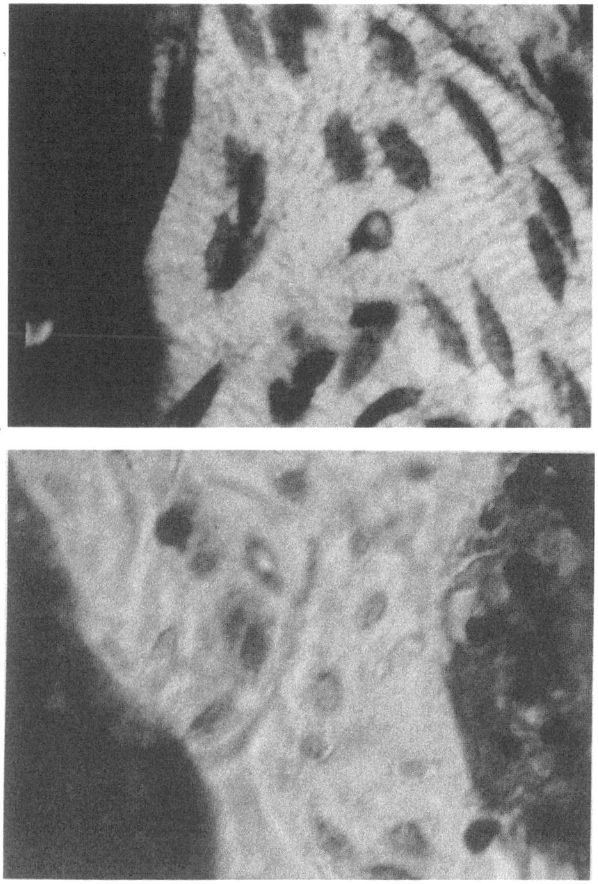

a

b

Fig. 5 a and b. Patency of the microcirculation to the osteocyte lacunae at 7 days post transplantation across a strong histocompatibility barrier (horseradish peroxidase-DAB, × 200). **a** Control knee, positive patency can be traced to the osteocyte lacunae as well as to the interosteocyte canaliculi. **b** Rejected graft, essentially no intraosseous circulation except for some shadows

numerous lacunae were empty. Acid phosphatase activity was barely perceptible (Fig. 4), and fluorochrome uptake was sparse. The intraosseal circulation was essentially absent (Fig. 5).

At 14 days, interstitial fibrosis replaced the bone marrow. All chondrocytes were dead in the growth plate and articular cartilage. Almost all the metaphyseal trabeculae and the diaphyseal cortices displayed empty lacunae (Fig. 6a). Micropaque injection into the femoral artery confirmed the patency of the femoral artery and vein (Fig. 6b) but showed little internal circulation. The absence of internal circulation was confirmed by peroxidase tracing. The extraosseous arterioles exhibited intimal proliferation with swelling and tearing of the media (Fig. 6c).

At 6 weeks, the femoral anatomoses had clotted. All bone and cartilage remained dead. There was no evidence of new bone formation.

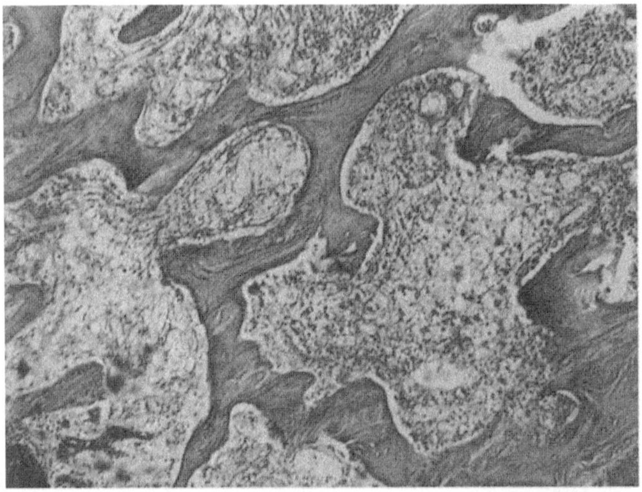
a

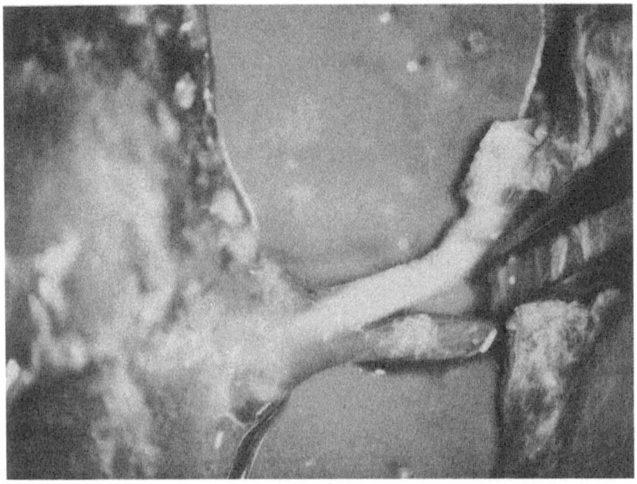
b

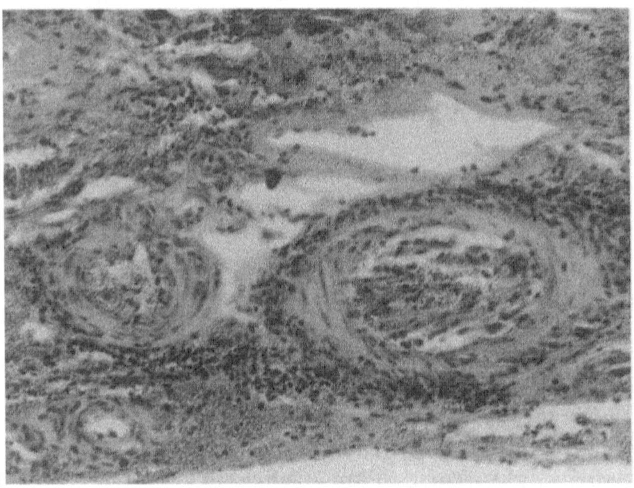
c

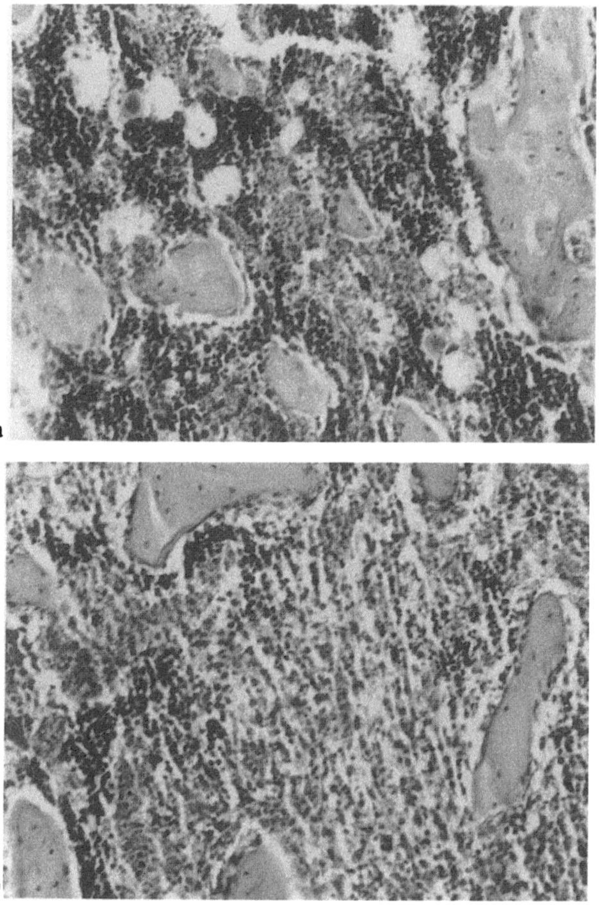

a

b

Fig. 7 a and b. Metaphysis of a vascularized allograft that was transplanted across a weak histocompatibility barrier, 7 days post transplantation (H&E, × 50). **a** Control, contralateral, nonoperated knee metaphysis. The general structural integrity of the marrow is maintained. **b** Transplanted graft metaphysis, reduction in bone marrow, absence of marrow fat cells

Fig. 6 a–c. Allograft across a strong histocompatibility barrier at 14 days post transplantation. **a** Interstitial fibrosis replaced the bone marrow. Empty lacunae predominate (H&E, × 20). **b** In spite of massive graft rejection, micropaque injection into the femoral artery confirmed the patency of the femoral artery and vein. **c** Extraosseous arterioles exhibit intimal proliferation, with swelling and tearing of the media (H&E, × 50)

a 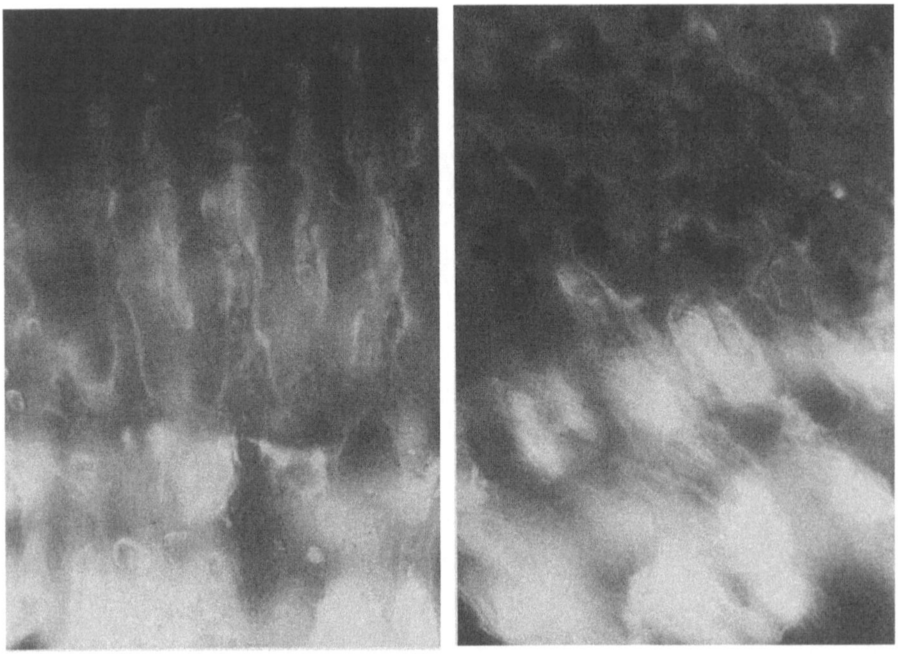 b

Fig. 8 a and b. Metaphyseal primary spongiosa of a vascularized allograft that was transplanted across a weak histocompatibility barrier, 7 days post transplantation (DCAF & Alizarin complex fluorochrome, × 50). **a** Control, contralateral, nonoperated knee. Incorporation of both fluorochrome labelling, the immediate postoperative DCAF (2,4-bis,N,N′dicarbomethylaminomethyl fluorescein) as well as the 6-day prekilling Alizarin complex. **b** Transplanted graft, the immediate postoperative DCAF fluorochrome label is entirely incorporated into the primary spongiosa. However, the prekilling 6-day label is sparse

Weak Histocompatibility Barrier. At 7 days, subtle changes were noted. The growth plate was thickened. In the primary spongiosa, the osteoblasts were slightly reduced in number. The general structural integrity of the marrow was maintained, however the marrow fat was absent, and there was a slight reduction in the number of marrow cells (Fig. 7). The immediate postoperative fluorochrome label was entirely incorporated into the primary spongiosa, but the prekilling 6-day label was sparse (Fig. 8).

At 14 days, graft damage remained confined to the marrow and the primary spongiosa. The capillaries and sinusoids were disrupted, and extravasation of red cells had taken place. Marrow cells had decreased in number, and fibrin deposition was noted. In the primary spongiosa, osteoblasts had disappeared (Fig. 9), and the prekilling fluorochrome label was absent. The growth plate had become enormously enlarged, with a dramatic increase in the number of cells in the hypertropic zone (Fig. 9). In 6-week specimens, the marrow showed evidence of reorganization with an abundance of fibroblasts and collagen formation. Fluorochrome labeling indicated that growth and calcification had ceased. Nonviable osteocytes were noted now only in the central metaphyseal trabeculae and

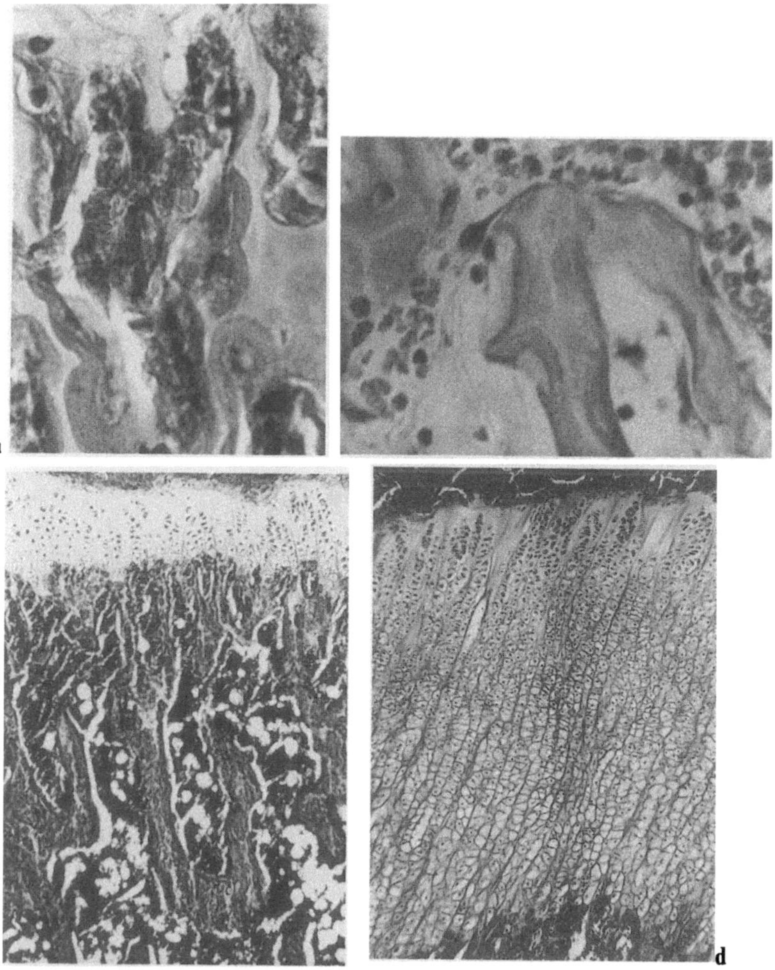

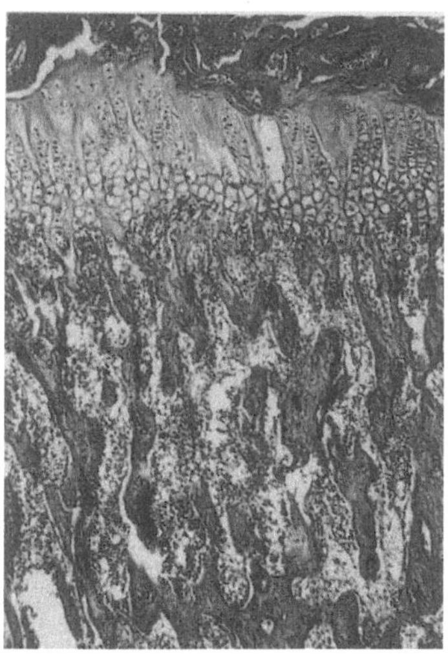

Fig. 9a–e. Metaphyseal primary spongiosa and growth plate of a vascularized allograft that was transplanted across a weak histocompatibility barrier, 14 days post transplantation (H&E, ×200 and ×20). **a** Control, contralateral, nonoperated knee, osteoblasts apposing new bone on calcified cartilage. No capillary or sinusoid damage (×200). **b** Transplanted graft, no osteoblasts are present on the calcified cartilage, and extravasation of red cells has taken place (×200). **c** Control, contralateral, nonoperated growth plate (×20). **d** Growth plate of a weak histocompatibility allograft: increased vertical height, particularly in the hypertrophic zone (×20). **e** Growth plate of a strong histocompatibility allograft: rejected bone marrow, partially damaged growth plate (×20)

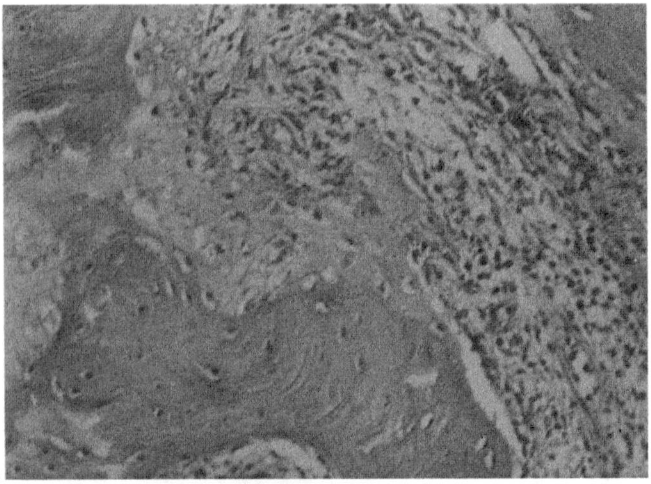

a

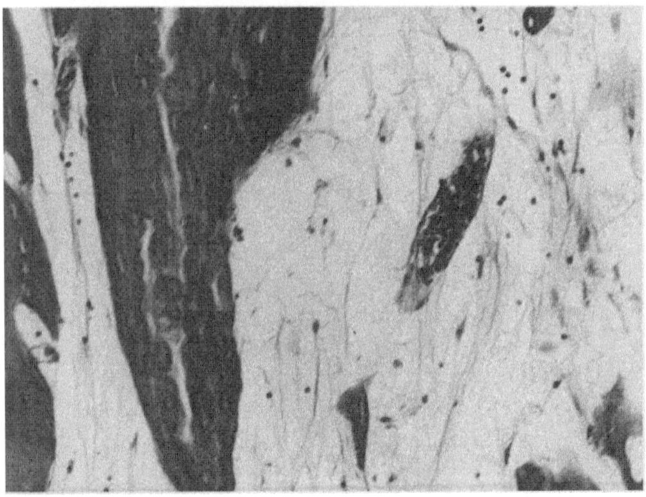

b

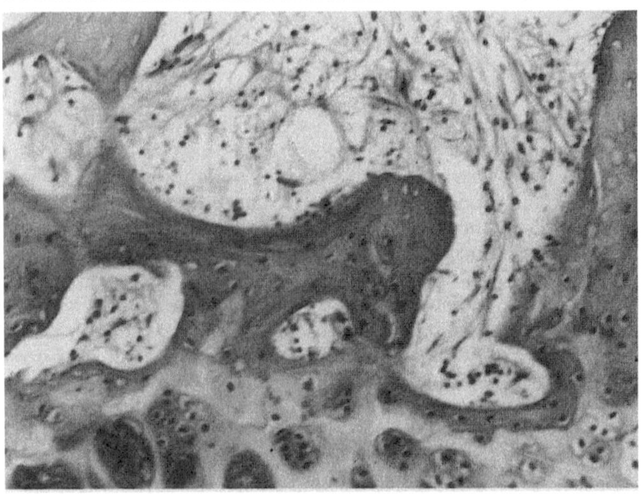

c

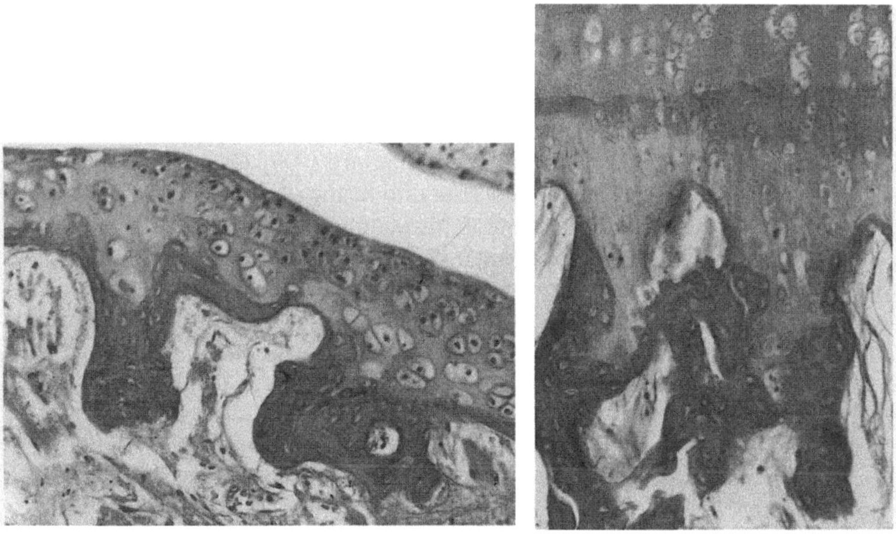

d e

Fig. 10 a–e. The basic differences between vascularized allografts transplanted across strong and weak histocompatibility barriers, at 12 weeks (H&E, × 50). **a** Diaphysis of a weak histocompatibility allograft, new bone formation along preexisting trabecular bone and neovascularization – all signs of reorganization. **b** Diaphysis of a strong histocompatibility allograft, dead bone and fibrotic marrow. No signs of reorganization. **c** Epiphysis of a weak histocompatibility allograft, nonviable osteocytes were noted only in the central trabeculae while the more peripheral portion remained viable. Growth plate cartilage remained viable as well. **d** Articular cartilage of a weak histocompatibility allograft, viable cartilage. Nonviable central bone trabeculae. **e** Articular cartilage of a strong histocompatibility allograft, nonviable cartilage and bone

occasionally in the endosteal portion of the cortex while the more peripheral portion of the cortex remained viable.

At 12 weeks, the bone marrow began to reorganize, and new bone formation was noted throughout. Neovascularization with medium-size vessels as well as capillaries had invaded most portions of the marrow cavity (Fig. 10).

Discussion

This study was designed to document the morphological events occurring during the acute rejection of vascularized bone allografts, since little or no fundamental information exists on the effect of primary vascularization of bone allografts by microsurgical anatomoses of donor and host arteries and veins, while extensive experimental data are well reported on the transplantation of nonvascularized bone allografts. Avascular grafts were used to discern changes due to ischemia from failed anatomoses and those due to immunologic rejection. These findings, shared by allografts and autografts, included fragmentation and necrosis of the marrow, a rapid decrease in osteocyte activity, subsequent osteocyte disappearance, and chondrocyte loss with proteoglycan depletion – all consistent with ischemic damage. Early different histological pictures were demonstrated by the vascularized bone allografts across a strong histocompatibility barrier. These included disruption of capillaries and sinusoids, with massive red cell extravasation, fibrin deposition, and endothelial damage with cessation of the microcirculation despite patency of the major vessels to the graft. Similar changes were observed in the acute rejection of vascularized renal allografts [5, 9]. Osteoblasts in the primary spongiosa and the marrow were found to be the early target of the rejection process in the transplants across a weak histocompatibility barrier. Whereas loss of osteocytes was always accompanied by loss of the microcirculation, osteoblasts were absent at a time when the microcirculation to this area remained intact. This suggests a direct immunologic attack on these cells. At a later stage normal osteocytes were present only where the microcirculation was intact, suggesting that ischemic damage secondary to presumed immune-related vascular compromise is a sigificant factor in graft loss, similar to the case in kidney allografting. Articular cartilage as well as growth plate cartilage survived, similar to the situation reported on nonvascularized grafts, which suggests that intact cartilage is weakly immunogenic [10, 11, 13, 17].

Summary

Using a genetically defined rat model for the heterotopic transplantation of a vascularized rat knee, histologic and histochemical studies of the acute rejection in vascularized bone allografts were carried out. Vascularized bone allografts transplanted across a strong histocompatibility barrier showed evidence of rapid rejection similar to that seen after visceral organ allograft transplantation. At 5 days, osteocyte necrosis, massive extravasation of red cells and fibrin deposition in the marrow were present. The large vessels demonstrated changes characteristic of vascular rejection. Transplants across a weak histocompatibility barrier showed a more gradually developing picture. The osteoblasts and marrow in the primary spongiosa of the metaphysis were early targets of rejection. Loss of osteoblasts from the surfaces of osteoid resulted in cessation of new bone formation. Chondrocyte proliferation and maturation in the zone of proliferating chondrocytes and upper hypertrophic zone continued and resulted in the formation of a thickened growth plate. Osteocyte loss in other areas of the graft occurred later and only in the areas where the microcirculation had been lost. These data suggest that ischemic damage, which may be secondary to an immune-related vascular compromise, is a significant factor in graft loss. New bone growth and host revascularization of the grafts transplanted across a weak histocompatibility barrier had occurred by 12 weeks; at the same time, no sign of regeneration could be observed in the strong histocompatibility transplanted allografts (Fig. 10).

References

1. Arata MA, Wood MB, Cooney WP III (1984) Revascularized segmental diaphyseal bone transfers in the canine. J Reconstr Microsurg 1(1):11–20
2. Bowen ID (1981) Techniques for demonstrating cell death. In: Bowen ID, Lockshin RA (eds) Cell death in biology and pathology. Chapman and Hall, New York, pp 399–418

3. Cotran RS, Karnovsky MJ (1968) Ultrastructural studies on the permeability of the mesothelium to horseradish peroxidase. J Cell Biol 37:123–137
4. Doty SB, Schofield BH (1972) Metabolic and structural changes within osteocytes of rate bone. In: Talmage RV, Munson PL (eds) Calcium, parathyroid hormone and calcitonins. Exerpta Medica, Amsterdam, pp 353–364
5. Foker JE, Najarian JS (1972) Section III: the pathobiology of organ rejection in transplantation. In: Najarian JS, Simmons RI (eds) Allograft rejection in transplantation, chap. 5. Lea and Febiger, Philadelphia, pp 122–144
6. Gomori G (1941) Distribution of acid phosphatase in the tissues under normal and under pathologic conditions. Arch Pathol 32:189–199
7. Gotfried Y, Yaremchuk MJ, Randolph MA, Weiland AJ (1988) Histological characteristics of acute rejection in vasularized bone allografts. J Bone Joint Surg [Am] already published JB35 *1988* (A)
8. Graham RC Jr, Karnovsky MJ (1966) The early stages of absorption of injected horseradish peroxidase in the proximal tubules of mouse kidney: ultrastructural cytochemistry by a new technique. J Histochem Cytochem 14:291–302
9. Herbertson BM, Millard PR (1971) The pathology of renal transplants, chap 7. In: Calne RY (ed) Clinical organ transplantation. Blackwell Scientific, Oxford, pp 292–329
10. Heyner S (1973) The antigenicity of cartilage grafts. Surg Gynecol Obstet 136:298–305
11. Heyner S (1969) The significance of the intracellular matrix in the survival of cartilage autografts. Transplantation 8:666–677
12. Jowsey J, Kelly PJ, Riggs BL, Bianco AJ Jr, Schole DA, Gershon-Cohen J (1965) Quantitative microradiographic studies of normal and osteoporotic bone. J Bone Joint Surg [Am] 47A:785–806
13. Langer F, Gross AE (1974) Immunogenicity of allograft articular cartilage. J Bone Joint Surg [Am] 56A:297–304
14. Laurence M (1974) The progress of six cases following allograft arthroplasty of the knee. Scand J Rheumatol 3:68
15. Kankin HJ, Doppelt S, Tomford W (1983) Clinical experience with allograft implantation. The first ten years. Clin Orthop 174:69–86
16. Mankin HJ, Fogelson FS, Tharsher AZ, Jaffer F (1976) Massive resection and allograft transplantation in the treatment of malignant bone tumors. N Engl J Med 294:1247–1255
17. McKibbon B, Ralis ZA (1978) The site of dependence of the articular cartilage transplant reaction. J Bone Joint Surg [Br] 60B:561–566
18. Ottolenghi CE (1972) Massive osteo and osteoarticular bone grafts. Clin Orthop 87:156–164
19. Parrish FF (1973) Allograft replacement of all or part of the end of the long bone following excision of a tumor. J Bone Joint Surg [Am] 55A:1–22
20. Parrish FF (1966) Treatment of bone tumors by total excision and replacement with massive autologous and homologous grafts. J Bone Joint Surg 48A:968–990
21. Rosenberg L (1971) Chemical basis for the histological use of safranin-O in the study of articular cartilage. J Bone Joint Surg [Am] 53A(1):69–82
22. Shaffer JW, Field GA, Goldberg VM, Davy DT (1985) Fate of vascularized and nonvascularized autografts. Clin Orthop 197:32–43
23. Volkov M (1970) Allotransplantation of joints. J Bone Joint Surg [Br] 52B:49–53
24. Weiland AJ, Phillips TW, Randolph MA (1984) Bone grafts – a radiologic, histologic and biomechanical model comparing autografts, allografts and free vascularized bone grafts. Plast Reconstr Surg 74(3):368–379
25. Wilson PD (1972) A clinical study of the biomechanical behavior of massive bone transplants used to reconstruct large bone defects. Clin Orthop 87:81–109
26. Yaremchuk MJ, Nettelblad H, Randolph MA, Weiland AJ (1985) Vascularized bone allograft transplantation in a genetically defined rate model. Plast Reconstr Surg 75(3):355–362

The Role of Histocompatibility in Bone Allografting *

V.M. Goldberg, A.Powell, J.W. Shaffer, J.Zika, S.Stevenson, D.Davy, and K. Heiple

Departments of Orthopedics and Surgery, Case Western Reserve University, Cleveland, Ohio 44106, USA

Clinical and experimental studies of large nonvascular osteochondral allografts and autografts suggest that they ultimately fail because of incomplete and inadequate revascularization and mineralization [4, 10, 15, 20]. It has been shown that bone allografts elicit an immune response by the host [2, 7, 12, 19]. Immune responses to fresh cancellous allografts are greater than to cortical bone and greater than to frozen or freeze-dried bone [7]. However, there still is controversy concerning the role of the immune system and the ultimate clinical outcome of bone allografts [10]. Since bone conforms to transplantation biology it would appear logical that transplantation antigens (histocompatibility) are important determinants of the success or failure of bone allografting.

It is important in light of the knowledge presently available in transplantation biology to explore the role of histocompatibility in bone transplantation. Previous studies in organ transplantation biology have shown that the transplantation antigens class I, class II, and minor H antigens stimulate an immune reponse from the host [5, 16, 17]. Data indicates that matching donors and recipients for histocompatibility antigens is important in renal and other organ transplants [14]. However, there are few data to suggest that this may be important in bone allografting.

Revascularization of bone appears to be an additional factor in determining the biologic outcome of autografts and allografts. Early experimental and clinical studies suggested that immediately vascularized autografts enjoyed improved osteocyte survival and bony incorporation [1, 6, 8, 11, 18, 21]. Studies using immunosuppressed animals in a vascularized osteochondral allograft model reported some long-term survivals [8, 18]. However, many complications were seen with the drugs used. Histocompatibility matching could be an important factor to improve the acceptance of vascularized allografts without toxic side effects and could have direct clinical application.

We have studied the effect of genetic relationships on the biological response of dogs to frozen bone allografts and have tested the effect of these relationships on the arterial anastomosis and early incorporation of fresh vascularized allografts. We have exchanged grafts between animals whose histocompatibility relationships were selected in advance so that we could study the importance of the histocompatibility antigens in bone allografting.

* Research supported by NIH grants AM 22166 and AM 30833.

Bone Transplantation
Eds.: M. Aebi, P. Regazzoni

Experimental Models

Pure-bred beagles weighing 10–12 kg were used. The animals were matched genetically by using a battery of serum antibodies directed against type I DLA antigens (histocompatibility). The serum panel defines at least 11 distinct specificities. This specific typing system has been previously described in detail [3, 5]. Animals were classified as closely matched if no antigenic differences were detected, and if they were considered disparate when one or more antigens were not shared by the potential recipient and were present on donor cells. Although these dogs may be considered closely matched and sharing major antigens, they are not considered truly syngeneic since, although they demonstrate doubling of skin graft survival times, these skin grafts will ultimately reject.

Two graft models have been studied, one a frozen cancellous bone ulnar segmental replacement model (model 1) and the other a fresh orthotopic vascularized fibular model (model 2). Model 1 consists of creating a segmental extraperiosteal defect of the dog ulna at the junction of the middle and distal third. This defect is made twice as long as the diameter of the bone at this level because of the observation that a defect in this area longer than 1.5 times the diameter of the bone results in a nonunion. This defect is repaired using a 1-cm core of cancellous bone from the donor animal's left femur, which is firmly wedged into the ulnar site without utilizing internal fixation. Control autografts were also removed from the distal femur and used to repair a similar contralateral defect. Each animal therefore donated and also received an allograft and had a contralateral control autograft. Initially, allografts were exchanged between animals that had either strong or weak differences at the DLA antigen site. Additional animals were used to further test the immune system and the effect of histoincompatibility by using a clinically adaptable immunosuppressive regimen in the same model. Allografts were exchanged between animals which had a strong disparity at the DLA locus. Three different programs of immunosuppression were utilized. In one, azathioprine and prednisolone at a dose of 3 mg/kg per day and 2 mg/kg per day, respectively, were given for 28 days after bone grafting; in another they were administered for 56 days after bone grafting. In the third program, these agents were administered for 28 days, and antilymphocyte globulin was used for 10 doses after surgery.

These dogs were evaluated clinically for signs of displacement of the graft, limp, infection, and instability of the involved limbs. In each of the experimental groups the animals were followed for 13 or 26 weeks after surgery. Periodic radiographs of both forelimb legs were made, and at the time of killing, final radiographs were made of the four legs using industrial fine-grain film and evaluated by a scoring system as shown in Table 1. Histologic evaluation was performed on decalcified specimens, cut longitudinally at 25 μm using a histological scoring system as shown in Table 2.

Model 2 used an orthotopic vascularized fibular graft. It is based on the anatomical concepts of isolating the proximal 8 cm of the fibula with its surrounding muscle cuff and its vascular pedicle, the caudal tibial artery and vein, without disturbing the blood supply to the distal limb. This technique protects the peroneal nerve. The proximal fibula is isolated and mobilized with its surrounding muscles,

Table 1. Radiographic scoring system

	Points
Appearance of graft	
Resorbed	0
Mostly resorbed	1
Largely intact	2
Reorganizing	3
Union (proximal and distal evaluated separately)	
Nonunion	0
Possible union	1
Radiographic union	2
Total points possible per category	
Graft	3
Proximal union	2
Distal union	2
Maximum score	7

the flexor hallucis longus and extensor digitorum lateralis. The pedicle artery and vein are transected, and the isolated fibula with its vascular pedicle either transplanted or replaced in its orthotopic site and fixed to the distal tibia. The pedicle vessels are repaired using microsurgical techniques and the remaining structures repaired using standard methods. The groups studied were: vascularized autografts, vascularized allografts exchanged between closely matched dogs, and vascularized allografts exchanged between histoincompatible dogs treated with cyclosporin A. This drug was administered at a dose of 20 mg/kg for 15 days. The opposite fibula served as either a nonvascularized or vascularized autograft control.

The blood flow through the pedicle was assessed immediately after the vascular repair and at the time of killing using the Whiteside hydrogen washout technique and by the electromagnetic flowmeter methods [9]. After surgery the animals were given fluorochrome markers periodically (alizarone complexone 30 mg/kg, DCAF 20 mg/kg, and tetracycline 25 mg/kg) to evaluate bone repair. However, because of the variability of fluorochrome uptake, qualitative data was obtained. At the time of killing, 3 months after surgery, further evaluation of the pedicle blood flow was performed by perfusing the hindlimb with a barium sulfate – Prussian blue mixture. The fibulae were removed, stripped of all soft tissue, and frozen for subsequent mechanical testing and histologic evaluation.

Mechanical testing was performed on thawed specimens embedded in methylmethacrylate grips and mounted in cylindrical grips in an Instron Model 1230 testing machine configured for torsional testing. All tests were performed as previously reported [9]. Following mechanical testing, the molded plastic ends were removed from the bones and the graft defatted, embedded, and sectioned to obtain transverse sections for fluorochrome analysis and microradiographs.

Table 2. Histologic scoring system

	Points
Union (proximal and distal evaluated separately)	
No sign of union	0
Fibrous union	1
Osteochondral union	2
Bone union	3
Complete reorganization of shaft	4
Spongiosa	
All resorbed, replaced by connective tissue	0
Mostly resorbed	1
Partly resorbed	2
No osseous cellular activity	3
Early apposition of new bone	4
Active apposition of new bone	5
Mostly reorganized spongiosa	6
Completely reorganized spongiosa	7
Marrow	
Dead	0
Replaced by fibrinous material	1
Some new fibrous tissue	2
Marrow $^{2}/_{3}$ replaced by new tissue	3
Less than $^{1}/_{4}$ adult marrow	4
Mostly adult marrow	5
Adult-type fatty marrow	6
Compacta	
None	0
Beginning to appear	1
Formation well underway	2
Completely reformed	3
Total points possible per category	
Proximal union	4
Distal union	4
Spongiosa	7
Marrow	6
Compacta	3
Maximum score	24

Results

Frozen Bones. The radiographic data demonstrated that at 13 weeks after transplantation there was no significant difference between transplants exchanged over strong or weak histocompatibility barriers. In general, autografts demonstrated nonunions at either the proximal or distal graft-host junction, and the extent of resorption seen was not significantly different between groups. However, at 26 weeks after transplantation, differences were quite clear. Disparate exchanges scored only one-fourth as well as their respective controls, in contrast to the close exchanges that averaged 95% of the control values. The disparate exchanges generally showed grafts which were mostly resorbed while the allografts exchanged between closely matched animals were mostly intact and already reorganized. Radiographic data at 13 weeks in the immunosuppressed groups again showed no real differences between any of the experimental groups, and there were no significant differences seen with any of the immunosuppressive regimens. However, at 26 weeks in the treated groups there was a significant improvement of frozen allograft characteristics by radiographic analysis, regardless of which immunosuppressive regimen was used. These grafts generally were intact and demonstrated early remodeling and only occasionally showed a proximal nonunion. There was no statistically significant difference in nonunions in these groups when compared to the control autografts.

The histologic evaluation at 13 weeks showed a significant difference between the strong and weak barriers groups, although neither group scored as well as their respective autograft controls. In general, the strong barrier group demonstrated which were either mostly or partly resorbed, marrow which was incompletely replaced, and numerous nonunions. At 26 weeks after transplantation, the differences between these groups were marked. The closely matched grafts scored almost as well as their control autografts while the disparate exchanges scored only 34% as well. In general, the closely matched grafts demonstrated either active apposition of new bone and reorganizing or mostly reorganized spongiosa. The marrow appeared to be replaced in many instances by adult-type normal marrow. The compacta was completely reformed in some animals. There were a few nonunions in the matched group but many more were seen in the disparate groups (Fig. 1).

There was significant improvement of allograft incorporation seen histologically in all the treated groups when compared with untreated, disparately matched animals at both 13 and 26 weeks after surgery. In addition, in the treated

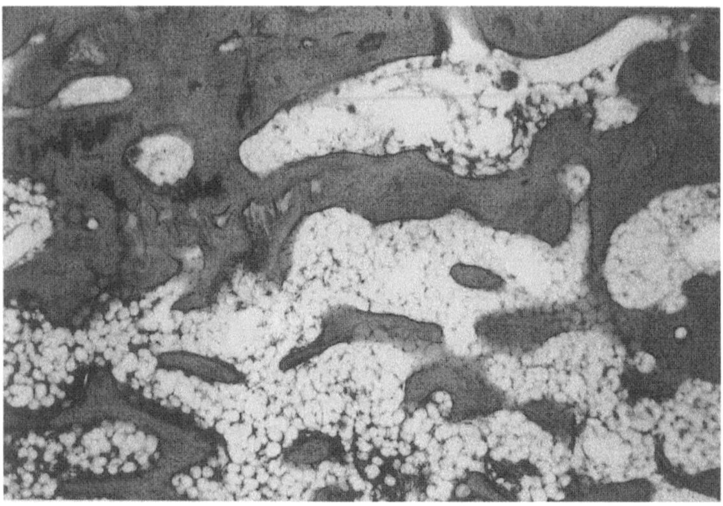

Fig. 1. Photomicrograph of a frozen allograft exchanged between closely matched animals 6 months after transplantation, demonstrating viable new bone reorganized spongiosa and normal marrow. (Hematoxylin and eosin ×16)

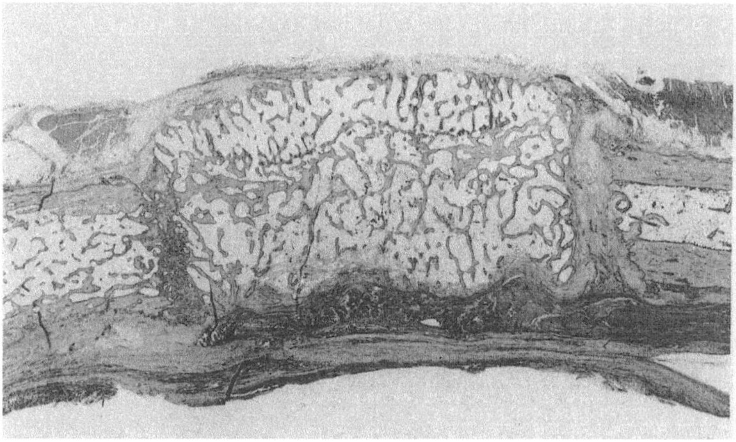

Fig. 2. Photomicrograph of a frozen allograft exchanged between disparate animals treated with azathioprine and prednisolone 6 months after transplantation. Active new bone and organizing spongiosa are seen although complete reorganization is not seen. (Hematoxylin and eosin ×4)

groups at both time periods, autograft incorporation was significantly better than allograft characteristics whether compared among themselves or with the autografts from the untreated groups. Treated allografts demonstrated organizing spongiosa, adult marrow in many instances, and reformed compacta (Fig. 2). Although there were nonunions seen in the allograft groups, they were not statistically different when compared to control autografts.

Fresh Vascularized Bone. All of the dogs survived the surgery and were weight bearing within 1 week. The fibular osteotomies all healed radiographically by 2 months following transplantation.

Both hydrogen washout and electomagnetic flowmeter assessment demonstrated excellent pedicle blood flow in the vascularized autografts which was not different when compared to the normal fibula. Hydrogen washout averaged 15.4 ± 10.6 ml/min per 100 ml tissue measured, while the flowmeter assessment averaged 5.72 ± 3.14 ml/min. The allografts exchanged between closely matched animals demonstrated excellent pedicle flow. In this group, the flow through the popliteal artery pedicle averaged 5.62 ± 0.5 ml/min while hydrogen washout averaged 14.4 ± 7.2 ml/min per 100 ml tissue at follow-up. There were no differences in pedicle blood flow between the autograft controls and the vascularized allografts exchanged between closely matched dogs or disparate animals treated with cyclosporin A.

The vascularized fibular grafts, whether autografts or treated or untreated allografts, showed Prussian blue staining of the arterial network in the periosteum, cortex, endosteum, and medullary canal. Barium sulfate was seen in the microradiographs within the arterial network in all anatomical locations in the vascularized grafts and not in the nonvascular grafts (Fig. 3). The three fluorochrome markers were seen in the entire vascularized specimens of both the original lamel-

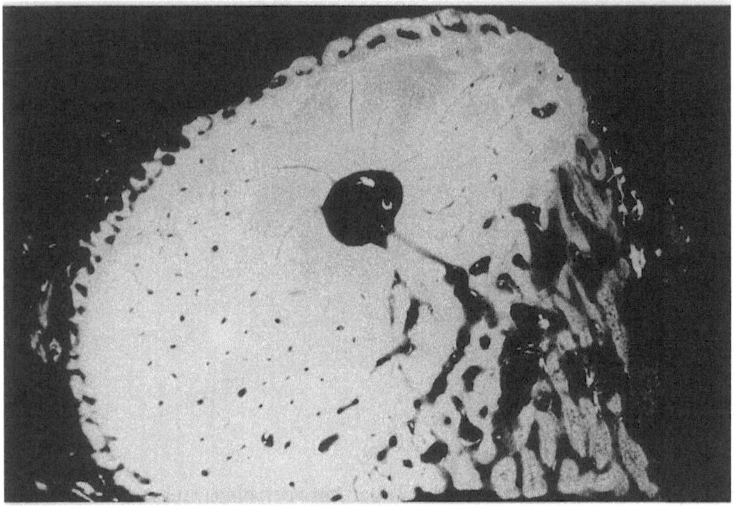

Fig. 3. Microradiographs of a successfully vascularized allograft exchanged between closely matched animals 3 months after surgery showing radioopaque dye in all anatomical locations

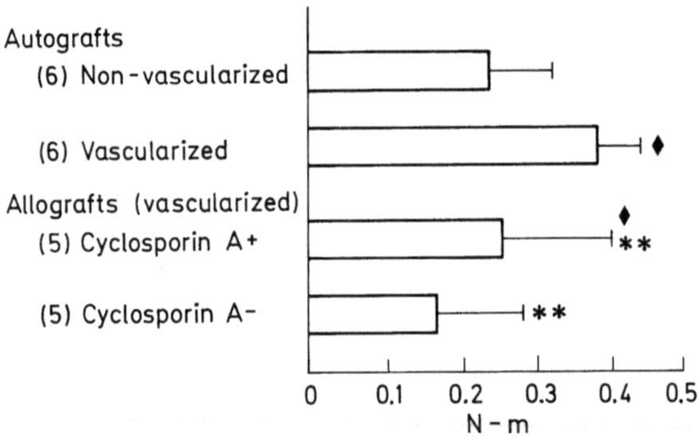

Fig. 4. Bar graphs illustrating the strengths of vascularized and nonvascularized autografts and allografts. Number of animals, in *parentheses*; **, $p<0.05$ (Mann-Whitney test); ◆, not significant

lar cortical bone and woven reactive bone. This pattern was present in the vascularized autografts, untreated closely matched allografts and treated disparate allografts. These fluorochrome markers were usually only seen in the woven cortical reactive bone of the nonvascularized grafts. There were no qualitative differences seen between all of the groups of vascularized fibulae, although there were degrees of variability between animals. Although detailed studies are presently being performed to evaluate the histomorphometric characteristics of the grafts, some general findings may be discussed. The vascularized fibulae showed a greater cross-sectional area of cortical bone compared to nonvascularized control grafts. The whole bone area was also generally greater, and this was reflected in the greater strength usually seen with these grafts.

Mean values for the vascularized and nonvascularized graft strengths are summarized in Fig. 4. The average midgraft strength for nonvascularized grafts was 40% less than that for vascularized grafts. Similar findings were seen for the vascularized fibular allografts exchanged between treated disparate animals. There was no significant difference between these treated grafts and control vascularized autografts.

Discussion and Conclusions

The results of these investigations indicate that frozen bone allografts exchanged between closely matched dogs are significantly better incorporated than are grafts exchanged across strong histocompatibility barriers. Additionally, histoincompatible grafts treated with clinically adaptable immunosuppressive regimens demonstrate significantly improved incorporation when compared with untreated animals. When vascularized fresh allografts were exchanged between closely matched beagles, without immunosuppression, pedicle blood supply was preserved for 3 months following transplantation. Blood flow and healing appeared to proceed in an orderly fashion, qualitatively similar to autografts. The preliminary mechanical test results indicate in addition that vascularized allografts exchanged between mismatched animals treated with cyclosporin A are as strong as vascularized autografts 3 months after surgery.

These findings in both frozen and fresh allografts suggest that the biologic outcome of bone allografts is determined by the immune system. In addition, although we have been unable in our initial studies to detect in vitro immunity in this canine allograft system, recent studies by Stevenson have demonstrated antibodies directed against donor-cell surface antigens when DLA-mismatched fresh grafts were exchanged [19]. Recent studies from our own laboratory have also confirmed these findings in fresh vascularized allograft exchanges, although clinical studies have been unable to show any direct relationship between an immune response and the clinical outcome of allografts. There is little doubt that the clinical failure rate of large osseous transplants is a result of inadequate revascularization and incomplete mineral accretion. This results in a structurally deficient construct which ultimately collapses. Muscolo et al. recently published clinical data using histocompatibility tissue frozen allografts [13]. No clear relationship could be established between the degree of histocompatibility of the donor and the recipient and the incorporation of the graft. Notwithstanding this preliminary clinical report, our experimental studies show clearly that the acceptance of bone allografts and the preservation of blood flow can be enhanced significantly by histocompatibility matching. The use of newer immunosuppressive agents such as cyclosporin A, along with major histocompatibility matching and immediate revascularization of preserved bone allografts, may be helpful to improve the clinical success of massive osseous replacements.

References

1. Berggren A, Weiland A, Dorfman J (1982) Free vascularized bone grafts: factors affecting their survival and ability to heal to recipient bone defects. Plast Reconstr Surg 69:19
2. Bonfiglio M, Jeter WS, Smith CL (1955) The immune concept: its relation to bone transplantation. Ann NY Acad Sci 59:417–432

3. Bos GD, Goldberg VM, Powell E, Heiple KG, Zika JM (1983) The effect of histocompatibility matching on canine frozen bone allografts. J Bone Joint Surg [Am] 65A(1):89–96
4. Burwell RG (1976) The fate of freeze-dried bone allografts. Transplant Proc 8[Suppl 1]:95–111
5. Dausset J, Rapaport FT, Cannon FD, Ferrebee JW (1971) Histocompatibility studies in a closely bred colony of dogs. III. Genetic definition of the DL-A system of canine histocompatibility with particular reference to the comparative immunogenicity of the major transplantable organs. J Exp Med 134:1222–1237
6. Doi K, Tominaga S, Shibata T (1977) Bone grafts with microvascular anastomoses of vascular pedicles. J Bone Joint Surg [Am] 59A:809–815
7. Friedlaender G, Strong D, Sell K (1976) Studies on the antigenicity of bone. I. Freeze-dried and deep-frozen bone allografts in rabbits. J Bone Joint Surg [Am] 58A:854–858
8. Goldberg VM, Porter BB, Lance EM (1980) Transplantation of the canine knee joint on a vascular pedicle. A preliminary study. J Bone Joint Surg [Am] A62:414–424
9. Goldberg VM, Powell AE, Shaffer JW, Zika J, Bos GD, Heiple KG (1985) Bone grafting: role of histocompatibility in transplantation. J Orthop Res 3:389–404
10. Mankin HJ, Gebhardt MC, TR, Tomford WW (1987) The use of frozen cadaveric allografts in the management of patients with bone tumors of the extremities. Orthop Clin North Am 18(2):275
11. Moore JR, Phillips TW, Weiland AJ, Randolph MA (1984) Allogeneic transplants of bone revascularized by microvascular anastomoses: a preliminary study. J Orthop Res 1:352–360
12. Muscolo DL, Kawai S, Ray RD (1976) Cellular and humoral immune response analysis of bone-allografted rats. J Bone Joint Surg [Am] 58A:826–832
13. Muscolo DL, Caletti E, Schajowicz F, Araugo ES, Makino A (1987) Tissue-typing in human massive allografts of frozen bone. J Bone Joint Surg [Am] 69A:583–595
14. Opelz G, Terasaki P (1973) Effect of blood group on relation between HLA match and outcome of cadaver kidney transplants. Lancet ii:220
15. Parrish FF (1973) Allograft replacement of all or part of the end of a long bone following excision of a tumor. Report of twenty-one cases. J Bone Joint Surg 55:1–22
16. Rapaport FT, Boyd AD, Spencer FD, Lower RR, Dausset J, Cannon FD, Ferrebee JW (1971) Histocompatibility studies in a closely bred colony of dogs II. Influence of the DL-A system of canine histocompatibility upon the survival of cardiac allografts. J Exp Med 133:260–274
17. Rapaport FT, Hanaoka T, Shimada T, Cannon FD, Ferrebee JW (1970) Histocompatibility studies in a closely bred colony of dogs I. Influence of leukocyte group antigens upon renal allograft survival in the unmodified host. J Exp Med 131:881–893
18. Reeves B (1968) Studies of vascularized homotransplants of the knee joint. In: Proceedings of the British Orthopaedic Association. J Bone Joint Surg [Br] 50:226
19. Stevenson S (1987) The immune response to osteochondral allografts in dogs. J Bone Joint Surg [Am] 69A:573–582
20. Volkov M (1970) Allotransplantation of joints. J Bone Joint Surg [Br] 52B:49–53
21. Weiland A (1979) The clinical importance of immediately vascularized bone grafts in surgery of upper extremity. J Hand Surg [Am] 4:129–144

Short-Term Immunosuppression and Dog Cortical Allografts

H. Burchardt

Pennsylvania Regional Tissue Bank, 814 Cedar Avenue, Scranton, Pennsylvania 18505, USA

Cortical segmental autografts and allografts have been used in the surgical reconstruction of large musculoskeletal defects. The use of allografts is an attractive alternative to autografts and metal implants because of their ready availability, their capacity to have soft tissues become attached to them, and their relative clinical usefulness in combination with implant devices. However, approximately 15%–25% of large allografts seem to be compromised by an apparent immunogenic disparity between donor tissues and the recipient.

To improve the clinical or functional incidence of allograft acceptablity, various techniques have been employed. Some techniques have merited consideration, such as the use of donor-recipient histocompatibility testing with or without the use of immunosuppression. The use of short-term immunosuppression alone is postulated in part on the ordered process of creeping substitutional repair: antigen deletion occurs in a host immunologically masked and incapable of recognizing the foreign components. As an allograft undergoes the normal piecemeal repair process, some immunogens decay quite naturally, some may be removed by osteoclasts, and others may persist yet be sequestered secondarily by host apposition of new bone. That is, allograft matrix is first resorbed and secondarily replaced by newly formed host bone apposed to the necrotic allogeneic surfaces that remain. Thereafter, normal physiologic remodeling occurs in viable host bone while the remaining necrotic allogeneic matrix is sealed off.

The above concept of decreasing antigenicity in an immunosuppressed host is more typically associated with fresh or viable allografts. The present study involves the use of freeze-dried allografts in immunosuppressed animals because of conflicting previous experimental data: studies by Friedlaender and coauthors demonstrated freeze-dried allografts to have reduced antigenicity [11]; freeze-dried immunoglobulins, cells, and vaccines retain their antigenic states, and in our laboratory, strong biological similarities were found between freeze-dried and fresh-frozen dog segmental allografts [5]. For the purpose of this study, it was concluded that freeze-drying does not reduce bone antigenicity. Hence, the following experimental project was designed to assess whether the rejection of a freeze-dried cortical allograft would be modified under the cover of 3 or 6 weeks of immunosuppression.

Experimental Approach

The dog was selected as the experimental animal because of its similarity to human osseous histology, its reparative process, and because of its outbred back-

Bone Transplantation
Eds.: M. Aebi, P. Regazzoni

ground, which simulates the immunologic disparity with randomly matched human donor-recipient combinations [7, 16]. In addition, the dog fibular model was selected because of previous work on autograft biodynamics [10], on autograft and allograft freeze-drying [4], and on short- versus long-term immunosuppression with fresh dog allografts [3, 4].

Fibular segmental grafts of 4 cm were chosen for the study because: (a) they provide a pure cortical material; (b) a segment could be excised and reinserted as an autograft or exchanged as an allograft in a simple reproducible fashion; (c) no internal fixation is required; (d) unrestricted activity could be resumed within hours after transplantation; (e) the opposite fibula functions as a valid internal control; and (f) the segments can be evaluated radiographically, tested biomechanically, and studied histologically.

The following groups of animals were assessed:

Group I: Assessed the inherent bilateral variability between fresh segmental autografts; 14 of 16 animals were previously reported [4, 5].

Group II: Assessed the effect of freeze-drying on autografts; 8 of 14 animals were previously reported [4].

Group III: Assessed the differences between fresh autografts and fresh allografts; 10 of 18 animals were previously reported [3–5].

Group IV: Assessed the effect of freeze-drying of allografts; 14 of 18 dogs were previously reported [4].

Group VA and VB: Assessed the effect of immunosuppression between fresh autografts and freeze-dried allografts. The group was subdivided into groups VA and VB to determine the differences between 3 weeks and 6 weeks of azathioprine immunosuppression.

A standard fibular segmental fresh autograft was performed in the left limb of each animal. Each transplant was removed subperiosteally, inverted, and then replaced in the defect. No internal fixation was employed. For the fresh allograft, identical procedures were performed in the right fibulae of paired dogs and exchanged. For the freeze-dried autografts or allografts, the segments were similarly removed, freeze-dried, inverted, and placed into the appropriate right skeletal defect. To optimize sterile technique, all surgical wounds were irrigated with 200 ml 0.5% solution of neomycin, normal saline-containing bacitracin (50 U/ml), and polymyxin B (0.05 mg/ml) [15]. The excised fibular segments were freeze-dried for a minimum of 24 h. After 24 h of freeze-drying, the fibular segments were rehydrated in a penicillin-streptomycin solution for 2 h prior to a second operative procedure, in which the surgical bed was again exposed and the grafts inserted using sterile operative technique. The residual moisture in all of the control segments was less than 5%. Seven of the 18 group IV allografts were freeze-dried at the United States Navy Tissue Bank in the Termovac model at −40 °C, for 57 h and had less than 3% residual moisture remaining [4]. All group II autografts and group V allografts were freeze-dried in a Virtis model at −30 °C for 24 h and had a residual moisture content of less than 3%.

Beginning on the day of surgery, all dogs were given 750 mg tetracycline each day in the standard laboratory dog food. Roentgenograms were made biweekly. Dogs in groups VA and VB received azathioprine in their food at a dosage of 4 mg/kg body weight each day starting 1 day before transplantation and continuing for 21 days. After 21 days, the immunosuppressed dogs in group VB received 2 mg/kg body weight of the drug each day until the 42nd day after transplantation [3, 5]. Peripheral white blood values were obtained every week to assess the effect of azathioprine as an indirect determinant of immunosuppression.

The roentgenographic features of repair recorded included the incidence of fatigue fracture and the time of union. All bone grafts were harvested at 6 months. The 6-month interval was chosen because previous studies demonstrated that internal repair and remodeling of cortical grafts in dogs is substantially completed by that time [5, 6, 10]. All persistent fibular grafts were tested with a rapid-loading torsional machine to determine torsional load to failure, as described in previous reports [3, 4, 10]. The physical properties, in terms of load to failure, were analyzed using actual failure torques (newton-meters) and a percentage difference between contralateral (homotypic) fibular segments of each dog in each group – $(L-R)/(L+R) \times (100)$ – and percentage differences between groups of dogs. After physical testing, the specimens were reassembled and vacuum-embedded in methylmethacrylate for sectioning and histomorphometric analyses. Contact microradiographs of each cross-section were made [3, 7, 12] to determine porosity and new bone formation. The cross-sectional area of the graft and of the surrounding callus was derived. The area data were obtained from every fifth contiguous cross-section, and the percentages for cumulative new bone formation and porosity were determined from every contiguous section.

The mean, range, and standard deviation of the biomechanical properties, porosity, new bone formation, cross-sectional areas, and encompassing callus were calculated for each specimen. A paired Students' t-test was performed on each experimental group to determine contralateral differences. Biomedical computer programs were also used for multivariable analysis of variance and for Fisher's randomization of the maximum t-statistic [1, 8, 13].

Experience with the Canine Model

In a previous study with freeze-dried cortical bone, the results suggested that freeze-drying does not eliminate the immunogenicity of allogeneic bone because the implants were similar to fresh allografts in roentgenographic appearance, mechanical strength, and microanatomy of repair [7]. In a second experimental study, using the same techniques, fresh segmental allografts were incorporated more as autografts when used in conjunction with azathioprine [3, 5]. It was postulated, therefore, that azathioprine could be used effectively with freeze-dried allogeneic material as it had previously been with fresh allografts.

This experimental study investigated the potentially useful employment of freeze-dried bone allografts with short-term immunosuppression, using the microanatomy of repair, appearance on roentgenograms, and physical strength as indicators of the graft being accepted or rejected by the host. To summarize, graft repair involves union of the graft to the host, creeping substitutional repair mechanisms, and the subsequent reshaping or remodeling of a graft along stress lines after creeping substitution has occurred. Thus, the incidence of union and creeping substitutional repair reflect biologic acceptance of the graft, and later remodeling of the template assures later functional usefulness of the graft.

Table 1. Roentgenographic results for union and fracture

Time (weeks)	I		II		III		IV		VA 3 Weeks AZ		VB 6 Weeks AZ	
	Auto L	Auto R	Auto L	FD Auto R	Auto L	Fresh Allo R	Auto L	FD Allo R	Auto L	FD Allo R	Auto L	FD Allo R
12	63	70	86	75	78	28	65	56	69	46	50	28
16	88	97	93	86	86	42	97	64	85	62	89	67
24	94	100	93	89	94	42	97	67	89	77	94	67
Failure (Fx) incidence	0/16	0/15	0/14	3/14	0/18	8/18	1/17	9/18	0/13	4/13	1/9	3/9

Auto, autograft; Allo, allograft; FD, freeze-dried; AZ, azathioprine therapy.

As a general overview of this study, 88 of 94 dogs, involving 174 transplants, were assessed. Five dogs in group VB and one in group VA died of upper respiratory disease. Two fresh autografts, one in group I and one in group IV, became septic and were therefore not assessed. All dogs treated with azathioprine had gradually decreasing white blood count (WBC) values, which tended to level off at 50% (range, 4000–5000 WBC) of the preoperative values.

The central question of the study was whether azathioprine effectively promoted freeze-dried allograft incorporation. The first variable to be addressed was whether freeze-drying itself effected graft incorporation. The data indicated that freeze-drying may impair the incorporation process: freeze-dried autografts were found to have fractured in 3 of 14 animals (group II, 21%), while 1 in 69 animals had a fractured fresh autograft (groups I–IV, 1.5%; Table 1); and freeze-dried autografts were more porous and had less graft material remaining than did the fresh autografted controls (Tables 3 and 4). In an earlier study we did not detect these differences between fresh and freeze-dried autografts [4], and the difference may reflect the increased numbers of animals used. The conclusion that freeze-drying itself is detrimental to normal autograft incorporation is not new: devitalization of a tissue modifies the incorporative process of the graft to the host tissue [9, 17].

Interestingly, the above modified course of repair for freeze-dried autografts was not reflected in their mechanical strength. Increased porosity and decreased graft cross-sectional area normally translates into decreased graft mechanical strength. Indeed, Pelker [14] and Bright and Burchardt [2] have shown that freeze-drying causes a significant reduction in mechanical strength due to microfractures of the bony matrix. Yet the mechanical strength values we observed for 6-month in vivo freeze-dried autografts were equal to the fresh autograft control (Table 2). The normal mechanical strength properties for the freeze-dried autografts was explained by noting that a bony callus had been placed about the periphery of the remaining material. This addition of host new bone made up for the loss of the original cortical graft material resorbed at the periphery. Thus, one may conclude

Table 2. Mechanical strength

Group	Left	Right	Paired t-test (left versus right) ($p<0.05$)
I Auto/Auto	0.30 (0.20)	0.33 (0.21)	L=R
II Auto/FD Auto	0.40 (0.18)	0.34 (0.26)	L=R
III Auto/Allo	0.43 (0.29)	0.19 (0.20)	L>R[a]
IV Auto/FD Allo	0.30 (0.13)	0.16 (0.12)	L>R[b]
VA Auto/FD Allo+3 weeks	0.39 (0.25)	0.22 (0.21)	L>R
VB Auto/FD Allo+6 weeks	0.29 (0.19)	0.13 (0.10)	L>R

Figures are means (SD) in newton-meters = kg × cm × 0.0981.
Auto, autograft; Allo, allograft; FD, freeze-dried; 3 and 6 weeks, interval of azathioprine therapy.
[a] $p<0.001$.
[b] $p<0.01$.

Table 3. Biologic data: graft porosity and new bone formation

Group	Mean % porosity ± SD			Mean % new bone ± SD		
	Right	Left	Paired t-test ($p<0.05$)	Left	Right	Paired t-test ($p<0.05$)
I Auto/Auto	7.4±4.5	8.7± 6.5	L=R	35.5±10.1	36.6±12.0	L=R
II Auto/FD Auto	10.7±4.1	25.1±24.6	L<R	42.0±15.2	35.9±19.6	L=R
III Auto/Allo	8.7±4.2	35.5±37.9	L<R	38.2±12.7	23.4±17.5	L>R[a]
IV Auto/FD Allo	9.5±7.4	31.0±24.9	L<R	46.7±13.2	39.5±17.1	L=R
VA Auto/FD Allo +3 weeks	10.7±5.6	15.8± 6.9	L<R	35.2±15.4	40.2±16.2	L=R
VB Auto/FD Allo +6 weeks	10.3±4.8	17.4± 5.3	L<R[a]	42.7±13.8	51.1±13.5	L=R

Auto, autograft; Allo, allograft; FD, freeze-dried; 3 and 6 weeks, interval of azathioprine therapy.
[a] $p<0.01$.

that freeze-drying leads to increased graft resorption in autogenous materials, but the secondary formation by the host of a bony callus suggests functional usefulness of the graft.

The combined effect of immunosuppression and freeze-drying of allogeneic grafts was not clearly resolved. Immunosuppression of animals with freeze-dried allografts (group VA, B) was seemingly effective because of the 50% reduction in WBC values. However, when allografts were compared in treated and untreated animals (group IV versus groups VA, VB), the equal percentages of fatigue failure, union, and porosity suggest that immunosuppression was therefore ineffective. The conclusions were further clouded by the results which also showed that the cross-sectional area of freeze-dried allografts in treated animals

Table 4. Biologic data: cross-sectional area (mm)

Group	Mean callus and graft area ± SD			Mean graft area ± SD		
	Left	Right	Paired t-test ($p<0.05$)	Left	Right	Paired t-test ($p<0.05$)
I Auto/Auto	6.7±2.8	7.1±2.8	L=R	4.9±1.9	5.0±1.8	L=R
II Auto/FD Auto	9.1±3.7	8.5±4.2	L=R	5.3±2.4	2.9±2.3	L>R[a]
III Auto/Allo	7.8±3.6	5.3±3.6	L>R	5.3±1.8	1.9±1.8	L>R[a]
IV Auto/FD Allo	7.4±2.2	5.2±3.1	L>R	4.6±2.0	1.8±1.4	L>R[a]
VA Auto/FD Allo +3 weeks	6.5±3.3	4.9±3.3	L>R	4.8±2.2	2.9±2.1	L>R
VB Auto/FD Allo +6 weeks	6.0±1.5	4.6±1.8	L>R	3.7±1.7	2.0±1.1	L>R

Auto, autograft; Allo, allograft; FD, freeze-dried; 3 and 6 weeks, interval of azathioprine therapy.
[a] $p<0.01$.

Table 5. % Difference of right limb compared to the internal control left limb

Group (L/R)	% Graft area remaining	% Total area: callus + graft
I Auto/Auto	0.0	0.0
II Auto/FD Auto	−45.3	− 7.0
III Auto/Allo	−62.3	−32.1
IV Auto/FD Allo	−60.9	−32.4
VA Auto/FD Allo + 3 weeks	−39.6	−24.6
VB Auto/FD Allo + 6 weeks	−48.7	−23.3

Negative sign indicates the right graft to be less than the left internal control. Therefore, in group II, FD autografts of the right limb had 45.3% less cross-sectional graft area remaining as compared to the internal left fresh autograft control.
Auto, autograft; Allo, allograft; FD, freeze-dried; 3 and 6 weeks, interval of azathioprine therapy.

was greater then in untreated animals: osteoclastic resorption of freeze-dried allografts was reduced in immunosuppressed animals (Table 5), and immunosuppression therefore effective.

In the comparison of freeze-dried allografts in treated animals with freeze-dried autografts in untreated animals, the percent reduction in graft cross-sectional area was the same, yet the amount of secondary bony callus formed was three times greater in the autografts. A possible explanation for this difference is that 3–6 weeks of azathioprine immunosuppression not only depresses resorption and recognition of a foreign material in a host, but it may also depress bone formation (directly and/or indirectly). On the other hand, freeze-dried materials combined with the retention of donor immunogens after immunosuppression has ceased may explain the reduced bony callus that was found for freeze-dried allografts in treated animals. Thus, increased resorption and decreased bone formation in fresh or freeze-dried allografts of treated or untreated animals, may reflect continued allogeneic antigenicity and the allograft's functional uselessness in this model.

The results of this study involving 3- and 6-week periods of azathioprine immunosuppression with freeze-dried fibular allografts in adult dogs are as follows:

1. The process of freeze-drying autogenous materials causes increased cortical graft resorption and fatigue fractures. However, secondary host bone formation makes up for this loss of material in time.
2. Freeze-dried allografts in azathioprine-treated animals did not improve the functional or biological state of the tissue when compared to freeze-dried allografts in untreated hosts. This does not necessarily imply that the concept of immunosuppression is unacceptable in as much as the experimental design of this study did not sufficiently clarify the variables.

References

1. Bradely JV (1968) Fisher's method of randomization. In: Distribution-free statistical tests. Englewood Cliffs, New Jersey, Prenticehall, pp 68–86
2. Bright RW, Burchardt H (1983) The biomechanical properties of preserved bone grafts. In: Friedlander GE, Mankin HJ, Sell KW (eds) Osteochondral allografts: biology, banking, clinical applications. Little, Brown, Boston, pp 233–247
3. Burchardt H, Glowczewskie FP, Enneking WF (1977) Allogeneic segmental fibular transplants in azathioprine immunosuppressed dogs. J Bone Joint Surg [Am] 59A:881
4. Burchardt H, Jones H, Glowczewskie FP, Rudner C, Enneking WF (1978) Freeze-dried allogeneic segmental cortical bone grafts in dogs. J Bone Joint Surg [Am] 60A:1082
5. Burchardt H, Glowczewskie FP, Enneking WF (1981) Short-term immunosuppression with fresh segmental fibular allografts in dogs. J Bone Joint Surg [Am] 63A:411
6. Burchardt H (1983) The biology of bone graft repair. Clin Orthop 174:28
7. Dausset J et al. (1971) Histocompatibility studies in closely bred colony of dogs: III. Genetic definition of the DL-A system of canine histocompatibility with particular reference to the comparative immunology of the major transplantable organs. J Exp Med 134:1222
8. Dixon WF (1973) BMD programm II V: Multivariate general linear hypothesis. In: Dixon WF (ed) BMD: biomedical computer programs. University of California Press, Los Angeles
9. Elves MW, Pratt LM (1975) The pattern of new bone formation in isografts of bone. Acta Orthop Scand 46:549
10. Enneking WF, Burchardt H, Puhl JJ, Piotrowski G (1975) Physical and biological aspects of repair in dog cortical-bone transplants. J Bone Joint Surg [Am] 57A:237
11. Friedlaender GE, Strong DM, Sell KW (1976) Studies on the antigenicity of bone: I. Freeze-dried and deep-frozen bone allografts in rabbits. J Bone Joint Surg [Am] 58A:854
12. Jowsey J, Kelly PJ, Riggo BL, Bianco AJ Jr, Scholz DA, Gershon-Cohen J (1965) Quantitative microradiographic studies of normal and osteoporotic bone. J Bone Joint Surg [Am] 47A:785
13. Morrison DF (1967) Multivariate statistical methods. McGraw-Hill, New York, pp 159–206

14. Pelker RR, Friedlaender GE, Markham TC, Panjabi MM, Moen CJ (1984) Effects of freezing and freeze-drying on the biomechanical properties of rat bone. J Orthop Res 1:405
15. Scherr DD, Dodd TA (1973) The effect of brief exposure of pathogenic bacteria to neomycin sulfate, bacitracin, and polymyx b sulfate. J Bone Joint Surg [Am] 55A:660
16. Vriesendorp HM et al. (1973) Joint report of first international workshop on canine immunogenetics. Tissue Antigens 3:145
17. Weiland AJ, Phillips TW, Randolph BS (1984) Bone grafts: a radiologic histologic and biomechanical model comparing autografts, allografts, and free vascularized bone grafts. Plast Reconstr Surg 74(3):368

Bone Banking

Organization, Legal Aspects and Problems of Bone Banking in a Large Orthopedic Center

W. W. Tomford, S. H. Doppelt, and H. J. Mankin

MGH Bone Bank, Massachusetts General Hospital, Boston, Massachusetts 02114, USA

Introduction

Banking bone and other tissues has become an important endeavor. Banked bone is now being used extensively in bone tumor surgery, failed joint replacement surgery, and trauma surgery. Hospitals around the world are beginning to bank femoral heads, and many centers have instituted programs utilizing large allografts in limb-sparing procedures. It is important therefore for bone banks to conform to high standards of sterility and safety in order to provide orthopedic surgeons the best possible bone allografts. This review discusses important aspects of bone banking as learned over 10 years of experience. Attention to the details outlined in this paper will help provide a solid base on which to build a bone bank that may provide the best possible bone allografts and build confidence in a bone bank supply.

Organization

The organization of a bone bank has several principles, but two are most important. The first is adherence to a set of accepted standards and practices of tissue banking. Standards have been published by and are available from the American Association of Tissue Banks, an organization whose individual members operate bone banks throughout the United States [1]. This association now has about 350 members and has adopted these standards as a guide for inspecting and accrediting tissue banks.

The second principle of bone banking is the appointment of a medical director with experience in bone banking procedures as well as knowledge of principles of sterility and control of infection. It is also advisable in an orthopedic center that the director have training in orthopedic surgery so that the choice of a banked bone can be made with detailed knowledge of its intended use in order to provide surgeons with the most feasible grafts.

Bone banking in some orthopedic centers may only involve banking of femoral heads. This can be easily accomplished by training orthopedists to place femoral heads into sterile packages at the time of procurement from living donors, storing the heads in a freezer, and keeping records on the bones. If, however, large bones are to be used, such as osteochondral allografts, a more extensive effort is necessary to select donors and procure bones on an on-call basis.

Bone Transplantation
Eds.: M. Aebi, P. Regazzoni

Medical Operations

The medical operations of a bone bank include donor recruitment and selection, tissue procurement, and packaging, storage, and record-keeping. Cadaver donor recruitment is difficult unless a bone bank is associated with a transplant center. The Massachusetts General Hospital (MGH) Bone Bank initially attempted to recruit donors by writing to neurosurgeons and orthopedists throughout the local Boston area. This effort did not meet with much success. Donors have become available in large numbers only through association with a regional organ bank which coordinates all organ procurements (kidney, liver, pancreas, heart) in the northeastern United States. Because medical personnel are much more aware of the need for kidneys than for bones, notification of potential donors from local hospitals are made almost exclusively to the organ bank. Educational efforts may alter this current pattern, but working with the organ bank has proven to be extremely helpful to our particular bone bank.

Donor selection is almost as important as donor recruitment. Once a donor is available, the medical director must make the decision of whether or not the donor is satisfactory. Criteria for donation are based on proven absence of transmissible diseases. These diseases include any bacterial or viral disease as well as diseases of unknown origin (Table 1). However, because there are false-negative tests for diseases such as AIDS and even hepatitis, the medical history is extremely important. For example, a patient with a sexual history suggesting a possible exposure to AIDS, even though a blood test for antibody to the AIDS virus is negative, would not be an acceptable donor to our bone bank. We feel strongly that because blood elements are present in the marrow which cannot be completely eliminated, and because we do not sterilize bones prior to transplantation, we would be at risk transplanting bones from such a donor. Consequently, our criteria exclude the potential presence of transmissible diseases.

A question has arisen recently over whether or not to procure tissue from patients who have had a transfusion within the past 6 months. Although blood donors are tested for the presence of antibodies to the AIDS virus, it is possible that for 6 months a donor may not react to the HIV (AIDS) antigen to produce a sufficient antibody titer that will result in a positive test. The cut-off date for previous transfusions, generally given as 6 months, is an arbitrary time limit, how-

Table 1. Laboratory tests for cadaver donors

Cultures
Bacterial (aerobic and anaerobic)
Fungal
Blood
Viral tests
Anti-HIV-I (AIDS)
HBsAg (hepatitis B surface antigen)
Anti-HBcAg (antibody to hepatitis B core antigen)
Other
Syphillis screen (RPR-R-reactive protein)

ever, in that patients may take longer than 6 months to respond. In addition, many donors would not be available to us because most of our donors are organ donors, and many are transfused at time of procurement of their solid organs. Therefore, we do not automatically exclude donors who have been transfused within the past 6 months. All relevant facts, including the transfusion history, are considered when evaluating a donor.

The technique of donor procurement is also important. Two methods of procurement are used: sterile and nonsterile. We prefer to perform sterile procurements because most methods of sterilization produce changes in a bone which may be a disadvantage to the use of that bone. For instance, ethylene oxide cannot sterilize thick cortical bone such as that of a femur [2] and may also inhibit bone formation [3]. The use of radiation produces heat in bone which destroys proteins, possibly including morphogenetic proteins. For these reasons, we procure bones in a sterile operating room using sterile techniques similar to those used in any orthopedic operation, and the bones are kept untouched until they are used, thereby minimizing the possibility of contamination. Some bone banks procure bones under semisterile conditons, such as in a morgue, and then sterilize them. In this circumstance, the sterilization procedure must be shown to sterilize the bone adequately.

Packaging bone, once it is procured, necessitates the use of a sterile material which will not disintegrate under conditions such as freezing. We use large thick plastic bags for an initial wrap followed by cotton cloth towels followed by an outer plastic bag to make certain that no water permeates through the cloth towels and to make certain that the outside of the package remains dry (Fig. 1). Other packaging methods include the use of a glass or plastic jar for femoral heads. A container which includes one plastic jar inside of another for this pur-

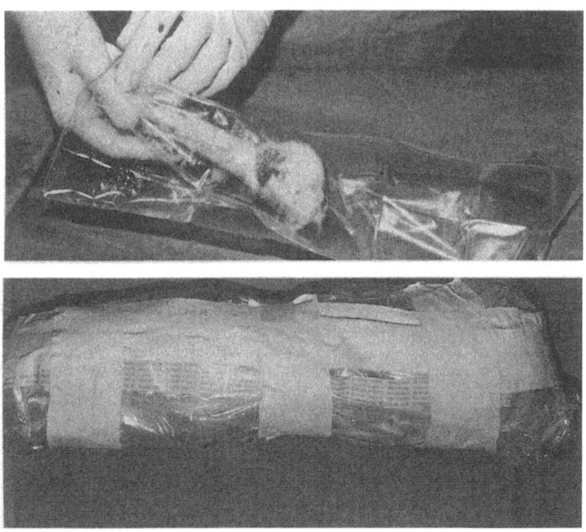
a

b

Fig. 1 a and b. Bone packaging. **a** Each bone is wrapped initially in a plastic bag and three cotton towels. **b** The final wrapping in another plastic bag which is taped for freezer storage

pose is currently available as a commercial product (Hydro-Med Products, Inc, Dallas, Texas 75220).

Bone storage is also important. The two most popular methods are freezing and freeze-drying. Our bone bank has experience with freezing, and we recommend this method for a large, in-house orthopedic center because it is much easier than freeze-drying. Freeze-drying necessitates the use of freeze-dryers which are expensive and require extensive monitoring if they utilize ethylene oxide for sterilization. Ethylene oxide is a toxic gas, and excessive exposure has been shown to result in spontaneous abortions [4]. Freeze-drying is a proven method of storage, however, and has been used for many years by tissue banks such as the United States Navy Tissue Bank and the University of Miami Tissue Bank. Our bone bank provides bone to surgeons only in our hospital. Given this circumstance, we do not feel that investment in a freeze-dryer is warranted. We use large freezers which operate on 210 v and keep the tissues frozen to approximately −80 °C. The freezers have alarms attached so that if the temperature varies 10° either below or above −80 °C, the alarm will sound.

The choice of the temperature of −80 °C is arbitrary. The decision to use −80 °C is based on work in the field of cryobiology which has shown that cells can be maintained at −80 °C with very little deterioration in viability. Banked bone is, of course, not viable, but deterioration is a concern. It is possible that enzymatic action may occur at temperatures warmer than −80 °C which will degrade bone proteins. Enzymes include collagenase and other proteinases. We have chosen the storage temperature of −80 °C in an attempt to diminish enzymatic activity as much as possible, and it has been shown in our laboratory that storage at −80 °C will successfully do this [5].

Keeping track of bones which are used by surgeons as well as bones which are stored in the bank requires compulsive record keeping. In a small bank, we have found the use of computers is helpful, but not mandatory. For several years we have used two books to keep these records manually. The first book is a demand book for recording requests by surgeons who call the bone bank a few days in advance of their need for bone. A record is kept of what the date of surgery will be, what the diagnosis is, who the patient is, who the surgeon is, and what type of bone is requested. Postoperatively, we record whether or not that bone is used, any bone that is returned to the bank, and the result of cultures taken of the bone at the time of use in the operating room. The second book is a supply book for recording the different types of bones available for use. Once a bone is known to be available for transplantation, a record of it is placed into the supply book along with the culture result, the result of AIDS and hepatitis testing, and the blood type of the donor. If the bone is a long bone, the length and width at each end are recorded. In sizing femurs at the time of procurement, the width at the femoral head, the midshaft and the condyles (anterior/posterior and medial/lateral) are measured. In addition, because degenerative disease is occasionally found in a patient's knee, comments are made on the status of the cartilage. From this information, the proper bone can be chosen for each particular demand.

Financial/Legal Considerations

The costs of banking bone vary depending on the methods of procurement and storage. Procurements in sterile conditions incur the cost of time spent in the operating theater, which varies from U. S. $600 to $900 per hour. Because a procurement averages around 2 h, the cost may be as much as $2000. The costs of storing the tissues include the costs of freezers, electricity, and maintenance (Table 2). This may become expensive during months when there is high electrical use, such as in summer. The monthly cost of electricity in our bone bank averages around $80 per freezer with a minimum being about $60 during the winter and a maximum of $100 during the summer. We have also installed an air conditioner in the bone bank to keep the room cool because the freezers have air-cooled compressors. Recently we have purchased freezers that have both air cooling and water cooling, which helps to minimize the use of electricity.

If bone is to be freeze-dried, it is usually procured sterile and then stored by freezing before processing. This adds an extra cost to the cost of freeze-drying. Once the tissues are freeze-dried, they of course do not have to be kept in a freezer but can be kept in vacuum-packed jars at room temperature. As long as the tissues are freeze-dried shortly after they are procured, only a small freezer is needed. Demineralization or manipulation of the bone, of course, adds another expense. This is dependent upon what type of manipulation is performed, such as grinding, chopping, or powdering. Once the bone is in its final form, it can be freeze-dried and kept indefinitely with minimal cost.

Because bone is an anatomical gift, no charge can be made for the tissue. However, because the bone bank incurs expenses in the procurement and processing of tissues, it should be able to recoup these losses by charging a processing fee. Most processing fees are paid by third-party insurance, and therefore the funds that the bone bank obtains should not be used to pay for research. These funds should be kept to pay solely for handling the bone.

In our bone bank, routine charges include $200 for a femoral head and $1500 for a whole femur. We base our charges for each new budget year on the previous year's expenses. The total expenses for the bone bank from the previous year are divided by the number of bone grafts that are transplanted. Each of the different

Table 2. Banking costs for massive allografts (U.S. $)

Procurement costs (per donor)	
Operating room rental	$ 2500
Labor	$ 1000
Supplies	$ 100
Storage costs	
Freezer (19-foot)	$ 8500
Electricity (per annum)	$ 3400
Record-keeping costs	
Computer (hard-disc)	$ 2500
Personnel (per annum)	$ 20000

types of bone grafts are weighted with different significance in order to make the charges more reflective of the cost of the procurement and storage of each type of bone. For instance, femoral heads cost around $200 because they are easily retrieved and stored and do not take up much freezer space. In contrast, whole femurs take more time and effort to retrieve and require more storage space. Therefore, charges for femurs are approximately $1500 per graft. In bone banks where there are other costs, such as freeze-drying, or in banks where procurements are performed in an operating room for which there are no charges, these costs are of course different.

The legal problems associated with bone banking are chiefly those of liability for the preparation (processing) of the bone. It is important to note that bone banks do not provide products. The donor provides the bone; the bank only processes it. There is no product involved because the bone is an anatomical gift for which no charge can be assessed. The bone bank provides a service, not a product, and therefore no product liability may be incurred, and no product warranty can be provided to the user. However, negligence may occur during processing, an event for which the bone bank would be responsible.

The legal ramifications of problems that may occur in banking bone also occur with other types of organs and tissues. In particular, blood is a similar type of tissue. Although blood to be used for transfusion is tested for AIDS, hepatitis, and other diseases, a blood bank may be responsible if these diseases are transmitted to a recipient because the blood bank is responsible for processing the blood, i.e., making certain that it is safe to use. The same is true for bone banks, which makes paramount the need for strict aseptic technique, compulsive tissue handling, and complete record keeping. The final step in protection in legal matters is to make certain that the patient who receives the bone understands that the bone has been obtained from another human, and that this bone, although culture-negative and test-negative, may still carry diseases which cannot be determined by current laboratory tests. If a bone bank is within a hospital, most hospitals will cover the bone bank liability on their insurance policy. However, if a bank is free-standing, it is important to obtain such insurance.

References

1. American Association of Tissue Banks (1984) Standards for tissue banking. (Private printing) Available from AATB, 1117 North 19th St., Suite 402, Arlington, VA 22209
2. Prolo DJ, Pedrotti MA, White DH (1980) Ethylene oxide sterilization of bone, dura mater, and fascia lata for human transplantation. Neurosurgery 6:529
3. Cornell CN, Lane JM, Nottebaert M, Klein C, Burstein AA (1987) The effect of ethylene oxide sterilization upon the bone inductive properties of demineralized bone matrix. Trans Orthop Res Soc 12:359
4. Hemminki K, Mutanen P, Saloniemi I, Niemi M-L, Viano A (1982) Spontaneous abortions in hospital staff engaged in sterilizing instruments with chemical agents. Br Med J [Clin Res] 285:1462
5. Ehrlich MG, Lorenz J, Tomford WW, Mankin HJ (1983) Collagenase activity in banked bone. Trans Orthop Res Soc 8:166

Bone Banking in Community Hospitals

A. A. Czitrom

Combined Orthopaedic Division, Toronto General Hospital and Mount Sinai Hospital, Department of Surgery and Immunology, University of Toronto, Toronto, Ontario, Canada

Introduction

It has become apparent that replacement of bone stock is necessary at an increasing rate during revision and reconstructive surgery after failed total joint arthroplasty [4, 5]. This requires the availability of banked bone. Since complex tissue banking is expensive, all large regional and institutional bone banks are limited to tertiary care centers. These institutions cannot supply sufficient banked allograft bone at a national level. On the other hand, patient access to tertiary care centers is limited and transfer of increasing numbers of patients to such centers is not practical. These considerations give a rationale for bone banking and the use of banked allograft bone at the local community hospital level. Although the logistics of bone banking in local community hospitals are different from those of complex banking procedures, the general guidelines that ensure reliable preservation, safety, and availability of banked bone apply in the same manner as established previously for regional and institutional tissue banks [1, 3]. Community bone banking requires safe, simple, and cost-effective methods or preservation. These criteria are best met by deep-freezing. Advantages of deep-frozen allografts (bank bone) over fresh autografts are: unlimited quantity, no donor site morbidity, and maintained osteoconductive function. Their disadvantages are: lack of osteogenic and osteoinductive function, slow healing rate, and potential to sensitize the recipient.

Donor Selection

There are no strict donor age limits for community banking. All disease-free bone can be used in some form or another. Female, postmenopausal bone should be used in morselized form only. Generally, bone is collected during surgery and is frozen immediately after removal. In the case of cadaver or spare-part (traumatic amputation) harvesting, bone should be collected within 24 h after death if the body or part is kept refrigerated (4 °C) and within 12 h if kept at room temperature (20 °C).

The most important single step in selection is the exclusion of donors that have the potential to transfer disease. General guidelines endorsed by the American Association of Tissue Banks [1] exclude all donors with the following conditions: infections (acute or chronic), malignancy, irradiation, systemic disease, venereal disease, hepatitis, slow virus disease, acquired immunodeficiency syndrome (AIDS), history of drug abuse, intoxications or toxic substances in tissues, pro-

Bone Transplantation
Eds.: M. Aebi, P. Regazzoni

longed steroid treatment, unexplained death. When a case is questionable or any doubt exists, exclusion is the safest way of preventing transmission of disease.

Laboratory screening of donor blood is another important step to assure safety of bone transplantation. In community hospitals the majority of donors are patients undergoing surgical procedures. Therefore, blood testing can be carried out preoperatively. The following tests are required: (a) syphilis (VDRL test), (b) hepatitis B (hepatitis B antigen and antibody), (c) AIDS (HIV antibody), and (d) blood group. In addition, in the case of cadaver harvesting, blood cultures (aerobic and anaerobic) must be obtained from three different sites. Harvested bone should be stored temporarily and must not be used until the results of blood tests are known. Bone from donors with positive serological tests must be discarded. The blood group result is important for the purpose of matching certain patients at risk (Rh-negative females of child bearing age) and thus avoid possible Rh sensitization [7].

Informed consent should be obtained from both donor and recipient. For live donors the consent should include the laboratory screening tests. Denial of consent for the screening tests outlined above disqualifies the donor (this may represent a problem because of the fear of AIDS testing).

Procurement

The major source of bone in community banking is the operating room because numerous orthopedic procedures require excision of bone. The most common source is that of femoral heads excised during hip arthroplasty. However, significant quantities of bone can be obtained from femoral condyles and tibial plateaus during knee arthroplasty, wedges removed at osteotomy, excisions of bone (patella, radial head), and ribs resected during thoracotomy. In addition, large amounts of bone become available in cases of traumatic amputation when replantation is not feasible. Cadaver harvesting permits the procurement of very large quantities of bone but is generally not within the capabilities of community hospital bone bank procedures. Methods of cadaver harvesting have been described in detail previously [3].

Donor bone must be screened meticulously prior to transplantation. This involves both microbiology and histopathology. After harvest and prior to storage, aerobic and anaerobic cultures are taken from the surface and marrow sections. A routine section of a representative area obtained by core biopsy is processed for histopathology. The results of these studies should be evaluated in the same manner as the serological tests prior to release of the bone for use. If pathology is detected the bone must be discarded.

Storage and Retrieval

The packaging of harvested bone is done under sterile conditions in the operating room. The triple-wrapping technique is recommended. It is acceptable to use glass, polyethylene, or plastic containers combined with towels. Labeling should be simple and informative, including: donor information, date of procurement, identification number. It is useful to add the surgeon's name, size of bone (small, large, medium femoral head), sex of donor (for simple quality estimate), and blood group.

Temporary storage of bones should be at −70 °C in a special area of the freezer or in a separate freezer if available. Upright freezers are recommended because of the convenience of sorting and retrieval. Bones in temporary storage are not used until screening (serology and bone) is complete. If screening tests are positive or if the living donor develops an infection after procurement, all bones from that donor must be discarded.

Final storage is also at −70 °C. Household freezers (−20 °C) are not recommended because of the possibility of slow autolysis at this temperature. The area of final storage should only contain bone that meets the criteria for use (i.e., is screening-negative).

When bones are removed from storage for use, the coverings should be removed under sterile conditions in the operating room. Repeat cultures (aerobic and anaerobic) are taken prior to thawing. The bones are placed into warm (50 °C) antibiotic solution (saline with 50000 U bacitracin or betadine solution) prior to use.

It is acceptable to store bones for 2–3 years at −70 °C. However, it is preferred to turn over bones more rapidly and to store them for less than 1 year in order to minimize the possibility of infection. Infection in the freezer should be monitored at 6-monthly intervals by (a) taking swabs from the inside freezer walls and (b) assessing random samples of stored bones (by submitting 5% of stored specimens in toto for microbiology and histopathology screening).

Sterilization is not obligatory for community bone banks, provided that all guidelines for exclusions, screening, and sterile procurement are met. However, sterilization is required for cadaver harvests done outside of operating rooms and can be an additional safety measure against infection in all cases. Gamma irradiation (2.5 Mrad from a ^{60}Co source) is the recommended method for hospitals where facilities exist. To date, clinical and experimental work in the author's institution has not shown any detrimental effects of this method on the biological and mechanical properties of bank bone. Sterilization is optional and by no means a substitute for proper screening and sterile procurement.

Simple manual record keeping is adequate for community banking. A local bone bank committee with involvement of a pathologist, microbiologist, and infection control nurse is very helpful. The use of radiographs and microcomputers for increased efficiency of record keeping is optional but not essential.

Cost and Safety

The guidelines given above are realistic in terms of the feasible range for most community hospitals. Evidence for the cost effectiveness and safety of these procedures is provided in Table 1. The table compares published data related to capital expenditures and complications from allografts in large, institutional banks and a small community bank [2, 6, 8]. It is clear from these data that community banking requires minimal expense and is as safe as institutional banking.

Table 1. Comparison of cost and safety of community bone banking with institutional banking. (From [2, 6, 8])

	Institutional bank	Community bank
Capital	U.S. $ 165000	U.S. $ 5000
processing	$ 2500/graft	3 h wages per week
Femoral heads	1983–1984	1982–1984
Total allografts	78	180
Discarded grafts	2	29
Implanted grafts	58	101
Procedures	47	77
Infections	1	0
Complications from grafts	0	0

References

1. American Association of Tissue Banks (1979) Guidelines for the banking of musculoskeletal tissues: Am Assoc Tissue Banks Newslett 3:2–32
2. Friedlaender GE (1976) Personnel and equipment required for a "complete" tissue bank. Transplant Proc 8:235–240
3. Friedlaender GE, Mankin HJ (1981) Bone banking: current methods and suggested guidelines. In: Murray DG (ed) AAOS instructional course lectures, vol 30. Mosby, St Louis, pp 36–55
4. Gross AE, Lavoie MV, McDermott P, Marks P (1985) The use of allograft bone in revision of total hip arthroplasty. Clin Orthop 197:115–122
5. Harris WH (1982) Allografting in total hip arthroplasty in adults with severe acetabular deficiency including a surgical technique for bolting the graft to the ilium. Clin Orthop 162:150–164
6. Hart MM, Campbell ED, Kartub MG (1986) Bone banking. A cost effective method for establishing a community hospital bone bank. Clin Orthop 206:295–300
7. Johnson CA, Brown BA, Lasky LC (1985) Rh immunization caused by osseous allograft. N Engl J Med 312:121–122
8. Tomford WW, Ploetz JE, Mankin HJ (1986) Bone allografts of femoral heads: procurement and storage. J Bone Joint Surg [Am] 63A:534–537

Bone Exposed to Heat

A. Kreicbergs and P. Köhler

Department of Orthopaedic Surgery, Karolinska Hospital, Sweden

Introduction

Properties of bone tissue after exposure to heat have been studied extensively for more than a century. The first major work in this research field was presented by Ollier in 1867 [31]. For several decades, interest was focused mainly on the feasibility of utilizing boiled bone for allo- and xenografting [2–4, 12–14, 22, 27]. Over time, several clinical studies seemed to substantiate the usefulness of boiled allografts [12, 24, 32, 33, 38]. However, with the development of new techniques for preparing and preserving allogeneic bone, such as freeze-drying and deep-freezing [6–8], the use of boiled allografts almost ceased. The last major clinical studies on boiled allografts were reported in the 1950s and early 1960s [24, 38, 45]. By then, more sophisticated methods were available for evaluating different types of bone grafts [6–8, 15]. Basic experimental works disclosed that boiled bone grafts were inert, devoid of osteoinductive capability and, moreover, poorly revascularized, resorbed and remodelled [5–8, 10, 19, 30, 34, 37]. Burwell, in his comprehensive review "The Fate of Bone Grafts" [7], concluded that boiled allografts were inferior to freeze-dried and frozen allografts. This opinion still prevails and, hence, these types of grafts are the most widely used for reconstruction of large skeletal defects [11, 26, 46]. Yet, bone devitalized by heat has been used occasionally in clinical practice until nowadays, however not for transplantation but for reimplantation [9, 16, 17, 20, 43].

To our knowledge, Orell in 1934 was the first to describe reimplantation of resected, boiled, autologous bone in the treatment of neoplastic bone disease and osteomyelitis [32]. The same principle, although later modified by the introduction of autoclaving, has been adopted by others as an alternative to modern allografting [17, 40, 41]. By its simplicity, reimplantation of devitalized, resected bone offers several advantages to allografting for reconstructing large skeletal defects. However, data on the applicability of the method are still scanty, in spite of several basic investigations on bone exposed to heat [1, 21, 23, 28, 39]. The physical properties of bone subjected to autoclaving and the biology of incorporation of autoclaved autologous bone has so far not been comprehensively investigated. Optimum autoclaving heat, which ensures complete devitalization, i.e. eradication of the lesion, but still preserves the mechanical properties of the bone, has so far only been studied to a limited extent [35, 36]. Hence, more research is needed to assess the validity of reimplanting autoclaved bone.

Bone Transplantation
Eds.: M. Aebi, P. Regazzoni

We investigated structural properties of diaphyseal bone after autoclaving and heat propagation in bone during autoclaving. In addition, bone-inductive capability of matrix prepared from autoclaved bone was investigated.

Material and Methods

Our study was based on examination of cadaveric bones from 38 adult rabbits. The material included 54 pairs of diaphyseal bone, 30 femoral, 14 humoral and 10 tibial pairs, for assessment of structural properties of bone after autoclaving. Another 16 femora were used for investigating heat propagation in diaphyseal bone during autoclaving. In addition, bone inductive capability of matrix prepared from autoclaved allogeneic bone was investigated in four young (1.5-kg) animals.

Autoclaving and Temperature Monitoring. The degree of sterilization (F0) obtained by autoclaving is a function of time (t) and temperature (T): $F0 = t \times 10^{(T-121)/10}$. In clinical practice the degree of sterilization applied for easily damaged goods such as rubber etc. is usually adjusted to an F0 value of 20. This degree of sterilization (F0=20), corresponding to approximately 33 h boiling, was consistently chosen in the present study. An autoclave (GE, 606, AR-1, Getingeverken, Sweden) was used, which Permitted alterations of time and temperature. Furthermore, it allowed continuous monitoring of temperature in both the autoclave and the autoclaved objects.

In the assessment of physical properties of autoclaved bone, time and temperature in the autoclave was varied, although the degree of sterilization was kept constant (F0=20). The bone specimens were divided into three groups: those autoclaved at 110 °C for 225 min, 121 °C for 20 min, and 131 °C for 2 min. The contralateral bone of each pair served as a non-autoclaved control. Heat propagation in bone was monitored at 121 °C and 131 °C by thermocouples inserted into the medullary canal through drill holes in the distal end of the specimens. Eight femora were autoclaved at 121 °C for 20 min and another eight at 131 °C for 2 min.

Torsional Test. Structural properties of the diaphyseal bones were investigated by means of a computerized torsion test machine previously described by Jonsson and Strömberg [18, 42]. Each specimen was twisted inwards at constant speed (6°/s) until fracture. Simultaneously, the torque-twist relationship was graphically registered. From each curve, strength (maximum torque capacity), stiffness (linear slope), linear deformation (linear phase) and total deformation (angle of fracture) could be derived.

Changes in structural properties of bone caused by autoclaving were assessed by determining the ratio between the autoclaved and non-autoclaved bone of each diaphyseal pair. The mean of the ratios for each group was subsequently calculated.

Bone Induction. Bone-inductive capability of allogeneic bone matrix prepared from autoclaved and non-autoclaved bone was compared in four young animals. Allogeneic bone matrix was prepared from fresh rabbit cadaveric bone as described by Urist [44]. Briefly, the long bones were demineralized in 0.6 *M* HCl, defatted in chloroform-methanol (1 : 1) and subsequently lyophylized.

Ten pieces of bone matrix (each approximately 50 mg) were prepared from autoclaved bone and non-autoclaved bone, respectively, and implanted in the muscles of the dorsal abdominal wall. The four animals were killed 6 weeks postoperatively and the specimens collected for histological examination.

Results

Heat Propagation. At both 121 °C and 131 °C the lag between autoclave temperature and intramedullary bone temperature proved to be short. Thus, the increase in temperature in relation to time proved to be almost as rapid in the autoclaved bones as in the autoclave at both temperatures (Fig. 1). However, at higher temperature the time needed for reaching the aimed temperature (131 °C) in the bones comprised a larger proportion of the whole autoclaving time.

Structural Properties. Ten pairs were excluded due to inadequate casting, as indicated by an atypical torque-twist curve and another two pairs because of computer processing errors.

Autoclaving of femoral specimens caused a decrease in strength and stiffness, which was most pronounced for those autoclaved at low temperature (110 °C) for a long time (255 min) and less pronounced for those subjected to standard autoclaving, i.e. 121 °C for 20 min (Table 1). The least decrease was noted for femora autoclaved at high temperature (131 °C) for a short time (2 min). Thus there was a relationship between autoclaving time and temperature, on one hand, and changes in structural properties of bone on the other, although the degree of sterilization was kept constant ($F0 = 20$).

Torsional test of bones of different size and form (humerus, tibia, femur) subjected to standard autoclaving (121 °C, 20 min) disclosed no significant differences in changes of structural properties (Table 2).

Bone Induction. Histological analysis disclosed that matrix prepared from autoclaved bone and implanted heterotopically had no bone-inductive capability. Control specimens, on the other hand, prepared from nonautoclaved bone consistently proved to have induced newly formed bone characterized by osteoid tissue containing abundant osteoblastic and bone marrow cells.

The present study on bone after autoclaving differs in several respects from other studies on bone exposed to heat. Amprino [1] studied the effect of dry heat on small pieces of cortical bone by the Brinell method and found increasing microhardness from 37 °C to 120 °C, followed by a clear decrease. Sedlin [39] investigated bending strength of boiled pieces of human cortical bone but could not with certainty demonstrate any changes. The difference in results between the present study and other studies should be attributed mainly to the fact that the type of heat exposure differed. Furthermore, other studies dealt exclusively with mechanical properties (pieces of bone), whereas the present study also took structural properties (whole bones) into account.

The observed changes in structural properties of diaphyseal bone after autoclaving are most likely related to collagen, which is known to alter its properties

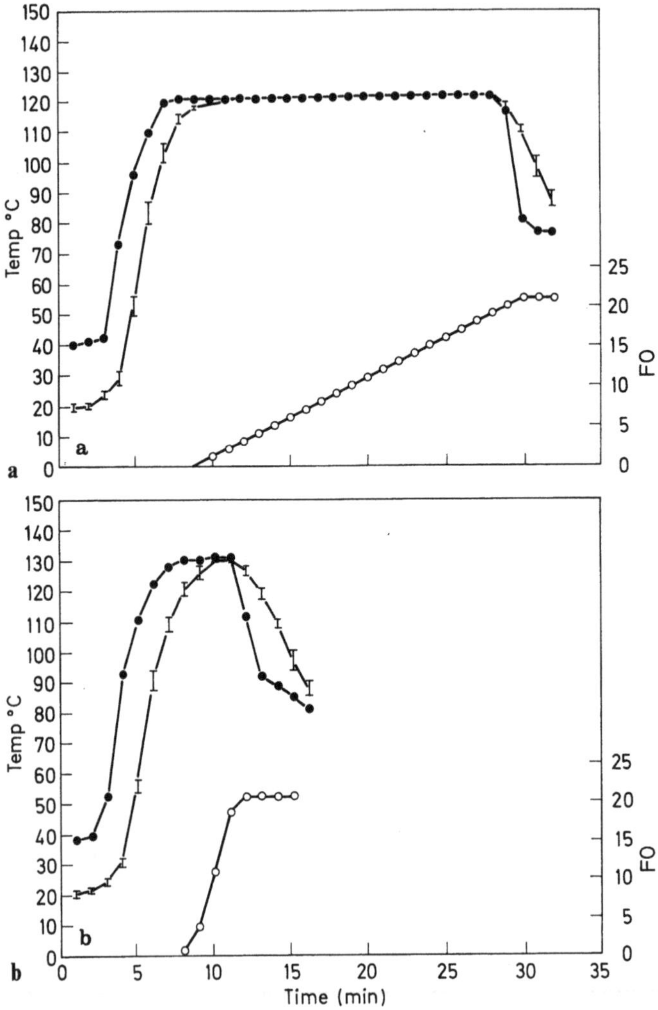

Fig. 1 a and b. Degree of sterilization (*F0*) and temperature over time. **a** Heating to 121 °C. **b** Heating to 131 °C. ●, Temperature of autoclave; I, temperature of autoclaved bone; ▲, F0 level. The two procedures produce the same degree of sterilization (F0 = 20)

when heated beyond 60 °C [29], probably by denaturation and degradation. The decrease in weight probably also applies to collagen (i.e. loss) since collagen is known to pass into solution as gelatin when bone is exposed to moist heat [7]. Loss of water seems less likely since autoclaving was performed in saturated water steam.

Since the least reduction in torsional strength (9%) was noted for specimens autoclaved at 131 °C for 2 min, this would seem to be the procedure of choice when using autoclaved bone for reconstruction of large skeletal defects. However, as mentioned previously, this procedure entails a very short period of optimum heat, which may be difficult to manage and control. From the devitalization point

Table 1. Structural properties of autoclaved bone by sterilization procedure

Temp. (°C)	Time (min)	*n*	Strength	Stiffness	Deformation changes		Weight
					Linear	Total	
110	255	7	0.65 (0.07)	0.73 (0.08)	0.74 (0.11)	0.97 (0.07)	0.88 (0.04)
121	20	9	0.77 (0.07)	0.80 (0.03)	0.86 (0.19)	1.05 (0.14)	0.95 (0.05)
131	2	9	0.91 (0.06)	0.80 (0.04)	0.85 (0.15)	1.05 (0.09)	0.92 (0.04)

Figures represent mean ratios (SD) of the level in autoclaved bone to the respective level in non-autoclaved bone.

Table 2. Structural properties of autoclaved bone by type of bone

Type of bone	*n*	Strength	Stiffness	Deformation changes		Weight
				Linear	Total	
Tibia	8	0.80 (0.10)	0.76 (0.07)	0.91 (0.12)	1.07 (0.17)	0.94 (0.04)
Femur	9	0.77 (0.07)	0.80 (0.03)	0.86 (0.19)	1.05 (0.14)	0.95 (0.05)
Humerus	10	0.77 (0.08)	0.77 (0.09)	0.86 (0.09)	1.07 (0.14)	0.94 (0.04)

Figures represent mean ratios (SD) of the level in autoclaved bone to the respective level in non-autoclaved bone.

of view it appears safer to expose tumorous bone to autoclaving at 121 °C for 20 min. The observed decrease (23%) in torsional strength of diaphyseal bone after autoclaving at 121 °C for 20 min may be considered moderate, since it has been reported that bone affected by a 50% reduction of its maximum strength still resists normal loads [25]. Furthermore, practical reasons also speak in favour of bone autoclaving at 121 °C for 20 min, since most standard surgical autoclaves are adjusted accordingly.

A main objection to using autoclaved bone as a graft is the total absence of osteogenic capability. Apart from being completely devitalized, there does not seem to remain the slightest bone-inductive capability, as demonstrated by testing allogeneic bone matrix prepared from autoclaved bone. Hence, there are reasons to assume that large autoclaved grafts require supplementation with an osteogenic promter to provide safe incorporation.

In summary, autoclaving causes clear, but moderate changes in structural properties of bone. By appropriate adjustment of time and temperature the physical effects of autoclaving may be minimized within limits consistent with normal mechanical loads and without compromising complete bone devitalization. Hence, resected, autoclaved, pathological bone may be used as a graft provided incorporation can be attained. In the reimplantation of major cortical segments this propably requires some type of osteogenic promotion.

Acknowledgement. Figure and Tables are published with the permission of *Acta Orthopaedica Scandinavica.*

References

1. Amprino R (1958) Investigations on some physical properties of bone tissue. Acta Anat (Basel) 34:161–186
2. Axhausen G (1908) Histologische Untersuchung über Knochentransplantation am Menschen. Dtsch Z Chir 91:388–396
3. Barth H (1893) Über histologische Befunde nach Knochenimplantationen. Arch Klin Chir 46:409–421
4. Baschkirzew P (1912) Beträge zur freien Knochenüberpflanzung. Dtsch Z Chir 113:490
5. Blaimont P (1960) Contribution expérimentale a' l'etude des greffes osseuses bouilles. Acta Chir Belg 59:871
6. Burwell GR (1966) Studies in the transplantation of bone. VIII. Treated composite homograft-autograft of cancellous bone, an analysis of inductive mechanisms in bone transplantation. J Bone Joint Surg [Br] 48B:532
7. Burwell GR (1969) The fate of bone grafts. In: Apley AG (ed) Recent advances in orthopaedics. Churchill, London, pp 115–207
8. Chalmers J, Lea L, Stewart L, Sissons HA (1960) Freeze-dried bone as grafting material. In: Parkes AS, Smith AU (eds) Recent research in freezing and drying. Blackwell, Oxford, pp 281–291
9. Chapchal, G (1970) Operative treatment of bone tumours. Thieme, Stuttgart
10. Deleu J, Trueta J (1965) Vascularization of bone grafts in anterior chamber of the eye. J Bone Joint Surg [Br] 47B:319
11. Friedlaender GE, Strong DM, Sell KW (1976) Studies of the antigenicity of bone freeze-dried and deep frozen allografts in rabbits. J Bone Joint Surg [Am] 58A:854
12. Gallie WE (1918) The use of boiled bone in operative surgery. Am J Orthop Surg 16:373
13. Groves EWH (1917) Methods and results of transplantation of bone in repair of defects caused by injury or disease. Br J Surg 5:185
14. Haas C (1921) Function in relation to transplantation of bone. Arch Surg 3:425–432
15. Heiple KG, Chase SW, Herndon CH (1963) A comparative study of the healing process following different types of bone transplantation. J Bone Joint Surg [Am] 45A:1593
16. Ikonomov I (1957) Surgical treatment of malignant tumours of bone: preliminary communication. Khirurgija (Sofia) 10:32
17. Johnston JO, Harries TJ, Alexander CE, Alexander AH (1983) Limb salvage procedure for neoplasms about the knee by spherocentric total knee arthroplasty and autogenous autoclaved bone grafting. Clin Orthop 181:137
18. Jonsson U, Strömberg L (1985) Torsional tests of long bones with computerized equippement. J Biomed Eng 7:251
19. Kiehn CL, Glover DM (1953) A study the revascularisation of experimental bone grafts by means of radioactive phosphorous. J Plast Reconstr Surg 12:233
20. Kirkup JR (1965) Traumatic femoral bone loss. J Bone Joint Surg [Br] 47B:106
21. Ku JL, Smith PA, Goldstein SA, Matthews LS (1985) An experimental investigation of the fate of autogenous autoclaved bone grafts. 31st Annual ORS Las Vegas, Nevada, January 1985
22. Levander G (1938) A study of bone regeneration. Surg Gynecol Obstet 67:705
23. Lundskog J (1972) Heat and bone tissue. Scand J Plast Reconstr Surg [Suppl] 9
24. Lloyd-Roberts GC (1952) Experience with boiled cadaveric bone. J Bone Joint Surg [Br] 34B:428
25. Låftman P, Sigurdsson F, Strömberg L (1980) Recovery of diaphyseal bone strength after rigid internal plate fixation. An experimental study in the rabbit. Acta Orthop Scand 51:215
26. Mankin HJ, Doppelt SH, Sullivan RT, Tomford WW (1982) Osteoarticular and intercalary allograft transplantation in the management of malignant tumors of bone. Cancer 50:613
27. Marchand (1901) Der Prozess der Wundheilung. D Chir 16:599

28. Molander H (1981) Revascularization and healing of stabilized nonvital cortical fragments. Thesis, University of Uppsala
29. Neustadt DH, Rotstein J (1963) In: Chemistry and therapy of collagen diseases. Thomas, Springfield
30. Odell RT, Mueller CB, Key JA (1951) Effect on bone grafts of radioactive isotopes of phosphours. J Bone Joint Surg [Am] 33A:324
31. Ollier L (1867) Traité expérimental et clinique de la régénération des os et de la production artificielle du tissu osseux. Manson, Paris
32. Orell S (1934) Studien über Knochenimplantation und Knochenneubildung, Implantation von „os purum“ sowie Transplantation von „os novum“. Acta Chir Scand 74[Suppl]:31
33. Orell S (1937) Surgical bone grafting with os purum, os novum and boiled bone. J Bone Joint Surg 19:873
34. Reynolds FC, Olliver DR (1950) Experimental evaluation of homogenous bone grafts. J Bone Joint Surg [Am] 33A:307
35. Rivard CH, Fallaha M, Labelle H (1981) The effect of autoclaving in normal and tumoral bone cells in the dog. Orthop Trans 5:474
36. Rivard CH (1984) The effect of autoclaving on normal and sarcomatous bone cells and on graft incorporation. In: Current concepts of diagnosis and treatment of bone and soft tissue tumours. Springer, Berlin Heidelberg New York
37. Ruf F (1954) Zur Vitalität von Knochenspänen. Untersuchungen mit Radiophosphor und Radiocalcium. Arch Klin Chir 279:829
38. Rocher HL (1953) Dead bone grafts in orthopaedic surgery. J Bone Joint Surg [Br] 35B:328
39. Sedlin EA (1965) A rheologic model for cortical bone. Acta Orthop Scand 36[Suppl]:83
40. Sijbrandij S (1978) Resection and reconstruction for bone tumours. Acta Orthop Scand 49:249
41. Smith WS, Simon MA (1975) Segmental resection for chondrosarcoma. J Bone Joint Surg [Am] 57A:1097
42. Strömberg LNE (1975) Diaphyseal bone in rigid internal plate fixation. Acta Chir Scand [Suppl]:456
43. Thompson VP, Steggall CT (1956) Chondrosarcoma of the proximal portion of the femur treated by resection and bone replacement. J Bone Joint Surg [Am] 38A:357
44. Urist MR, Silverman BF, Buring K, Dubuc FL, Rosenberg JM (1967) The bone induction principle. Clin Orthop 53:243
45. Williams G (1964) Experiences with boiled cadaveric cancellous bone for fractures of long bones. J Bone Joint Surg [Br] 46B:398
46. Volkov MV, Imamaliyev AS (1976) Use of allogenous articular bone implants as substitutes for autotransplants in adult patients. Clin Orthop 114:192

A Method for the Investigation of Bone Transplants, Ceramics, and Other Material in a Human Bony Layer

M. Roesgen

Berufsgenossenschaftliche Unfallklinik, Duisburg-Buchholz, 4100 Duisburg, FRG

Surgical literature includes a wide variety of models for systematic research into the process of bony ingrowth, the rebuilding of bone, and the various reactions of bone. All such studies have been carried out on animals as the only object of research [2, 4, 8]. Depending on the specific reaction of the bone being investigated, different methods are described, such as hole drilling, segmental resections comparing sides, fenestration of bone segments, and transplanting complete parts of bones and joints. To the present, however, there has been no research model of this kind with regard to the specific reactions in man. Any clinical research, i.e., research in man, is justified only if it shows therapeutic effects. The handicap is thus that, while investigating the scientific problem, the research itself must be a success in a therapeutic sense.

To investigate the regeneration of human bone in a suitable firm layer, we introduced a model developed by us out of therapeutic necessity. This is to be continued in the course of further investigations, independent of specifically therapeutic considerations. The iliac crest offers an ideal area for such investigation. In order to carry out a successful treatment in bone diseases it is often necessary to use cancellous bone, usually obtained from the iliac crest. Cancellous bone grafting is a method that can be used repeatedly as a specific means of therapy in cases of delayed bone healing, pseudarthrosis, bony defect, corrective osteotomy, or for filling up a defect in chronic osteomyelitis [1].

In preparing the iliac crest for therapy associated with obtaining cancellous bone, the layer can simultanously be prepared for scientific investigation. We make use of the empty iliac crest itself. This does not entail a departure from therapeutic standards as conventionally observed. A lid of the iliac crest is chiseled in a tangential manner and tipped medially. Between medial and lateral cortex the cancellous bone is easily accessible and is removed by a hollow chisel and spoon, if the range of the spoon is long enough in both anterior and posterior directions. In the anterior direction one reaches the anterior iliac spine, in the dorsal direction the borderline for the dorsal approach to the cancellous bone area [5, 7]. In the medial direction there is a borderline defined by the convergence of the medial and lateral cortex in the iliopectineal line.

The location provided by this therapeutic procedure is a bony layer ideal for investigation. The substance to be examined is inserted here, for example, ceramics, collagen or allogenous bone. This layer, well supplied with blood, offers bony contact from all sides. When closing the hole, the bony lid is refixated through suture of the periosteum.

Bone Transplantation
Eds.: M. Aebi, P. Regazzoni

Especially in patients with complicated bone healing or osteomyelitis, in whom repeated operations are necessary, a later operation allows simultaneously taking a specimen from the previously prepared iliac crest. This can accompany further cancellous bone grafting, corrective operation, reosteosynthesis, change in procedure of osteosynthesis, or removal of metal. The biopsy is done by a stab incision in the former scar. A hollow drill with inner diameter of 4 mm is used. Transverse drilling of the iliac crest in the prepared region through the lateral to the medial cortex can provide a bony cylinder for histological examination [6].

This model has now been used for half a year to investigate the regenerative capacity of bone in a firm layer. We have implanted various materials in such a bony layer of the iliac crest of 49 patients. Biopsies have been carried out on 15 patients to date. There were no complications caused by this procedure. All wounds healed by first intention. The rate of complications while obtaining cancellous bone from the iliac crest did not rise over normal levels. In the literature the rate has been reported at less than 7% [3], while among our patients there were 65 complications in about 1600 bone grafts from the anterior and posterior iliac crest – a complication rate of 4.3%.

The period until biopsy can be taken cannot be predetermined. This depends on the time required for regeneration of the injured bone, which bears no relation to the aim of scientific investigation but only to the treatment of the fracture.

This model allows further investigations under comparatively standardized equivalent conditions. Obtaining cancellous bone for therapy is the basic condition for clinical research with this model. Relevant ethical considerations here include the following:

1. No specific complications at the region of interest caused by the implanted material.
2. No additional risk for the patient.
3. No influence on the therapy (e.g., prolonged anesthesia).
4. No disadvantages caused by biopsy.
5. No additional traumatization.
6. The biopsy must be performed in conjunction with another operation.
7. Informed consent must be given by the patient.

The aims of investigation do not correspond to the aims of therapy, and the former must always be secondary to the latter. All investigations and biopsies hitherto carried out on a great number of patients give hope for concrete results. These we will evaluate in future research.

References

1. Burchardt H (1983) The biology of bone graft repair. Clin Orthop 174:28–41
2. Faensen M (1981) Die Knochenneubildung durch komprimierte autologe und homologe Spongiosatransplantate im kortikalen Lager. Habilitationsschrift (thesis), FU Berlin-Steglitz
3. Gerngroß H, Burri C, Kinzl L, Merk J, Müller G-W (1982) Komplikationen an der Entnahmestelle autologer Spongiosatransplantate. Akt Traumatol 12:146–152
4. Maatz R, Lentz W, Graf R (1954) Spongiosa test of bone grafts. J Bone Joint Surg [Am] 36:721–731

5. Popkirov S (1981) Entnahme autologer Knochentransplantate und gleichzeitiger osteoplastischer Ersatz des Donorknochendefektes. Zentralbl Chir 106:455–462
6. Rao DS (1982) Practical approach to bone biopsy. In: Recker RR MD (ed) Bone histomorphometry: techniques and interpretation. CRC, Boca Raton
7. Sarvary A, Berentey G (1981) Die Behandlung von Defektpseudarthrosen mit „autologisierter“ heterologer Spongiosa. Akt Traumatol 11:228–230
8. Schweiberer L (1970) Experimentelle Untersuchungen von Knochentransplantaten mit unveränderter und mit denaturierter Knochengrundsubstanz. Z Unfallheilkd 103

Perforated Demineralized Bone – A Highly Osteoinductive Allograft

E. Gendler

Pacific Coast Tissue Bank, University of Southern California and Orthopaedic Hospital, 2500-19 So. Flower St., Los Angeles, California 90007, USA

This communication reports the development of a new material with a high osteoinductive capacity that can be used as a research model for osteoinduction as well as for practical purposes in orthopedic and reconstructive surgery.

Long bones from Long-Evans rats were dissected free of soft tissue. The bone marrow was removed. Multiple perforations were made with a drill 0.35 mm in diameter. The perforated bone was demineralized in 0.6 *N* hydrochloric acid, washed in water, and cut into plates measuring 5 × 20 mm. The perforated, demineralized bone matrix (PDBM) was treated sequentially with ethanol and ethyl ether, then air-dried and stored in plastic containers.

Four-week old Long-Evans rats were used for the experiment. An incision was made in the skin over the thorax. Two subcutaneous pockets were made by blunt dissection; one plate of PDBM was deposited in each pocket, and the skin was closed. After various intervals the rats were killed. One implant from each animal was used to demonstrate alkaline phosphatase activity; the second implant was embedded in nitrocellulose. Alternate longitudinal serial sections were stained with hematoxylin and eosin, carmine-Bismarck brown-indigo carmine, toludine blue, Masson's trichrome stain, and von Kossa method.

Four days after the implantation the perforations were filled with undifferentiated mesenchymal cells. The cells adjacent to the surface of the bone matrix exhibited weak alkaline phosphatase activity. The same cells stained with Bismarck brown, indicative of accumulation of sulfated mucopolysaccharides. The core of the perforations contained loose connective tissue and capillaries. Seven days after implantation the mesenchymal cells within the perforations changed from spindle-shaped to oval and showed an increase in alkaline phosphatase activity. Ten days after implantation the mesenchymal cells within the perforations transformed into typical chondrocytes. Resorption of calcified cartilage occurred with ingrowth of blood vessels, leading to deposition of bone. Fourteen days after implantation, cartilage within the perforations underwent resorption and was replaced by endochondral bone that was covered with active osteoblasts. Three and four weeks after implantation the perforations were enlarged and filled with trabecular bone, bone marrow cells, and capillaries. Six and eight weeks after implantation, resorption of bone matrix and its replacement by newly formed bone and bone marrow continued. Three months after implantation the bone matrix had undergone considerable resorption and was replaced by a thin layer of compact bone encircling a structure similar to medulla and which contained trabecular bone and marrow.

Bone Transplantation
Eds.: M. Aebi, P. Regazzoni

It appears that the creation of multiple artificial perforations in demineralized bone highly enhances its osteoinductive and osteogenic potential. Perforations become synchronous centers of endochondral osteogenesis, from which the matrix resorption and bone apposition spread centrifugally.

Segmental Femoral Defect Model in the Rat

G. F. Muschler, J. M. Lane, J. Werntz, M. Gebhardt, H. Sandu, C. Piergentili, M. Nottebaert, C. Baker, and A. Burstein

Hospital for Special Surgery, 535 E. 70th Street, New York, New York 10021, USA

A segmental defect model has been developed in the rat and used to evaluate a variety of bone graft materials both alone and as part of composite graft materials. These include: fibrillar collagen (FC), lyophilized fibrillar collagen (LFC), air-dried fibrillar collagen (ADFC), trypsinized demineralized bone powder (TBP), 0.5 mm hydroxyapatite-tricalcium phosphate ceramic granules (HA/TCP), bone marrow (BM), and cancellous bone (CB). In addition, a bone-derived protein fraction (15–30K) which includes bone morphogenetic protein (BMP) and transformation growth factor beta was combined with TBP to form a reconstituted demineralized bone matrix (RDBM) material (approximately 1 mg/defect).

A 5-mm segmental defect in the midshaft of the femur of a 250 to 300-g Lewis rat serves as the testing bed for the graft material. Fixation is maintained using a four-hole polyethylene plate and 0.062-treaded wires as screws. Local marrow was flushed from the intramedullary cavity. When left untreated, 8% of these defects unite. Graft materials are added to fill the defect. Bone marrow (0.75 cc) is harvested from the femur and tibia of a syngeneic donor rat. Cancellous bone is harvested from the distal femur and proximal tibia of a syngeneic donor.

Serial radiographs are obtained, as well as faxitron radiographs at sacrifice. A modified Bos-Heiple system for bone formation, union, and remodeling at the defect site is used (scores 0–4).

Biomechanical testing is performed at sacrifice (12 weeks) by rapid torsion to failure, as described by Burstein. This method allows quantification of four mechanical parameters: stiffness, maximum torque, angular deformation to failure, and total energy absorption. Comparison between defects is made by reporting the measurement of each defect femur as a percent of the normal contralateral side.

Radiographic observations (Table 1) were the following:

1. The presence of live bone marrow significantly enhanced all measured parameters of fracture healing ($p<0.01$). Killed marrow was not effective.
2. The presence of bone matrix derived proteins of 15K–30K significantly enhanced all measured parameters of fracture healing ($p<0.01$).
3. Adding fibrillar collagen to bone marrow significantly increased union rate ($p<0.05$).
4. Addition of HA/TCF ceramic granules to FC and BM significantly decreased the remodeling observed ($p<0.01$).

Bone Transplantation
Eds.: M. Aebi, P. Regazzoni

Table 1. Radiographic scoring

	n	Formation	Union	Remodeling	% Union
Autogenous bone	11	3.5	3.1	2.4	82
Live marrow (0.75 cc)	16	3.4	2.0	1.5	50
Freeze-killed marrow	5	1.2	0.2	0.0	0
TBP	9	2.1	0.3	0.0	11
TBP+BM	12	3.7	3.5	1.7	92
RDBM	12	3.9	3.3	2.2	92
RDBM+BM	8	4.0	4.0	2.9	100
FC	12	2.1	0.6	0.5	8
FC+BM	12	3.9	3.9	2.0	100
10% HA/TCP+90% FC+BM	13	3.4	2.8	0.9	61
25% HA/TCP+75% FC+BM	11	3.6	2.9	0.6	72
50% HA/TCP+50% FC+BM	13	3.8	3.0	0.2	61
LFC	7	2.3	1.3	0.6	43
LCF+BM	12	3.8	2.8	1.3	75
33% HA/TCP+67% ADFC	4	1.0	0.0	0.0	0
33% HA/TCP+67% ADFC+BM	15	3.9	3.6	0.9	100

Numbers represent means at 12 weeks after fracture.
TBP, Trypsinized demineralized bone powder; BM, bone marrow; RDBM, reconstituted demineralized bone matrix; FC, fibrillar collagen; LFC, lyophilized fibrillar collagen; HA/TCP, hydroxyapatite-tricalcium phosphate ceramic granules; ADFC, air-dried fibrillar collagen.

Table 2. Results of biochemical testing

	n	Stiffness	Maximum torque	Maximum defect	Total energy
Autogenous bone	7	91 (28)	66 (26)	71 (23)	44 (25)
Live marrow	4	90 (20)	66 (11)	100 (22)	51 (19)
FC+BM	12	85 (22)	81 (24)	107 (37)	73 (50)
LFC+BM	7	73 (28)	74 (40)	68 (26)	54 (30)
TBP+BM	10	96 (13)	66 (18)	64 (20)	52 (27)
RDBM	6	104 (63)	86 (21)	88 (21)	75 (24)
RDBM+BM	7	104 (50)	77 (11)	72 (26)	56 (25)
FC+BM	12	85 (22)	81 (24)	107 (37)	73 (50)
10% HA/TCP+FC+BM	8	58 (19)	64 (23)	87 (27)	59 (35)
25% HA/TCP+FC+BM	6	98 (41)	74 (22)	94 (51)	68 (49)
75% HA/TCP+FC+BM	8	114 (56)	62 (18)	85 (44)	67 (30)
LFC+BM	7	73 (28)	74 (40)	68 (26)	54 (30)
33% HA/TCP+LFC+BM	9	59 (37)	41 (30)	72 (28)	41 (34)

Numbers represent percent of respective values for normal femur. Only groups with radiographic scores not different than cancellous bone are listed. For abbreviations key, see Table 1.

5. Addition of bone marrow to LFC alone was not as effective as with other materials, presumably because the marrow cells were excluded from the defect site by the lyophilized material.

Biomechanical findings (Table 2) were:

1. In general, equal radiographic scores predicted comparable biomechanical properties.
2. Unions resulting from RDBM had significantly higher total energy absorption than cancellous bone ($p<0.05$).
3. Adding ceramic to FC and BM (0%–10%) decreased stiffness ($p<0.01$), but additional ceramic (10%–75%) increased stiffness ($p<0.02$). It did not significantly change other parameters, however.

Bone Bankin – Experience with 1175 Donors

T. I. Malinin, M. D. Brown, W. Mnaymneh, O. Martinez, R. E. Marx, and S. N. Kline

Tissue Bank, Departments of Surgery, Orthopaedics and Rehabilitation, University of Miami, Jackson Memorial Medical Center, Miami, Florida, USA

Massive osteoarticular and intercalary allografts used for reconstruction of extremities as well as allografts used for the arthrodesis and stabilization of the spine, filling of bone defects, maxillofacial reconstruction, and the reconstruction of ligaments and tendons of the knee were prepared from 1175 consecutive donors during a 14-year period. Clinical results with these allografts have been encouraging and included over 80% satisfactory results with intercalary and osteoarticular allografts in selected groups of patients, as well as high rates of fusion in the cervical and lumbar spines. A large number of donors allowed for selection of anatomically matched grafts for given recipients. Results with allogeneic grafts supplemented with autologous bone marrow in mandibular reconstructions have been likewise satisfactory. Histological examination of these grafts demonstrated early incorporation, revascularization, resorption of freeze-dried component, and formation of bone ossicle that continued to remodel and form lamellar bone.

To safeguard the recipients, donors were subjected to a variety of studies and screening tests. These included determinations of HBsAg, HBcAb, HBsAb, HIV Ab, STS, serum chemistries, blood cultures, a postmortem examination, and special histological study of lymph nodes. Bone allografts were also subjected to repeated microbiological testing. On the average, 203 microbiologic cultures were performed per donor.

The authors supplied over 900 massive allografts for reconstruction of the extremities and several thousand allografts used in elective surgical procedures in several institutions on the premise that banking and transplantation of bone constitute a clinical service. This assumption of joint responsibility for the patients established a close relationship between cooperating institutions and surgeons and allowed for the accumulation of clinical data on a large pool of bone allograft recipients.

All bone allografts were excised aseptically and were processed under sterile conditions. These were stored either frozen or freeze-dried. Controlled-velocity freezing of osteoarticular allografts was carried out after exposure to glycerol. However, the majority of bone allografts prepared at the University of Miami were freeze-dried.

Freeze-dried cortical and cancellous bone allografts maintain normal histological structure. Biomechanical properties of freeze-dried shafts of human femurs and tibias were similar to frozen and fresh shafts of femurs and tibias. Laboratory animal studies showed freeze-dried bone to be osteogenic.

The current trends in orthopedic surgery suggest that reliance on bone allografts will probably become a more common practice than it has been in the past.

Bone Transplantation
Eds.: M. Aebi, P. Regazzoni

Initially, massive allografts were used primarily for tumors. In the past few years the use of allografts in nontumourous conditions, particularly in revision hip arthroplasties, has increased dramatically. These developments can be partially explained by the ready availability of allografts made possible by the advent of modern tissue-banking techniques and by the awareness of the patients of the limb-saving procedures. With the current practices of allograft preparation, the patients can be assured that the potential for transmitting an infection or other disease with an allograft is remote.

Organisation of a Bone Bank: Experience over 16 Years

P. Kalbe, A. Illgner, and W. Berner

Department of Traumatology, Hanover Medical School, Hanover, FRG

Since 1971 there has been a bone bank at the Department of Traumatology of Hanover Medical School. Since 1975 bone preservation has been carried out exclusively by deep-freezing at -80 °C. This is today the only generally accepted method (Tomford et al. 1983).

Femoral heads and cancellous wedges are used, which are obtained by reconstructive surgical intervention. Also femoral condyles, tibial heads, femoral heads and iliac crests are procured from organ donors. Donors with hepatitis, lues, AIDS and sepsis, as well as neoplasms, systemic diseases and those on long-term steroid therapy are excluded. The procurement of bones is carried out not later than 6 h after circulatory arrest in aseptic operating theatre conditions. The same strict criterion for sterility should apply for this operation as for aseptic joint surgery. A bone sample is taken from every donor site for bacteriological culture.

The fundamental requirement for organisation is careful documentation. On a special form, in addition to transplant specifications, the personal data and diagnosis of the donors and recipients, the kind and the origin of the bone material as well as the results of the serological and bacteriological investigations are recorded. As long as these are not completely available, the bones remain set apart in the deep-freezer. Only after their release by the responsible organiser can they be transplanted. Matching of the blood groups or the HLA system is not carried out. All data are stored in a relational data bank on a personal computer.

Between January 1, 1975 and December 31, 1986, a total of 1845 transplants in 1371 operations on 1201 patients were used. Most frequently, allogeneic transplants are used for fracture treatment ($n=777$). In exceptional cases bank bone is also transplanted for non-unions if autogeneic reserves are exhausted ($n=133$). A frequent indication is in the reconstruction of bone defects, especially revision arthroplasty of the hip ($n=296$). A classic indication for bank bone is the filling up of bone cavity after resection of bone tumours and cysts, especially in children ($n=165$).

A total of 101 transplants (5.2%) from 43 donors were abandoned because of bacterial contamination, 12 as a result of positive lues reaction and 8 as a result of positive Hbs-AG-titre. Since September 1985 the ELISA test on HIV antibodies has been carried out; this has so far been negative in all cases. With the bacterially contaminated transplants, skin organisms almost without exception were cultivated. Although most of these germs cannot be regarded as potentially infectious, for the reason of safety all contaminated transplants were rejected. Strict asepsis and bone procurement as soon as possible after circulatory arrest has led to a reduction of the contamination rate.

Bone Transplantation
Eds.: M. Aebi, P. Regazzoni

References

Tomford WW, Doppelt SH, Mankin HJ, Friedlaender GE (1983) 1983 bone bank procedures. Clin Orthop 174:15–21

Control of Sterility in Bone Banking with Irradiation

P. Hernigou, G. Delepine, and D. Goutallier
Hôpital Henri Mondor, 94010 Creteil, France

Among all the complications of bone allografts surgery, infection is the most frequent and one of the most devastating. One of the major problems experienced by those who collect and store humoral tissues for clinical transplantation is the control of sterility [3, 4]. This report studies the incidence of sterilization by irradiation in 90 massive allografts (of more than 7 cm) with a follow-up of at least 6 months.

Bone allografts were removed from selected donors (victims of trauma). The donor was always a multiorgan donor; bone excision followed in the same operative room as removal of heart and kidneys. Bones were removed after a simple sterile skin preparation and draping, the donor placed in a supine position. Bones were placed in a freezer at −30 °C where they remained for no more than 6 months. A dose of 2.5–3.5 Mrad beta irradiation [2] was administered. The allografts were used for reconstruction in 85 patients from which highly malignant bone tumors had been resected and in 5 patients with severe failed total hip replacement. They were used either alone (31 grafts) or in combination with metallic prostheses (54 grafts).

Culturing a portion of the graft at the time of transplantation showed no contamination of the graft after sterilization. Prophylactic antibiotics were used for 10 days after surgery. The cement used with prostheses contained antibiotics. After surgery, there was no complication of wound healing, such as erythema and delayed epithelization. Temperature usually became normal by days 7–10 following surgery. At follow-up (between 6 months and 3 years) three infections are noted: in one patient with an intercalary graft, the wound separated 45 days after radiotherapy and remained separated, necessitating removal of the graft; in the two other cases, infection occurred in an allograft in combination with a prosthesis, but at the follow-up it did not necessitate removal of the graft and prosthesis. Evaluation of effects of irradiation on the graft is difficult because no satisfactory objective measure of a specimen's biologic activity is currently available. In this series, the rate of bone union with the host does not seem very different from that in other series: with supplemental autografts used regularly at the host-graft interface 85% of osteosynthesis sites showed radiological healing between 3 and 6 months by a peripheral callus. Technetium scans used in evaluating rèvascularization and biologic incorporation of the graft showed that at 3 months the processes of revascularization and bone turnover within the grafts had begun. When revision was necessary (six nonunions, three fractures, four recurrences of the tumor, two lengthenings in children, one infection, and one removal of osteosynthesis material), gross observations showed that after 6 months muscles had to be strip-

Bone Transplantation
Eds.: M. Aebi, P. Regazzoni

ped from the outer surface of the grafts, and that under muscles the cortical surface appeared to be vascularized. Biopsy specimen of the graft showed that some minimal focal new bone formation was present near the site of interfaces and under muscles. Five patients developed antibodies against HLA specificities represented in a pooled preparation of 20 lymphocytes. This immune response did not cause an adverse clinical result.

Clinical experience with large bone allograft implants that are merely frozen has demonstrated that infection represents a serious problem. Sterilization by irradiation [1] is a simple method of decontamination which provides a safe source of allografts. In this series, the incidence of infection was only 3%. Sterilization is not perhaps the only cause of such a low incidence of infection, but with the increasing demand for allografts by surgeons and with the increasing use of bone allografts with metallic prostheses, the importance of multiplying potential sources of bone and ensuring their sterility has become paramount.

References

1. Bright R, Smatsh J, Gambill V. Sterilization of human bone by irradiation; in oesteochondral allografts. Little, Brown, Boston, pp 223–232
2. Hernigou P, Delepine G, Goutallier D (1986) Allogreffes massives cryoconservées et stérilisées par irradiation. Rev Chir Orthop 72:403–413
3. Dopplet S, Tomford NW, Lucas A, Mankin H (1981) Operational and financial aspects of a hospital bone bank. J Bone Joint Surg [Am] 63:1472–1481
4. Tomford NW, Starkweather RS, Goldman MH (1981) A study of the clinical incidence of infection in the use of banked allograft bone. J Bone Joint Surg [Am] 63:244

Conservation of Bone Homografts in Cialit: 5 Years Clinical Experience

F. Ghisellini, G. Palamini, and G. Brugo

Department of Orthopedics and Traumatology; Ospedale Magiore della Carità; Novara, Italia

The technique that we use for conserving bone homografts requires the chemical substance 2-(ethyl 1-mercuro-mercapto)-5-benzoxazole-carbonate-sodium, known commercially as Cialit. This white powder carbonizes when heated, without melting; it is used in water solution with bidistilled water in various dilutions. Bone segments are placed into air-tight glass containers filled with a solution of Cialit (1 : 5000) stored at +4 °C and sheltered from light. After 15 days the bone can be used for grafts. The solution must be changed regulary every 15–20 days. The maximum period of conservation advised by its manufacturers is about 12 months. The only caution necessary when using segments in Cialit is that they should be thoroughly washed in a physiological solution before clinical use so as to eliminate completely the conversation solution.

As suitable parts, we use principally proximal femoral epiphyses (obtained during the treatment of femoral neck fractures). Before putting them into Ciliat, the bones are carefully cleaned of all fleshy parts, cartilaginous tissue, and corticals and are rapidly washed in physiological solution.

From February 1982 to December 1986, we used bone allografts for the treatment of 84 patients suffering from the following pathologies: depressed factures of the tibial upper end (50 cases), depressed calcanei (26 cases, 2 of which were operated bilaterally), excessively thin acetabula in patients bearing hip protheses (6 cases), ankle fractures with loss of fibula substance (1 case), finger enchondromas (1 case: Fig. 1). The patients have been followed up from clinical, radiographic, and laboratory points of view at regular intervals, and at the beginning we also considered the T-lymphocyte cell-mediated immune reaction using a technique suggested by Lennert. Moreover, we have always confirmed microbiological sterility on a sample of the conserved bone, before and at the moment of its grafting.

We have found no local reactions at the site of its grafting due to host rejection or to possible contact with the solution used for conservation (as noted above, the bone is washed thoroughly before use to eliminate Cialit). Frequently conducted radiographic controls, necessary for clinical supervision of the patient, have always shown perfect incorporation of the graft. We have observed no weakening of the graft (e.g. fractures); even after immediate loading, and consider this a confirmation of the validity of the conservation method used. In regard to microbiological controls, the grafts have always proven to be perfectly sterile. And, finally examination of T-lymphocytes has shown no notable signs of activation.

Bone Transplantation
Eds.: M. Aebi, P. Regazzoni

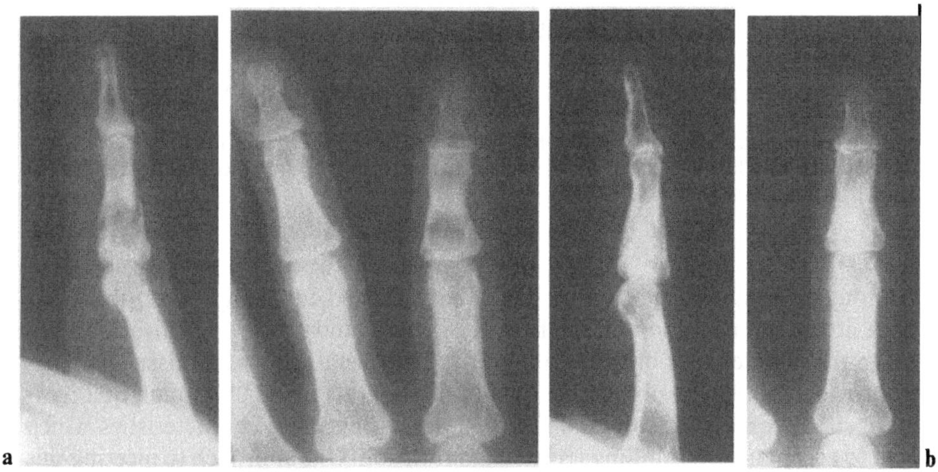

Fig. 1. **a** Finger enchondroma before treatment. **b** Same case, 3 months later, after treatment

We are satisfied with this conservation method for the following reasons:

- It is extremely simple
- It does not require the use of special equipment, which can often be very expensive.
- It has proven to be safe from an immunological and a bacteriological point of view.
- It allows a remarkable shortening of the time necessary to perform the operation, diminishing postoperative morbidity and avoiding further surgical incision.

In contrast to autografts, which we use when the osteoinductive effect is required, the allograft has no limits as to volume.

References

1. Friedlaender G, Mankin HJ (1979) Guidelines for the banking of musculoskeletal tissues. Newslett Am, Assoc Tissue Banks 3:2
2. Triantafyllou N, Sotiropoulos E, Triantafyllou J (1975) The mechanical properties of the lyophilized and irradiated bone grafts. Acta Orthop (Belg) 41:35
3. Urist MR, Dawson E (1981) Intertransverse process fusion with the aid of chemosterilized autolyzed allogeneic (AAA) bone. Clin Orthop 154:97–113

Procedures and Practices for Aseptic Processing of Sterile Bone for Banking

D. A. Present [1], D. W. Anderson [1], F. A. Glowczewskie [2], and W. J. Vanjonack [1]

[1] Hospital for Joint Diseases, Orthopedic Institute, New York, New York, USA
[2] University of Florida School of Medicine, Department of Orthopedic Surgery, Gainsville, Florida, USA

Although musculoskeletal tissue banks have existed for many years, there has been little documentation on method, equipment, and process certification critical to the maintenance of sterile allografts. The overall goal of all tissue banks is to provide the highest obtainable quality of allograft tissue. Although quality is an abstract concept, it can be defined as possessing those characteristics which lead to acceptance in fulfilling its intended function. Our approach to meeting this overall goal of obtaining the highest achievable quality level was to develop programs and specifications based on state of the art technologies and scientifically sound principles. This challenge was met through design of the facility, process control and conformance, and training of personnel. By controlling these variables and validating the systems and processes, one can produce tissue that is uniform and conforms to preestablished specifications. Integral to this system, is an independent quality control function. This group is responsible for testing of tissue for compliance to specifications, assuring processing conformity, and developing quality systems and controls.

One aspect of the integration of quality systems is the purpose of this paper, which is to present data and discussion on guidelines for facilities, clean room design, components, processing, validation, laboratory control, and sterility testing for aseptic processing of allogeneic tissues. In addition, it is intended to expand on the technical aspects of aseptic processing of sterile allograft tissues.

There are major differences between the processing of sterile tissue by aseptic processing and the use of terminal sterilization. For processors utilizing terminal sterilization, the tissue, container, and closure system should be of a microbiological quality so as to minimize the bioburden to help assure that the subsequent sterilization process is successful. In the arena of sterile procurement and aseptic processing of allogeneic tissue, it is critical to the maintenance of sterility that the tissue is procured, processed, filled into containers, and sealed in environments designed specifically to maintain sterility. Aseptic processing requires distinctly separate areas for each step of the operation to preclude opportunities for contamination. Air must be supplied through high-efficiency particulate (HEPA or ULPA) filters under positive pressure and monitored with systems for evaluating the environment and maintaining processing equipment.

The particulate content in controlled areas is of critical concern, since it can contaminate the bone physically or act as a vehicle for microorganisms. Therefore, our aseptic area is designed to allow no more than 10 particulates in a size range of 0.3 micron or larger percubic foot (class 10). The air is of such high quality that no viable organisms are allowed. The air flow should be sufficient to

Bone Transplantation
Eds.: M. Aebi, P. Regazzoni

achieve a minimum of 70 air changes per minute (vertical laminar flow) and maintain a pressure differential of at least 0.05 in. water between the controlled areas and the outside environs. Once the aseptic area, equipment, and methods are in place and performing to specification, a validation of the systems must be conducted to assure sterility. Microbiological growth nutrient medium is utilized to provide artificial stimulus to the aseptic processing area. The nutrient medium is manipulated and exposed to personnel, equipment, surfaces, and environmental conditions to simulate the same exposure which the tissue undergoes. The nutrient medium in conjunction with comprehensive environmental monitoring provides valuable information necessary to monitor the control of the process.

All autoclaves that impact upon the aseptic area have established loading patterns, and cycles that are validated as different configurations may affect patterns of heat distribution and the effect of the sterilization cycle. The environmental monitoring program establishes the effectiveness of cleaning and sanitizing of equipment and surfaces which contact the tissues. The monitoring program includes a comprehensive standardized sampling schedule. Maximum microbial limits are established and a definitive course of action prescribed if abnormal results are obtained. All filters utilized are validated on their ability to prevent the passage of microorganisms (maximum mean porosity 0.2 micron) into the filtrate. The microorganism *Pseudomonas diminuta* is used for this purpose. Mandatory sterility testing on representative samples of tissue is performed throughout the processing. All positive results are thoroughly evaluated. Any investigation includes an analysis of the organism's origin. Each organism must be evaluated as to: (a) identification, (b) source, i.e., facility/quality control laboratory environment, etc, and (c) review of all records to detect signs of failures or anomalies in the environment or support systems/personnel.

Although aseptic processing of allograft tissue is very difficult to achieve, the problems are not insurmountable with the proper facility design, equipment, and knowledgeable, dedicated personnel.

Center for Drugs and Biologics and Office of Regulatory Affairs, Food and Drug Administration (1987) Guideline on sterile drug products produced by aseptic processing.

Bone and Soft Tissue Banking: The University of Florida Experience

C. Reinecke, F. Glowczewskie, Jr., and D. Springfield

Department of Orthopaedics, University of Florida, Gainesville, Florida, USA

The University of Florida (UF) Bone Bank was established in July 1983 to supply frozen allograft bone for the reconstruction of large segmental defects created by wide excision of musculoskeletal tumors in UF patients. In July 1985, with increasing demand for freeze-dried bone and soft tissue grafts, the Bone Bank became the UF Tissue Bank and began processing and distribution of freeze-dried bone, frozen large segmental, and soft tissue grafts, including fascia lata, Achilles tendon/calcaneus, and patella/tendon/tubercle units to requesting centers. All procedures were delineated in accordance with American Association of Tissue Banks guidelines, with additional UF standards.

From the initiation of the bank through October 14, 1986, grafts from 109 donors were procured in a sterile manner, with an average of 27.2, each, aerobic and anaerobic cultures taken per bone to ensure sterility. A total of 1018 tissues were obtained from these donors (10 per donor); of these, 409 were freeze-dried and processed, to provide 1571 items (3.84 per tissue). Of these, 161 (16%) tissues were discarded for not meeting quality control guidelines. The UF Tissue Bank has provided service to 81 hospitals and 120 physicians in ten states.

The clinical results of allografts used in UF orthopedic patients are being evaluated. In one group of patients receiving large segmental frozen intercalary and osteochondral grafts, there are 49 patients with 55 grafts. Of these, 40 are considered to have good results and 9 poor results in a follow-up of 7–42 months. Of 30 patients with freeze-dried corticocancellous bone used to fill 37 bony defects created by curettage, there are no significant complications in a follow-up of 1–34 months (mean, 12). Eight show complete union of their grafts. Anterior cruciate ligament reconstruction with patella/tendon/tubercle allograft (Jones' type) has been performed on 60 patients at UF with no immediate postoperative or early complications thus far. Maximum follow-up on these patients is 1 year. There have been 163 anterior cervical fusions accomplished by the neurosurgery service using freeze-dried allograft iliac wedges over a 2-year period. They report one incident of graft fracture, radiographically apparent resorption of the graft in one patient, and one postoperative infection. Follow-up on the use of UF grafts at outside hospitals is poor. As of October 14, 1986, 919 grafts had been distributed elsewhere. Of these, 742 (81%) were freeze-dried, and 177 (19%) were fresh-frozen. Nine (1.02%) complications were reported, with three (0.4%) in freeze-dried grafts and six (3.4%) in fresh-frozen grafts.

The experience at the UF Tissue Bank is reflective of an increasing tendency by orthopedists to use allograft bone and soft tissue for musculoskeletal reconstruction. The successful application of allogeneic tissue as an alternative to autogenous graft is evident in the results of current clinical trials.

Bone Transplantation
Eds.: M. Aebi, P. Regazzoni

Organizational Aspects of a Hospital Bone Bank

C. Delloye and E. Munting

Department of Orthopedics, St. Luc University Clinic, 10 avenue Hippocrate, 1200 Brussels, Belgium

As a result of the expanding role of bone allograft in reconstructive surgery, a bone bank has been established to support a bone and cartilage allograft transplant program. Three types of allografts are delivered: (a) small, freeze-dried alloimplants used in various conditions; (b) dia/epiphyseal bone segments (−80 °C) for skeletal reconstruction or for supporting long-stemmed prosthesis; and (c) cryoprotected osteochondral grafts (−80 °C). The aim of this report is to survey the procedures we have followed to obtain and manage bone allografts since 1983.

Donors are evaluated by history, physical examination, and laboratory studies to rule out transmission of potential disease. In addition, blood tests are sampled for hepatitis, syphilis, and AIDS. When osteochondral or massive bone allografts are procured, lymph nodes are taken for histocompatibility group determination. Deep-frozen bone and cartilage allografts are procured in a sterile manner from young donors (<40 years) in an operating room by a trained surgeon. Three to four samples of soft tissues for each segment are taken for contamination control, including research for tuberculosis. These are cultured for 8 days. The joint is usually incised medially. Cartilage is protected from freezing injury by an 8% dimethylsulfoxide solution kept at 4 °C. Implants are then placed in three sterile plastic bags and wrapped in waterproof labeled paper before being frozen at −80 °C. Finally, implants are registered if bacteriologic control and laboratory tests are negative.

Small freeze-dried bone allografts are recovered from lower limb epiphyses of young donors after skin preparation. The bone implants, freed from soft tissues, are sawed in standard shapes. They are washed thoroughly under a jet of distilled water to eliminate bone marrow and blood cells. Lipids are further extracted by a chloroform-methanol solution (1 : 1), renewed three times for at least 2 days. Implants are rinsed with methanol and finally with demineralized water before being freeze-dried. They are packed in two peel-off bags, wrapped in a polyethylene bag and are gamma-irradiated (25 kGy).

Deep-frozen allografts are stored at −80 °C, while freeze-dried ones are kept at room temperature. They are classified according to the type of bone. Frozen allografts are thawed for 1 h in saline at 37 °C prior to implantation. Freeze-dried ones are reconstituted in saline. This effort is necessary to identify cause of failure. Data on each donor and receiver are entered in a computer program. A radiograph of each graft is recorded.

The rate of bone contamination at sterile procurement was 10.4% ($n = 77$). Most contaminations were caused by *Staphylococcus epidermidis*. To date, more

Bone Transplantation
Eds.: M. Aebi, P. Regazzoni

than 700 freeze-dried bone implants have been supplied to 330 patients; 17 massive bone allografts have been implanted after tumor resection, and 9 osteochondral grafts including total joint replacements (elbow and knee) have been performed. No infection after graft implantation has been reported.

A bone bank appears to be a valuable service to the community. It spares the patient autograft procurement, allows limb-salvage surgery after tumoral resection, and provides the surgeon with a convenient filling material or anatomic bone components.

Bone Alternatives

Bone Morphogenetic Protein Induced Bone Formation and the Bone – Bone Marrow Consortium *

M. R. Urist

Bone Research Laboratory, University of California at Los Angeles, Los Angeles, California 90024, USA

A low molecular weight component named bone morphogenetic protein (BMP), chemically isolated from the organic matrix of bone, induces postfetal connective tissue cells (pericytes) surrounding small blood vessels to differentiate into cartilage and bone. The sequence of biochemical and morphological pre-, para-, and postdifferentiated events indicate that BMP initiates an organized process of diverse means to an end. The end product is a spherical ossicle of lamellar bone filled with red bone marrow. The process is morphogenetic because a preliminary phase of 24 h of hyaluronate accumulation followed by 24 h of hyaluronidase activity, characteristic of embryonic skeletal tissue anlagen formation, precedes the cytodifferentiation phase of development. Cytodifferentiation culminates in the formation of a complete ossicle (Figs. 1, 2). It is not known whether BMP is endocytosed and transferred to the nucleus to derepress one key gene, or a tandem-linked chain of genes, regulating the biosynthesis of various skeletal products.

Supported by grant-in-aid from the USPHS, NIH number DE2103 and in part by the Max Factor Foundation.

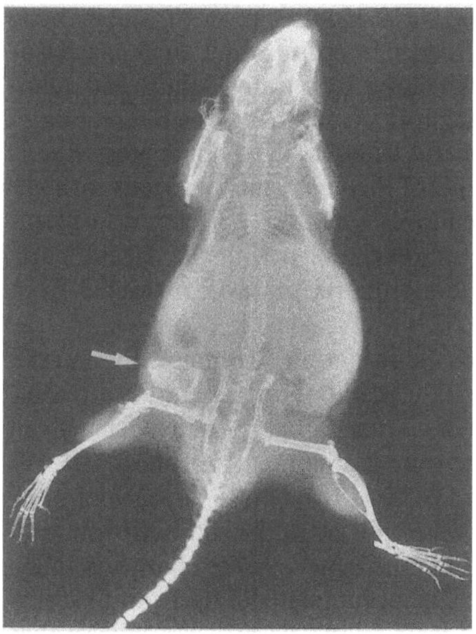

Fig. 1. Roentgenogram of an ossicle (*arrow*) developed in response to bovine BMP as associated bone matrix noncollagenous proteins shown in Figs. 2, 3, 4

Bone Transplantation
Eds.: M. Aebi, P. Regazzoni

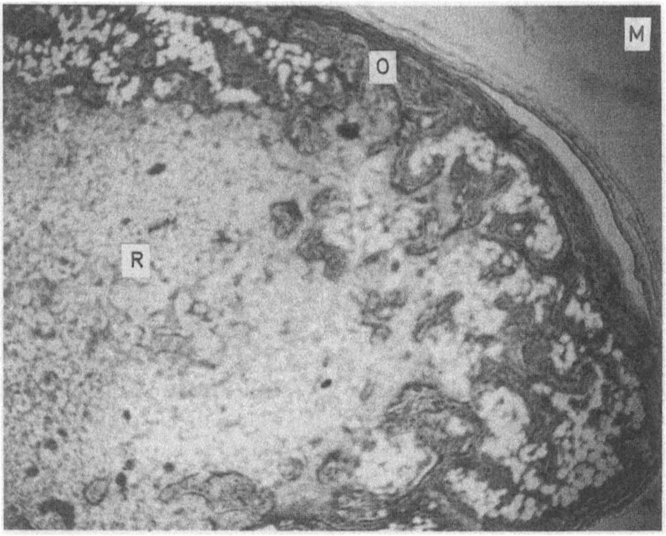

Fig. 2. Photomicrograph of a section of an ossicle (*O*) developed in the mouse quadriceps muscle (*M*), 4 weeks after implantation of 5 mg BMP and associated bone matrix noncollagenous proteins. *R*, marrow cavity

The history of inductive factors before and after the uncovering of BMP, dating back to the 1950s, has been reviewed in detail [1]. The reader is referred to the original literature by others and by our group for a more detailed survey than can be presented in this book. In the recent literature, BMP is presented with three objectives. The first objective is purification and physiochemical characterization, including gene cloning. The second objective is identification of biosynthetic products of cells developing under the influence of either whole bone matrix or BMP; this objective includes experiments which systematically identify and quantitate nutritional, hormonal, and metabolic products synthesizd by interaction of cells of subcutis with powders of allogeneic rat demineralized bone; biosynthetic products are used for assays of the response of mesenchymal-type cells to BMP in implants in a muscle pouch or in tissue cultures. The third objective is augmentation of bone regeneration in repair of craniofacial or peripheral skeletal parts implanted with xenogeneic or allogeneic bone matrix or BMP extracted from bone matrix.

Until BMP is completely characterized, the reader may assume only that the bone morphogenetic proteins are the same if the methods of preparation are comparable, and bioassay results are identical in vivo and in vitro even when a given name is different. If BMP is present in the sample, the bone morphogenetic response is all or none. In the interval from 1965 to 1970, before histochemical or biochemical evidence of an isolated BMP was reported, induced bone formation was hypothetically viewed as a reaction to change in net surface charge on internal and external surfaces of bone matrix. The accumulated data from observations since the 1970s on whole matrix and isolated matrix proteins suggest that the physicochemical property associated with induced bone cell differentiation is a function of the BMP.

Before BMP was isolated, induced bone cell differentiation was attributed to a bone induction principle in the intact bone matrix. The term "matrix-induced bone formation" was proposed to indicate that bone collagen and the whole structure might be essential. Currently, the preferred term is "BMP-induced bone formation" because synthetic delivery systems have been observed to substitute as a carrier for bone matrix. Early in the 1970s, a lipid- and carbohydrate-depleted bone matrix was prepared and interpreted to suggest that the bone induction principle could be a morphogen, a discrete entity with morphogenetic activity. Soluble, locally diffusible BMP was demonstrated with the aid of diffusion chambers to support the concept of a BMP that regulates the same sequence of developmental events as observed in an implant of whole matrix, culminating in the formation of an entire new ossicle. Cortical bone extracellular matrix, with or without apatite mineral, was the storage or servo mechanism system for BMP.

A group of noncollagenous proteins isolated from cortical bone, dentin, and osteosarcoma tissues with high levels of BMP activity was partially purified and characterized as an acidic protein with a relative migration rate (M_r) or 17.5–19 k, pI of 4.9–5.1, and a blocked N-terminal amino acid. Purification of all traces of nonmorphogenetic noncollagenous proteins has been difficult owing to the high affinity of BMP for other proteins that form highly insoluble aggregates. Several other bone matrix proteins, thousands of times more abundant than BMP, require the use of chaotropic denaturants to dissociate one from another. The problem is recounted in detail in a recent article on methodology [2]. A sensitive serum or culture medium BMP radioimmunoassay (RIA) [3, 4] is available to substitute for bioassay when there is no longer a requirement for verifying induced cartilage cell differentiation in vitro and induced bone formation in vivo in the mouse. Isolated by electroelution from polyacrylamide gels, almost free of other bone matrix proteins, and identified by BMP RIA, the molecule has low or no morphogenetic activity. To restore activity lost by denaturation from electroelution, BMP may be renatured in acetone.

Chemical Isolation of BMP

The starting material for isolation of BMP from bone is bone matrix gelatinized at room temperature. BMP can be isolated from whole HCl demineralized bone matrix, but the process is greatly facilitated by converting whole demineralized bone matrix into gelatinized bone matrix by separating the hydrophilic proteins lacking BMP activity from the hydrophobic proteins containing BMP activity. The hydrophilic noncollagenous proteins are soluble in aqueous media. Gelatinized bone matrix is prepared from whole demineralized bone matrix by sequential extraction of non-BMP, noncollagenous components with: (a) chloroform methanol to extract lipids, lipoproteins, proteolipid, and various transplantation antigens including dendogenous proteolytic enzymes with BMPase activity; (b) HCl to demineralize the matrix and extract acid soluble proteins; (c) calcium chloride to extract low molecular weight proteoglycans; (d) EDTA to extract sialoproteins, osteonectin, and GLA-proteins; (e) lithium chloride to shrink collagen fibrils and transform bone collagen into gelatin and extract high molecular weight

Table 1. Estimated percentages (w/w) of the major proteins in relation to BMP, in a partial list of bone matrix noncollagenous proteins

	(%)
1. Residual proteins	
a) Collagen	88
b) Structural glycoprotein	1
2. Bone tissue specific proteins	
a) γ-Carboxyglutamic acid rich protein	2
b) Osteonectin	2
c) Bone morphogenetic protein (BMP)	0.001
d) Bone derived growth factor	0.1
3. Extracellular matrix protein under investigation with respect to the calcification mechanism	
a) Proteoglycans	0.8
b) Proteolipid	0.3
c) Bone sialoprotein	0.9
d) Phosphoprotein	0.2
e) Phosphopeptides	0.1
f) Acid soluble peptides	0.6
4. Lipids	0.9
5. Plasma proteins accumulating in extracellular matrix	
a) Albumin	0.3
b) α_1 Acid glycoprotein	0.4
c) α_2 HS-glycoprotein	0.4
6. Immunoglobulins, unassociated and associated with bone tissue specific protein	
a) IgE, including anti-BMP	1.0
b) IgD	Trace
7. Unaccounted for	0.999

proteoglycans; and (f) warm water to extract denatured fractions of the bone matrix gelatin. All the extractant solutions were employed at 2 °C, except the first and last. The sequential extraction of soluble noncollagenous proteins lacking BMP activity reduces the fat-free dry weight of demineralized bone matrix approximately 20% and at the same time significant increases specific activity of the residual matrix with respect to the bone morphogenetic properties. Under neutral or acidic conditions, the various solvents for noncollagenous proteins described above do not reduce bone morphogenetic activity, but under alkaline conditions, even at 2 °C, as for example in 1.0 *N* sodium hydroxide, all of the BMP activity in the matrix is lost presumably by alkaline hydrolysis; in 0.02 *N* sodium hydroxide, about 20% is lost; in 0.05 *N* sodium hydroxide, more than 80% is lost. The loss from exposure to alkaline conditions is approximately the same from bone matrix gelatin as from whole bone demineralized bone matrix. Another mechanism of loss of BMP activity is from degradation by endogenous proteases following incubation in phosphate buffers at pH 7.4 at 37 °C for 48 h. Before sequential extraction of the matrix, incubation in phosphate buffer degrades all of the BMP activity. After sequential extraction, more than 90% of the activity survives incu-

Table 2. Characteristics distinguishing BMP from many other bone matrix proteins

Acidic protein, pI 5.0 ± 0.2
M_r 18.5 K (bBMP)
M_r 17.0 ± 0.5 K (hBMP)
No carbohydrate detected
Soluble in aqueous media under dissociative conditions in 6 *M* urea or 4 *M* GuHCl
Expelled from solution by formation of complexes with other hydrophobic molecules
Insoluble in acetone, absolute alcohol, chloroform methanol
Insoluble in Triton X-100
Forms insoluble complexes with matrix gla protein (M_r 14 K)
Disulfide bonded
Inactivated by:
Heat >70 °C
Deamination in HNO_3
β-ME reduction
Lathyrism
Pencillamination
Ultrasonification
Binds to OH apatite
Resistant to:
Collagenase
Chondroitinases ABC
Amylase
Neuraminidase
Hyaluronidase
Hyaluronidase
Alkaline phosphatase
Acid phosphatase
Chymopapin
Tyrosinase
Thermolysin

bation (Tables 1, 2). The degradation is attributed to the action of endogenous proteases, BMPases, removed by chemical extraction. Digestion with pepsin gradually reduces while collagenase increases the specific activity of BMP in bone matrix gelatin. The advantage of converting bone collagen to insoluble bone matrix gelatin is to open up the densely packed structure of bone matrix for infusion of solvents for hydrophobic protein and thereby to prepare the matrix for quantitative extraction of the BMP. Although in nature collagen is a part of the matrix as a carrier for BMP, the two are separable.

Another method of removing the BMP from bone matrix gelatin is by dissociation with agents that produce reversible denaturation of BMP, such as 4 *M* guanidinium HCl (GuHCl), 7 *M* urea, 10 *M* KCNS, 2.5 *M* GuCNS. Biochemically, BMP is more directly associated with other bone matrix noncollagenous proteins, i.e., matrix carboxyglutamic acid rich proteins (MGP) than with collagen. When

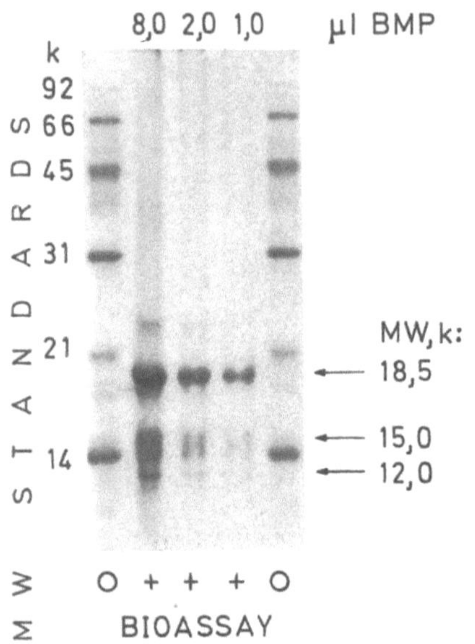

Fig. 3. Sodium dodecylsulfate polyacrylamine gel electrophoresis (SDS-PAGE) pattern of bovine BMP isolated by hydroxyapatite chromatography. Note that when the gel is overloaded with 8.0 µl, the BMP component with M_r of 18.5 K is associated with the components with M_r of 34 K, 24 K, 15 K, 14 K, and 12 K

GuHCl-extracted bone matrix is solubilized and reprecipitated within matrix residues for bioassay in rats, the BMP component has a greater affinity for the residual GuHCl-insoluble noncollagenous proteins than for collagen. In experiments with a composite of soluble BMP obtained from collagenase digests of bone matrix gelatin, the new bone forms on external surfaces of the implant. This surface location reflects the region of the reprecipitated BMP rather than reconstitution of the original matrix. In the original matrix BMP is distributed throughout the interior structure, possibly in part even in intracellular sites. If the matrix had been reconstituted, the products of interaction with host mesenchymal cells would begin with formation of cartilage in the interior and with bone on the vascularized exterior of the implant.

Table 2 is a list of some basic biochemical characteristics of BMP. The N-terminal amino acid is blocked. Knowledge of the amino acid sequence comes from peptide maps of the interior structure and is incomplete. Figure 3 demonstrates an SDS-PAGE pattern of bovine BMP with an M_r of 18.5 k, isolated by hydroxyapatite chromatography. Figure 4 is a diagramatic representation of a supramo-

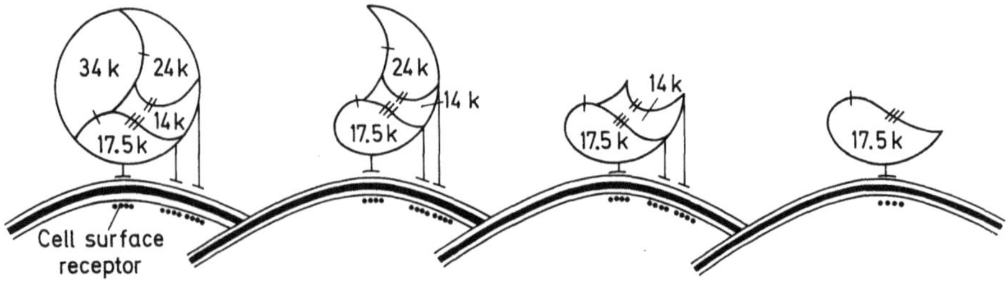

Fig. 4. Diagrammatic representation of successive stages of dissociation of BMP from a hypothetical, supramolecular aggregate of the bone matrix proteins, isolated by methods shown in Fig. 3

Table 3. Hypothetical partition of BMP in cortical bone

Mineral-bound interface BMP	6%
Matrix BMP	
Extracellular osteocytes	88%
Other	6%
Coated pit receptors	
Coated vesicles	
Endosomes	
Chromatin-bound nucleosomes	

lecular aggregate of human BMP with an M_r of 17.5 k and associated bone matrix noncollagenous proteins to show successive stages of a hypothetical transfer from bone matrix to membrane receptors in the surface of a target perivascular connective cell. The possible loci of BMP, determined by bioassay observations on solvents, residues, and broken cell preparations, are shown in Table 3. Attempts to demonstrate BMP-induced heterotopic bone formation in dogs and humans, comparable to heterotopic ossification in human beings, have been unsuccessful owing either to undefined inhibitors or to various factors described below.

Factors Determining or Influencing BMP-Induced Bone Formation: Competence, Determination, and the Bone–Bone Marrow Consortium

The not yet activated state of readiness to respond to BMP is defined as osteogenetic or bone morphogenetic competence. Muscle-derived mesenchymal cells of rodents possess competence because, although muscle injury or transplantation does not initiate bone formation, exposure to BMP does. The proto- or predifferentiated state is called determination. Bone marrow stroma cells are determined with respect to bone morphogenesis because transplantation alone without any exposure to BMP initiates bone formation. The perisinusoidal cells of bone marrow stroma include cells with bone morphogenetic competence as well as cells with osteogenetic determination. The evidence is that bone marrow produces more new bone after than before exposure to BMP in a heterotopic site. Levels of determination and degrees of competence have been more thoroughly investigated in plants than in animals.

The capacity of implants of allogeneic bone matrix to induce bone formation depends upon the concentration gradient of BMP; the degree to which this influences the recipient's level of competence is not known. The most reliable information available about osteogenetic competence of the mesenchymal cell populations comes from implants of bone matrix or BMP in various species of rodents. The rat produces consistently higher levels of induced bone formation than the rabbit in response to implants of bone matrix in a muscle pouch. However, the rabbit's response to an implant of bone matrix in a long bone segmental defect is the same as in the rat. The guinea pig response to bone matrix in either a muscle pouch or a bone defect response to bone matrix in either a muscle pouch or a bone defect is so low that it is possible to detect induced bone formation only when autogeneic bone marrow was added in the form of a composite graft. Without the activity of supplemental bone marrow stroma target cells for BMP, bone matrix in dogs, monkeys, or human beings induces only scanty deposits of bone and then only after a lag phase of several weeks or months. Interaction of bone marrow stroma cells with bone establishes a bone–bone marrow consortium in which one tissue enters into the service of the other in the bone regeneration process.

Quantitative data on matrix-induced bone formation in muscle pouches show yields of new bone in laboratory species in the following descending order: rat, rabbit, mouse, guinea pig. Corresponding data on the yield of new bone from implants of equal doses of purified BMP, with and without specified volumes of autogeneic marrow, have not yet been published. When such data become available, an understanding of the biochemistry of bone morphogenesis organized by a bone–bone marrow consortium may emerge. The homing of blood-borne bone marrow-derived cells to sites of bone formation, precisely wherever woven bone is being or has been remodeled into lamellar bone, may be a function of the BMP content of the bone, and another example of the operation of the bone–bone marrow consortium.

The evidence for a bone–bone marrow consortium is presented in a recent interview of the literature as follows. Scintimetry measurements of blood flow through bone (uptake of ^{18}F by bone mineral, correlated with ^{52}Fe uptake) demonstrate preferential formation of marrow around blood vessels that pass through bone. This is interpreted to suggest that a hematopoietic stem cell differentiation factor would be carried from bone to marrow via a system comparable to the portal system between the pituitary and hypothalamus glands. In oviparous animals, estrogen treatment stimulates bone cell proliferation only on endosteal surfaces adjacent to hematopoietic marrow. Marrow-derived monocyte-macrophages resorb cortical bone that could release BMP and induce new bone formation. During the process of the remodeling of woven bone into lamellar bone, in heterotopic bone outside as well as normal bone inside the skeleton, blood-borne bone marrow-derived stem cells colonize areas of new bone formation. Bone marrow DNA does not recover from irradiation damage of even less than 1 Mrad (1000 mdl), while BMP resists doses greater than 1 Mrad; when rat bone marrow is transplanted into an isogeneic individual whose bone marrow has been destroyed by irradiation therapy for malignancy, hematopoietic stem cells preferentially migrate out of the circulating blood only toward BMP-storing lamellar bone surfaces. Even though unequivocal evidence has not been found for a stem cell in common for bone and bone marrow, the highest concentration of both hematopoietic and osteogenetic stem cells resides in endosteum cells at the interface between bone marrow and bone. No single chemotactin or factor thus far has been isolated from bone and proven to perform the function of organizer of the bone–bone marrow consortium. However transplants of composite grafts of allogeneic bone or bone matrix and bone marrow yields of new bone greater than comparable transplants of marrow alone. Inasmuch as labeling with [^{3}H]thymidine show osteocytes in sites of induced bone formation with no labeled nuclei, the negative evidence may be interpreted to indicate that a preferred target for

BMP released from either bone or bone matrix is not the osteoprogenitor cells but the preprogenitor cells or pericytes of the bone marrow stroma.

Studies with parabiotic animals demonstrated that the release of BMP from bone matrix coincides with the fusion of blood-borne monocytoid cells to form matrix clasts. In some autoimmune disorders of the bone-bone marrow consortium may initiate overproduction, while others cause underutilization of BMP stored in cortical bone matrix.

The bone and bone marrow consortium is exhibited in the bone morphogenetic response to rat bone matrix in muscle exposed to low dose X-ray therapy (900–1800 rad) for the first 48–72 h after implantation. In response to radiation damage, the DNA of host bed perivascular cells recovers and proliferates but does not differentiate into bone. If radiation is administered 4 days after implantation, at the conclusion of the morphogenetic phase of development, the recovery from radiation damage occurs, and cell proliferation culminates in differentiation of cartilage and bone. Thus when irradiation is delayed until after the cytodifferentiation phase of bone, development occurs as if no irradiation had been given. Once osteoprogenitor cells appear, as indicated by higher levels of incorporation of [^{3}H]thymidine into DNA than are displayed by predifferentiated mesenchymal cells, the DNA is relatively resistant, and recovery from irradiation damage includes further development of cartilage and bone. For this reason, if heterotopic ossification is to be prevented, irradiation therapy should be prescribed as early as possible after injury or total hip arthroplasty operations. Early therapy is indicated especially in predisposed individuals, i.e., males with osteoarthritis.

The role of the bone marrow in bone regeneration is demonstrated by treatment of mice with busulfan to produce anemia. The hematopoietic stem cells but not muscle-derived mesenchymal cell receptors of BMP were suppressed when busulfan was administered in sublethal doses. Implants of bone matrix in mice given busulfan induce formation of large, relatively avascular deposits of cartilage. Since the matrix BMP-induced bone morphogenetic process is dependent upon circulatory systemic bone marrow-derived cells for resorption and remodeling, bone development is incomplete in anemic mice. Thus a continuous influx and interaction with bone marrow-derived blood-borne cells are essential for the progress of normal bone development and regeneration. Systemic factors, including BMP, may be released but have not yet been measured during regeneration of new pools of bone marrow.

Bone and bone marrow are so interdependent that for many years de novo bone development in tissue culture or diffusion chambers, isolated from circulating blood-borne, bone marrow-derived cells, was thought not to be possible. Bone marrow organ cultures, including osteogenetic precursor cells with high alkaline phosphatase activity, differentiate into bone-like tissue. This tissue calcifies in media supplemented with Na-beta-glycerophosphate. In a variety of experimental systems, bone is so dependent upon bone marrow stroma cells that development may fail or end in disarray if the precursors of these tissues are separated from one another.

Growth Factors

The discovery of a wide selection of growth factors stored in bone matrix and synthesized by bone cells in tissue culture has raised important questions about whether BMP is a single entity or one of a group of polypeptides regulating both the occurrence or the act in succession and are coefficient in action. A working hypothesis assumes that several growth factors associated with bone contribute synergizing activities by stimulating receptor acquisition and proliferation in cells, which then become responsible to a terminal differentiating agent in an orderly, hierarchical manner. Alternatively, a commitment progression mechanism acts on cells with multiple potentialities and within one cell cycle may induce commitment to new lineages. Synergizing activities may regulate either competence or progression factors in concert with other known hormones, nutrients, metabolites, and respiratory conditions. The question of whether synergistic action of various growth factors found in bone matrix are an essential requirement for BMP-induced bone formation may be investigated by experiments with a single ubiquitous macrophage-derived growth factor (MDGF). MDGF is a protein (40–50 k) partially purified from a conditioned medium of peritoneal macrophages in tissue cultures. MDGF also increases the yield of new bone formed in response to a composite transplant of bone marrow macrophages and gelatinized bone matrix. The macrophages were collected by adherence to plastic and classified as perioxidase-staining bone marrow mononuclear phagocytes with inspecific esterase activities. Bone formation, measured by ^{45}Ca incorporation in newly calcified tissues, suggests that macrophages secrete a mitogen for osteoblast-like cells. The literature has been reviewed [1] to reconsider the frequently discussed problem of extrapolation of in vitro observations to conditions in the intact animal.

Chemotactic Factors

The morphogenetic phase of induced bone formation is characterized by disaggregation and migration of cells. Using the same solvents as used for extraction of BMP, bone matrix yields a 60–70 k protein that has chemotactic activity for mouse calvarial osteoblast-like cells, but not for monocytes. Comparable experiments with muscle-derived predifferentiated cells with osteogenetic competence showed diffusion of BMP toward areas of migrating cells along a concentration gradient. Macrophages and other cells inside and beneath porous membranes remained in areas outside differentiating cartilage and bone cells (unpublished observations). Thus further investigation of the predifferentiated mesenchymal cell population rather than postdifferentiated cells is required to clarify the role of chemotactins in the response to BMP.

Metabolic Activity Index, Aging, Growth Factors and Angiogenesis

A useful parameter of the physiology of some laboratory mammalian species is metabolic activity index (MAI). The MAI of man is 1.0. The dog is remarkably similar, 1.5. In comparison, the rat is 5.15, and the mouse is 15.60. The time of appearance and the quantity of induced bone formation in response to implants of BMP appears to be inversely proportional to the level of MAI.

The quantity of BMP in bone matrix, as reflected in the quantity of induced bone in implants in muscle or subcutis, declines with aging in rats, rabbits, and human beings. The quantity of bone obtained in implants of bone matrix from senile individuals is significantly lower than obtained in young adults. The bones of women show a decline in BMP content after the fifth decade in life. As a matter of policy, many bone banks collect bone only from young and previously healthy individuals, less than 45–50 years of age. Other than age, and transmissible disease, the donor tissues have not been tested for biologic properties conducive to incorporation of a bone graft. The first clue of a biologic factor came from the observation that incorporation was slow when the donor tissue had been irradiation sterilized. These deleterious effects have now been attributed to the decline in BMP activity and correlated with the extraordinarily high levels of irradiation (3.0 Mrad) required for sterilization of bone. Irradiation sterilization has now been eliminated for all allogeneic bone except in some institutions where bone is in short supply and use is limited to filling small bone cysts in children.

As a consequence of exposure to BMP, including the synergizing activities of various growth factors such as FGF, MDGF, TGF-B, angiogenin, etc., angiogenesis becomes a prominent part of the bone morphogenetic process. Angiogenesis and antiangiogenesis factors may be secreted at various levels in successive stages of development. In the morphogenetic phase, in the first 3 days, BMP incites localized swelling and hyperemia. Early in the cytodifferentiation phase, by 4–14 days, cartilage cells differentiate and grow in the avascular interior of the implant. Antiangiogenesis factors are elaborated by cartilage cells. In the same interval, sprouting capillaries grow across the interface between the host bed and the BMP. The most profuse ingrowth of blood vessels begins in areas of formation deposits of woven bone on the surface of an implant of either bone matrix or BMP. By 5–20 days, when blood-borne marrow derived factors enter the system, monocytoid cells and macrophages including capillary sprouts penetrate the cartilage. The highest levels of influence of angiogenin and growth factors with angiogenetic effects begin with the growth of preosseous tissue. At peak levels when bone growth is most rapid, the development of a new ossicle is supplied by a rich network of blood vessels, with tributaries to and from the nearby arteriovenous system.

Applied Surgery of the Bone–Bone Marrow Consortium

The population of osteogenic stem cells of bone marrow is contiguous with endosteum and functionally committed to the bone–bone marrow consortium. Investigations of BMP in cell surface receptors in vitro would be of great interest and could explain why osteogenetic determination (but not competence) may be lost in repeated subcultures of a clonogenic line of osteogenic stem cells.

Missing substance of the entire midshaft of a long bone is reparable by means of a novel method of circumferential cortical osteotomy and extension by Ilizarov. Since the method depends upon slowly stretching the stromal attachment of endosteum to bone on the outer surface and to marrow on the inner surface, the process would appear to activate the bone–bone marrow consortium. A new diaphysis is regenerated when endosteal proliferation begins, and differentiation of bone marrow stroma into woven bone progresses. By stretching a sleeve of endosteum along with a column of marrow, a fraction of millimeter per day from the proximal to distal ends of the bone, the defect becomes filled with new bone. Throughout the process, the bone ends are rigidly stabilized in a circular frame, equipped with fine-caliber Kirschner wires transfixing and rigidly immobilizing the upper and lower fragments inside the frame. The extension process is delayed for 10–14 days until the completion of the morphogenetic phase, progression of the cytodifferentiation phase to callus formation, and sealing of the marrow cavity. The slow process of extension and tension or strain on endosteum would institute cortical bone resorption and facilitate transfer of BMP from bone to bone marrow stroma. Cell populations adjacent to endosteum are rich in determined or predifferentiated osteogenic stem cells. Bone marrow stroma cells also include perivascular cells that are highly receptive to BMP. The hematopoietic stem cells degenerate while the stroma cells proliferate. As the bone ends separate, the marrow cavity becomes filled with a cord of intramedullary woven bone, aligned parallel to the long axis of the diaphysis. The skin, fascia, muscle, and neurovascular structures accommodate to the wires, slowly cutting through the tissues, provided that the extension is applied in a proximodistal direction. Extensive experimental and clinical observations have been reported in the Russian literature for over 10 years [5].

Bioassay Systems

A noncollagenous protein component of bone matrix is designated BMP if it induces chondrogenesis in vitro. In vivo, a preparation is BMP if it induces differentiation of *both* cartilage and woven bone within 10 days, remodeling of woven bone to lamellar bone by 20 days, and formation of a spherical ossicle filled with functional bone marrow by 30 days. Since isolated bovine or human proteins produce exactly the same activities as implants of whole bone matrix gelatin or aggregates of bone matrix noncollagenous proteins or whole tumors, or isolated bone tumor cells, induced bone formation may be viewed as a function of the BMP constituent. This includes BMP preserved in alcohol-fixed undemineralized bone or associated with old deposits of dystrophic calcification. BMP adsorbed onto apatite mineral surfaces may induce bone formation. Apatite mineral is therefore one of several delivery systems in nature.

GuHCl soluble proteins with an M_r of less than 50000 or proteins with M_r of 23000 (16) have been precipitated on residues of bone matrix and implanted as a composite for bioassay in rats. A more direct method is implantation of BMP with M_r of 19000, either isolated or aggregated with other matrix noncollagenous proteins in a quadriceps muscle pouch in mice [2].

Implants of the products of limited proteolysis indicate that a fragment of the internal structure of the BMP molecule, which could be the active domain, may be sufficient to transfer BMP activity. A more complete characterization of BMP and associated growth factors (including preparations of recombinant BMP that are more homogenous than the natural form of BMP in bone matrix) should appear in the literature before the end of the 1980s.

References

1. Urist MR (1988) Bone morphogenetic protein, bone regeneration, heterotopic ossification, and the bone body fluid consortium. In: Peck WA (ed) Bone and Mineral Research, vol 6. Elsevier, New York, (in press) pp
2. Urist MR, Chang JJ, Lietze A, Huo YK, Brownwell AG, DeLange RJ (1987) Methods of preparation and bioassay of bone morphogenetic protein and polypeptide fragments. In: Barnes D, Sirbaska DA (eds) Methods in enzymology, vol 146. Academic, New York, pp 294–312
3. Urist MR, Hudak RT (1984) Radioimmunoassay of bone morphogenetic protein in serum: a tissue-specific parameter of bone metabolism. Proc Soc Exp Biol Med 176:472–475
4. Urist MR, Huo YK, Chang JJ, Hudak RT, Rasmussen JK, Hirota W, Lietze A, Brownwell AG, Finerman GAM, DeLange RJ (1987) Hydroxyapatite affinity, electroelution, and radioimmunoassay for identification of human and bovine morphogenetic proteins and polypeptides. In: Sen A, Thornhill T (eds) Development and diseases of cartilage and bone matrix. Liss, New York, pp 149–176
5. Ilizarov GA (1983) Bianchi-Maiocchi (ed) Experimental, theoretical, and clinical aspects of transosseous osteosynthesis by the method of ilizarov. Medi Surgical Video, Milan

Reconstruction of Large Diaphyseal Defects by Autoclaved Reimplanted Bone: An Experimental Study in the Rabbit

A. Kreicbergs and P. Köhler

Department of Orthopaedic Surgery, Karolinska Hospital, Sweden

Introduction

Limb-preserving surgery by local resection has become increasingly applied in the treatment of malignant bone tumours as an alternative to ablative surgery [5, 12, 13, 16]. However, the mandatory requirement for radicality often leads to extensive resections causing considerable problems of reconstruction. Several means of substituting skeletal defects have been tried both experimentally and clinically [1, 5–7]. At present, the methods most widely used in clinical practice seem to be endoprosthetic replacement and bone transplantation, either autologous or allogeneic [5, 12, 16].

Autologous bone grafting represents beyond doubt the most physiologic procedure for reconstructing skeletal defects [4, 5]. However, when using autologous grafts with a major cortical component in the reconstruction of long diaphyseal defects, late fatigue fractures often occur in spite of osteotomy healing [5]. Although microvascular surgery may improve the results [13], autologous bone almost never offers congruent skeletal substitution, i.e. grafts of exact size, form and osteotomy fit. However, the most important limitation of autologous bone grafting for major skeletal reconstructions is the amount of material available. Allogeneic bone grafting offers a means of obtaining almost unlimited amounts of material for skeletal reconstruction [12]. However, it is a most elaborate and expensive procedure [2]. Moreover, follow-up of patients subjected to allografting has shown a rather high rate of complication, with infection, graft non-union and resorption [16, 22]. These failures should be attributed mainly to low, if any, osteogenic capability [3]. Nevertheless, speculations about the presence of a potentially active osteogenic factor in non-viable bone have since long prevailed [9, 14].

Urist et al. have shown that bone demineralized by HCl, i.e. bone matrix, induces new bone formation, even heterotopically [25]. However, in the reconstruction of large skeletal defects, particularly diaphyseal, the mere substitution by allogeneic bone matrix does not meet the immediate demand for skeletal continuity and mechanical stability. Hence, Urist introduced the principle of AAA bone, which entails reconstruction by a chemosterilized, antigen-extracted, autodigested, allogeneic bone graft [26, 27]. Although AAA bone probably represents the optimum allograft, it still involves a most elaborate complicated and expensive procedure. Occasional reports indicate that reimplantation of tumorous bone after autoclaving may afford a combined means for tumour devitalization and skeletal reconstruction [7, 10, 17, 19, 23]. The procedure, although seldom ap-

Bone Transplantation
Eds.: M. Aebi, P. Regazzoni

plied, seems to offer several advantages by its simplicity [11, 15, 20]. The major objection to the procedure is the anticipated low osteogenic capability of the graft. However, a combined graft procedure, analogous to the AAA bone principle, involving a bone-inductive substance and a non-viable bone graft, may offer a system with high osteogenic capability.

The aim of the present study in the rabbit was to investigate the fate of autoclaved reimplanted bone supplemented with bone matrix. Frozen allogeneic bone was used for comparison.

Material and Methods

The study included 40 adult rabbits (New Zealand White). Bilateral osteo-periosteal defects (20 mm) of ulna were substituted by (a) autoclaved reimplants in ten animals, supplemented with allogeneic bone matrix (ABM) on one side and non-supplemented on the other; (b) autoclaved reimplants versus frozen allografts in ten animals; and (c) autoclaved reimplants versus frozen allografts, both supplemented with allogeneic bone matrix in ten animals. No internal fixation was used. The animals were sacrificed 16 weeks postoperatively. In another ten animals, diaphyseal humeral defects (mid third) were reconstructed by autoclaved reimplants supplemented with allogeneic bone matrix. The reconstructions were stabilized by two intramedullary AO pins, the longer of which was extracted at 6 months. The animals were sacrificed 2 months later. All 40 animals were allowed full weight-bearing postoperatively.

Autoclaving of resected ulnar and humeral specimens was performed in a standard autoclave Citomat (16LS) at 121 °C for 20 min. The allogeneic ulnar grafts were obtained from adult female rabbits (different breeder) immediately after sacrifice and stored in a deep freeze (−70 °C) under sterile conditions. Allogeneic bone matrix was prepared from fresh rabbit cadaveric bone as described by Urist [25]. Briefly, the specimens were demineralized in 0.6 *M* HCl, defatted in chloroform-methanol (1 : 1) and subsequently lyophylized. At grafting the substance was placed both as fragments in the osteotomy gaps and as pieces along the reconstruction.

The fate of the ulnar grafts was followed for 4 months by conventional radiography, scintimetry (^{99}Tc-labelled methylene diphosphate) and bone mineral determination ^{125}I absorption) [21]. Numerical data from scintimetry and bone mineral determination of the ulnar reconstructions were used to assess changes in relation to time by calculating the mean values of each type of implant at 2, 4, 8, 12, and 16 weeks. Post-mortem the ulnar specimens were investigated by high-resolution radiography, autoradiography (^{45}Ca) and histological analysis [18]. The humeral reconstructions were followed for 8 months by conventional radiography and scintigraphy. Post-mortem they were further analysed by high-resolution radiography and torsional test [8]. Strength and stiffness of the reconstructed humeri compared to the contralateral intact humeri were determined by calculating the ratio for each pair and the mean of the ratios. For statistical analysis, the two-tailed Student's *t*-test was used. Values at $p > 0.05$ were considered non-significant.

Results

Out of 30 animals subjected to bilateral ulnar resection 8 were sacrificed because of unilateral fracture of radius and one because of infection. Statistical analysis of numerical data from scintimetry disclosed significantly higher uptake in ABM-supplemented reconstructions. Comparison of non-supplemented reconstructions with autoclaved reimplants and allogeneic transplants disclosed no significant difference, nor was there any significant difference between the two types of reconstructions when ABM-supplemented (Fig. 1). The bone mineral content was significantly higher in the ABM-supplemented reconstructions compared to the non-supplemented at 4 and 8 weeks, but later equalized. No consistent difference could be demonstrated between non-supplemented autoclaved reimplants and allogeneic transplants (Fig. 2).

Serial radiography of non-supplemented reconstructions with autoclaved reimplants and allogeneic transplants disclosed some new bone formation around the osteotomies between 4 and 16 weeks, but almost none along the implants. There were signs of non-union (at least one osteotomy) in 13 out of 21 non-sup-

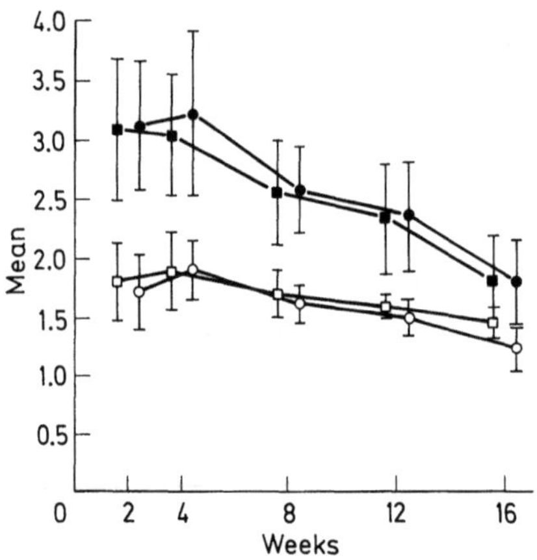

Fig. 1. Uptake of ^{99m}Tc-labelled MDP in relation to time. Mean uptake of autoclaved reimplants (*squares*) and allogeneic transplants (*circles*). *Filled symbols* represent implants supplemented with bone matrix

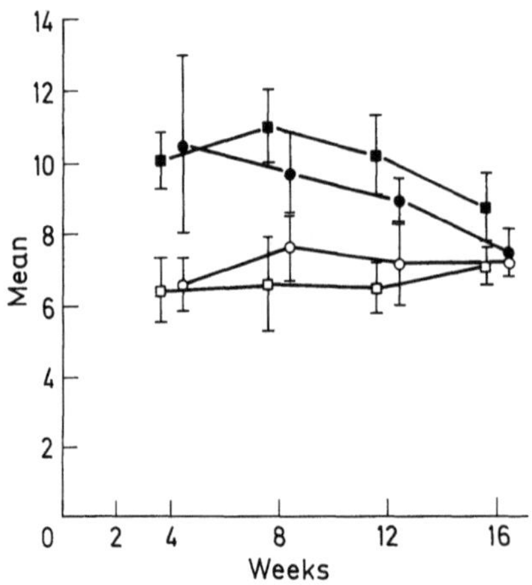

Fig. 2. Bone mineral content in relation to time. Mean content of autoclaved reimplants (*squares*) and allogeneic transplants (*circles*). *Filled symbols* represent implants supplemented with bone matrix

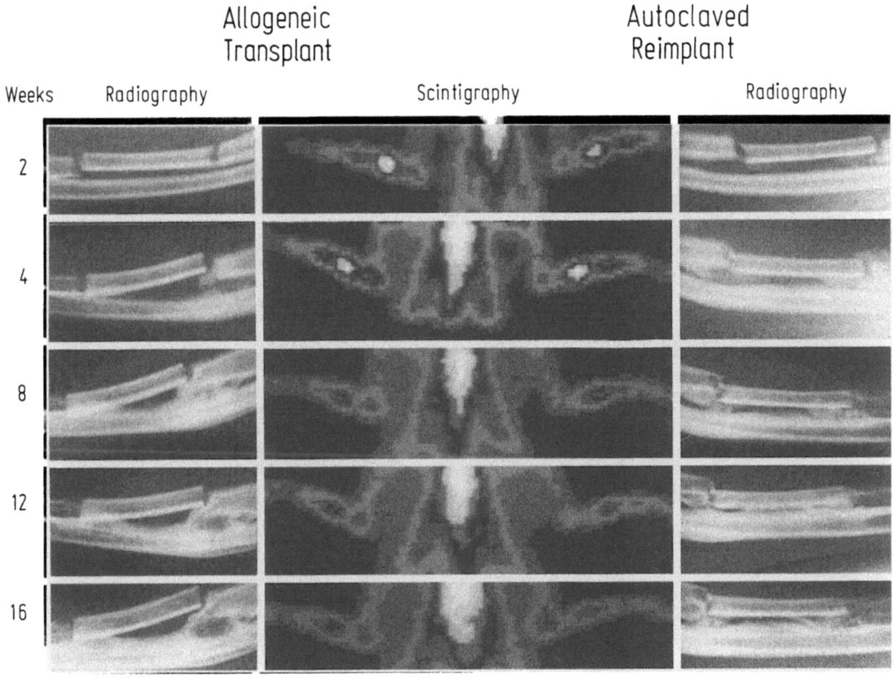

Fig. 3. Serial radiography and scintigraphy of a rabbit with non-supplemented ulnar implants

plemented reconstructions: in 8/14 with autoclaved reimplants and in 5/7 with allogeneic transplants (Fig. 3). When ABM-supplemented, both types of reconstructions exhibited new bone formation already at 2 weeks in the osteotomy areas. From 4 to 8 weeks the implants were gradually covered with abundant new bone, followed by complete consolidation of the reconstructions between 12 and 16 weeks. Not one single non-union was observed in any of the 21 ABM-supplemented reconstructions corresponding to 42 osteotomies (Fig. 4).

High-resolution radiography confirmed that there was non-union in as many as 13 of the 21 non-supplemented reconstructions, but none in the 21 ABM-supplemented. Autoradiography of the non-supplemented reconstructions showed that there was some deposition of ^{45}Ca in the osteotomy areas and a thin layer along the implants, regardless of whether autoclaved autologous or frozen allogeneic (Fig. 5). However, when ABM-supplemented the entire reconstructions, equally exhibited abundant ^{45}Ca deposition (Fig. 6).

Histologic analysis of the non-supplemented ulnar reconstructions disclosed no major differences between those with autoclaved reimplants and allogeneic transplants. Both types of implants appeared non-viable, as no cell nuclei in the lacunae nor any distinct vessel structures could be demonstrated. Along both types of implants there was a thin, irregular, appositional layer of presumably new viable bone in intimate contact with implant bone (Fig. 7). In those osteotomies that radiographically appeared healed there was some cancellous bone showing sprouty ingrowth into the cortical ends, which, however, still were dis-

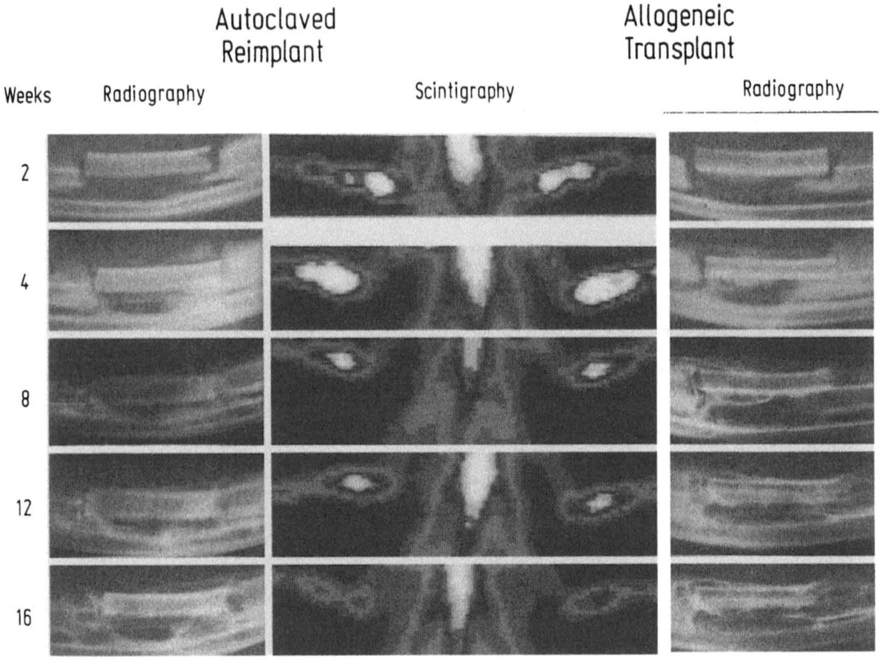

Fig. 4. Serial radiography and scintigraphy of a rabbit with ABM-supplemented ulnar implants

cernible. In those osteotomies that radiographically showed non-union there was abundant, transversely arranged fibrous tissue, without signs of osseous bridging. In the ABM-supplemented ulnar reconstructions there was abundant new cancellous bone along the entire length of the implants, the cortices of which to a large extent were replaced by new bone (Fig. 8). The remainders of the grafts appeared

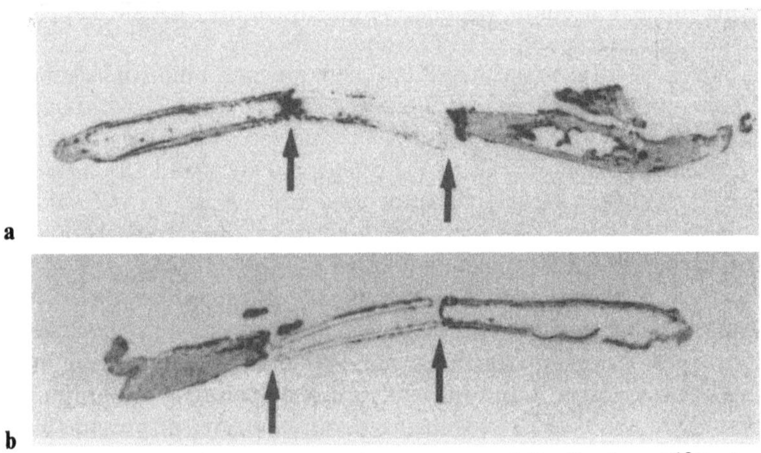

Fig. 5 a, b. Autoradiography showing amount and distribution of ^{45}Ca deposit in non-supplemented reconstructions. **a** Autoclaved reimplant. **b** Allogeneic transplant. Implant area between *arrows*

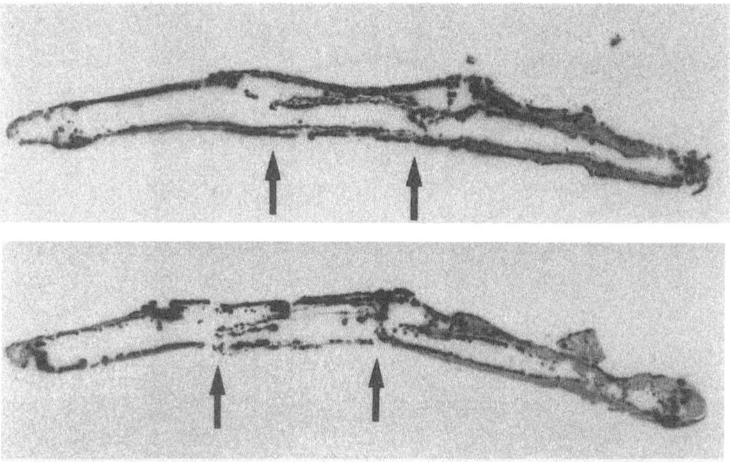

a

b

Fig. 6 a, b. Autoradiography showing amount and distribution of ^{45}Ca deposit in ABM-supplemented reconstructions. **a** Autoclaved reimplant. **b** Allogeneic transplant. Implant area between *arrows*

non-viable. In the osteotomies, all radiographically healed, there was abundant cancellous bone almost completely replacing the cortical ends of the implants.

In the series of ten animals subjected to humeral reconstruction by reimplantation of autoclaved bone supplemented with allogeneic bone matrix, two were sacrificed because of radial nerve injury and infection. One animal developed non-union because of upward pin dislocation. Hence, out of eight animals completing the whole experiment, seven with healed reconstructions were subjected to evaluation. Radiography showed abundant new bone along the entire length

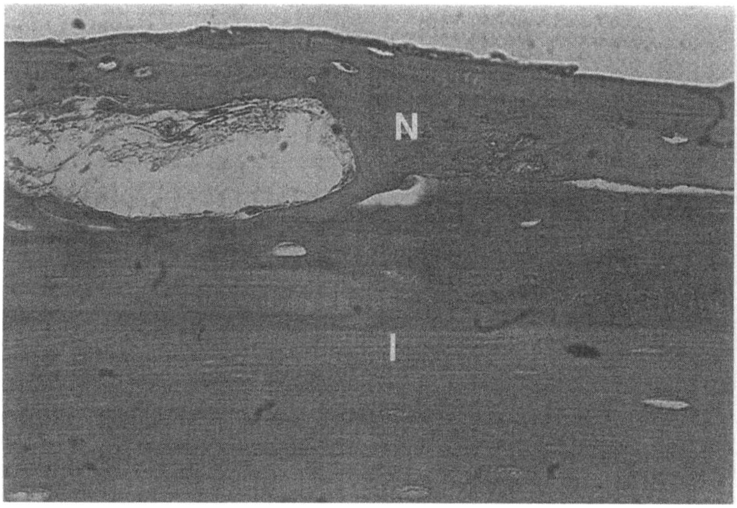

Fig. 7. Non-supplemented autoclaved reimplant (*I*) with thin layer of appositonal new bone (*N*) (× 300)

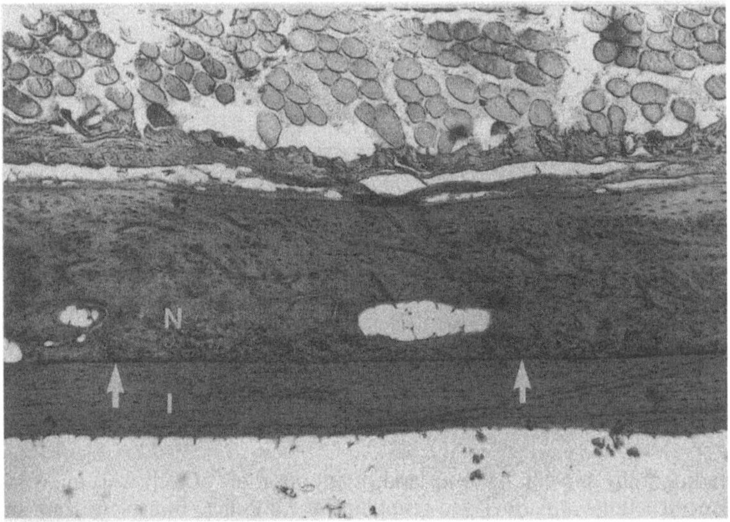

Fig. 8. ABM-supplemented autoclaved reimplant showing thickness of new appositional bone (*N*) in relation to cortex of implant bone (*I*) (×30). Junction denoted by *arrows*

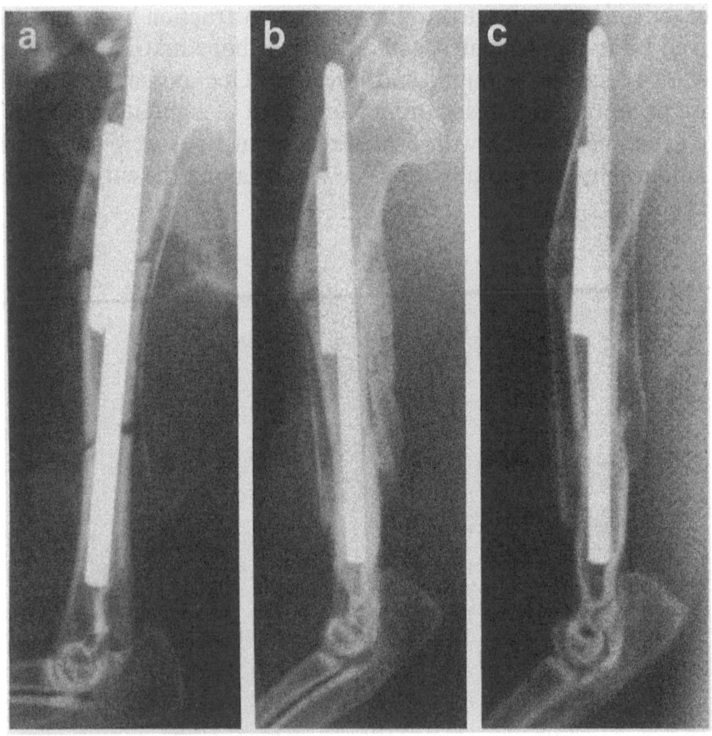

Fig. 9 a–c. Serial radiography showing the incorporation process of reimplanted autoclaved bone in humeral reconstruction supplemented with allogeneic bone matrix immediately, (**a**), 6 weeks (**b**) and 3 months postoperatively (**c**)

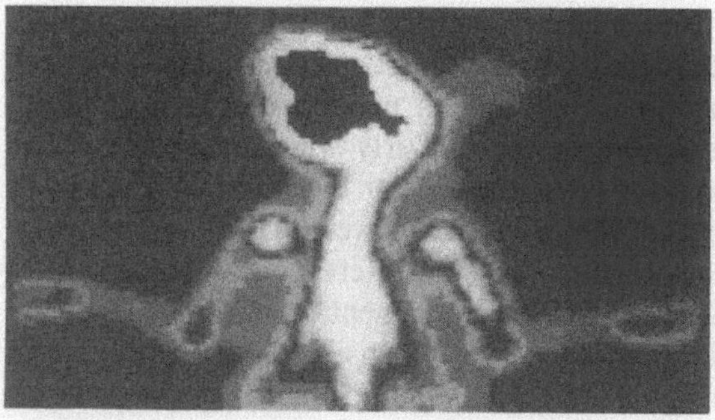

Fig. 10. Scintigraphy showing increased uptake of ^{99m}Tc-labelled MDP 8 months postoperatively in a humerus reconstructed by reimplantation of autoclaved bone supplemented with allogeneic bone matrix

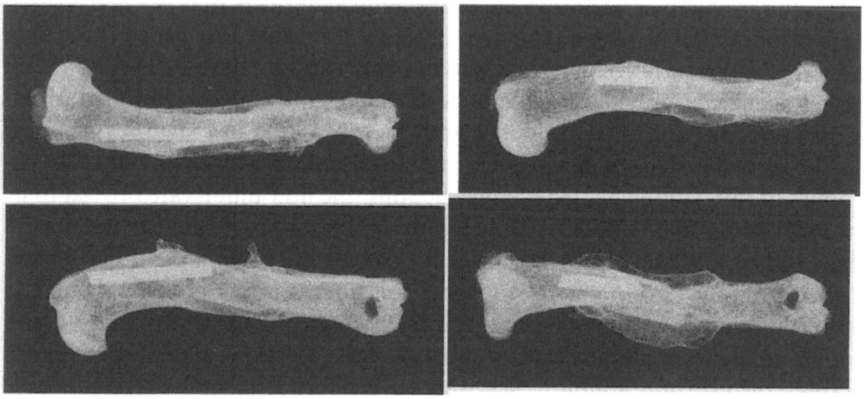

Fig. 11. High-resolution radiography of four different humeral specimens at 8 months postoperatively showing complete incorporation of autoclaved reimplants supplemented with allogeneic bone matrix

of the humeral reconstructions at 6 weeks. Incorporation was observed at 3 months (Fig. 9). Scintigraphy disclosed increased uptake in the reconstructed humeri compared to the contralateral intact at both 6 and 8 months postoperatively (Fig. 10). High-resolution radiography of the collected specimens showed abundant new bone surrounding the whole length of the reconstructions including the osteotomies (Fig. 11).

The mean torsional strength of the reconstructed humeri was found to be 84% (range, 71%–96%; SD, 0.10) of the normal contralateral. Stiffness, on the other hand, was 40% higher (range, 17%–81%; SD, 0.21).

Discussion

Incorporation of bone grafts may be defined by osseous fusion between recipient and implant bone in the osteotomies or by complete osseous integration of the entire implant. Integration provides viable osseous continuity which is probably of decisive importance for the permanence of skeletal reconstructions. In the present study, not only ABM-supplemented reconstructions but also non-supplemented reconstructions exhibited signs of viable osseous continuity, although there was a significant difference in the amount of new bone covering the implants. The importance of this difference, particularly when using non-viable bone grafts, may be assumed to be greater, the greater the skeletal defect to be bridged. Another important aspect of the difference between ABM- and non-supplemented reconstructions applies to the observed difference in replacement of implant bone by new viable bone. Thus, ABM-supplementation seems to increase the amount of new bone, to a large extent at the expense of implant bone. This would seem to suggest that the original defect may in the long run become almost completely replaced by new viable bone.

Presumably, new bone observed around the non-supplemented autoclaved reimplants should be attributed exclusively to recipient bone, i.e. to bone conduction. Since no significant difference in new bone formation was found between autoclaved reimplants and allogeneic transplants, it appears that not even frozen allogeneic bone has any bone inductive capability, or only very little. There may be a subtle difference in osteogenic capability between autoclaved autologous and frozen allogeneic bone which could not be detected by the methods applied. However, this does not appear to influence graft incorporation in a significant way.

Although clear signs of new bone formation were consistently found in the osteotomies of non-supplemented reconstructions, the non-union rate proved to be high. This should be attributed mainly to the fact that the recipient can not always be expected to form sufficient new bone for osteotomy healing. Another important factor for the development of several non-unions in the non-supplemented ulnar reconstructions applies to the surgical technique. In a study by Albrektsson [1] on internally fixed allografts after subperiosteal resection of ulnar segments in the rabbit, the rate of non-unions was only 10%. Thus, it appears that non-viable implants incorporate better if recipient periosteum is preserved, and if the grafts are properly stabilized. However, in bone tumour surgery for reasons of radicality local resection should include the periosteum [12]. In the present study, therefore, it was removed. Nevertheless, all ulnar ABM-supplemented implants, in spite of periosteum removal and deficient fixation, consistently incorporated as opposed to the non-supplemented. The observed difference in incorporation may be assumed to reflect the quantitative significance of new bone formation for graft incorporation. When using large non-viable bone grafts, it appears that osteogenic promotion is more important for incorporation than type of graft chosen.

There are reasons to believe that the combination of two grafts, i.e. a non-viable bone implant and a bone inductive substance, is superior to either of the two alone for reconstructing large skeletal defects. Mere substitution with allogeneic or autologous bone matrix without a bone implant has been reported to be associated with incomplete osseous bridging in 19% and 25%, respectively [24, 28]. However, other experimental studies applying an analogous principle to the one being now presented – a combination of a bone inductive substance and a skeletal substitute – using surface decalcified allogeneic bone have reported similar good results [26, 27].

In the study on reconstruction of humeral defects, mechanical stability during the initial postoperative period depended substantially on internal fixation. The fact that one out of eight reconstructions developed non-union should be attributed mainly to inadequate internal fixation causing pin dislocation. Provided appropriate surgical technique is applied, however, it appears that the described principle for diaphyseal reconstruction represents a safe procedure for obtaining viable osseous continuity and permanent mechanical stability.

Our combined results show that ABM-supplemented autoclaved bone may be used to obtain a physiologic skeletal reconstruction. Resected, autoclaved and reimplanted bone represents a graft that is obviously easily accessible, sterile, cheap, congruent with the resected specimen and, moreover, mechanically supportive. Supplementation with allogeneic bone matrix seems to yield a reconstruction with high osteogenic capability. The procedure, by its simplicity, appears to offer several advantages to other procedures such as endoprosthetic replacement and allografting.

Acknowledgement. Figures published with the permission of *Acta Orthopaedica Scandinavica.*

References

1. Albrektsson B (1971) Repair of diaphyseal defects. Experimental studies on the role of bone grafts in reconstruction of circumferential defects in long bones. Thesis, Gothenburg
2. American Association of Tissue Banks (1980) Guidelines for the banking of musculoskeletal tissues. Am Assoc Tissue Banks Newslett 4:30
3. Burwell GR (1969) The fate of bone grafts. In: Apley AG (ed) Recent advances in orthopaedics. Churchill, London
4. Carnesale PL, Spankus JD (1959) A clinical comparative study of autogenous and homogenous bone grafts. J Bone Joint Surg [Am] 41:887
5. Enneking WF, Eady JL, Burchardt H (1980) Autogenous cortical bone grafts in the reconstruction of segmental skeletal defects. J Bone Joint Surg [Am] 60:1039
6. Friedlaender GE, Strong DM, Sell KW (1976) Studies of the antigenicity of bone freeze-dried and deep frozen allografts in rabbits. J Bone Joint Surg [Am] 58:854
7. Johnston JO, Harries TJ, Alexander CE, Alexander AH (1983) Limb salvage procedure for neoplasms about the knee by spherocentric total knee arthroplasty and autogenous autoclaved bone grafting. Clin Orthop 181:137
8. Jonsson U, Strömberg L (1985) Torsional tests of long bones with computerized equippement. J Biomed Eng 7:251
9. Key AJ (1934) The effect of a local calcium depot on osteogenesis and healing of fractures. J Bone Joint Surg 132:176
10. Kirkup JR (1965) Traumatic femoral bone loss. J Bone Joint Surg [Br] 47:106
11. Ku JL, Smith PA, Goldstein SA, Matthews LS (1985) An experimental investigation of the fate of autogenous autoclaved bone grafts. 31st Annual ORS Las Vegas, Nevada, January 1985
12. Mankin HJ, Doppelt SH, Sullivan RT, Tomford WW (1982) Osteoarticular and intercalary allograft transplantation in the management of malignant tumors of bone. Cancer 50:613
13. Moore RJ, Weiland AJ, Daniel RK (1983) Use of free vascularized bone grafts in the treatment of bone tumors. Clin Orthop 175:37
14. Orell S (1934) Studien über Knochenimplantation und Knochenneubildung, Implantation von „os purum“ sowie Transplantation von „os novum“. Acta Chir Scand 74 [Suppl]:31
15. Orell S (1937) Surgical bone grafting with os purum, os novum and boiled bone. J Bone Joint Surg 19:873

16. Ottolenghi CE (1972) Massive osteo and osteo-articular bone grafts. Clin Orthop 87:156
17. Rivard CH (1984) The effect of autoclaving on normal and sarcomatous bone cells and on graft incorporation. Current concepts of diagnosis and treatment of bone and soft tissue tumours. Springer, Berlin Heidelberg New York
18. Rohlin M, Larsson Å, Hammarström L (1977) Distribution of Tc-99m labelled phosphorous compounds, Ca-45 and 85-Sr in diphosphonate-treated rats. Acta Radiol Phys Biol 16:513
19. Sijbrandij S (1978) Resection and reconstruction for bone tumours. Acta Orthop Scand 49:249
20. Smith WS, Simon MA (1975) Segmental resection for chondrosarcoma. J Bone Joint Surg [Am] 57:1097
21. Sorenson JA, Cameron JR (1967) A reliabel in vivo measurement of bone-mineral content. J Bone Joint Surg [Am] 49:481
22. Stabler CL, Eismont FJ, Brown MD, Green BA, Malinin TI (1985) Failure of posterior cervical fusion using cadaveric bone graft in children. J Bone Joint Surg [Am] 67:370
23. Thompson VP, Stagall CT (1956) Chondrosarcoma of the proximal portion of the femur treated by resection and bone replacement. J Bone Joint Surg [Am] 38:357
24. Tuli SM, Singh AD (1978) The osteoinductive property of decalcified bone matrix. J Bone Joint Surg [Br] 60:116
25. Urist MR, Silverman BF, Buring K, Dubuc FL, Rosenberg JM (1967) The bone induction principle. Clin Orthop 53:243
26. Urist MR, Mikuliski A, Boyd SD (1975) A chemosterilized antigen-extracted autodigested alloimplant for bone banks. Arch Surg 110:416
27. Urist MR, Dawson E (1981) Intertransverse process fusion with the aid of chemosterilized autolyzed antigen-extracted allogeneic (AAA) bone. Clin Orthop 154:97
28. Wittbjer J (1983) Bone matrix and bone formation. An experimental study of demineralized bone reimplanted in bone defects. Thesis, Malmö

Histological Response to Natural Bone Mineral and Synthetic Hydroxyapatite

H. Bereiter[1], A. H. Huggler[1], K. Kita[2], and M. Spector[2]

[1] Rätisches Kantons- und Regionalspital, Orthopaedic Dept. 7000 Chur, Switzerland
[2] Emory University School of Medicine, Atlanta, Georgia, USA

Many recent investigations have focused on synthetic calcium phosphate ceramics as replacements for allogeneic bone for grafting procedures. However, nonresorbable synthetic hydroxyapatite (HA) may be problematic in many applications because its high stiffness significantly alters the stress distribution in the surrounding bone, which can resorb as it undergoes remodeling. Synthetic calcium phosphates which degrade in vivo (e.g., tricalcium phosphate) do so in a nonphysiologic manner, often interfering with the osseous response required for initial incorporation of the implant.

Many investigations performed over the past decades have shown anorganic xenogeneic bone (particularly bovine bone) to be an adequate substitute for allograft. Poor clinical results with this material can be attributed to incomplete deorganification of the substance and to inappropriate use in highly stressed applications. The objective of this study was to compare the osseous response to a new anorganic bovine bone substance with the response to a synthetic HA material.

Anorganic bovine bone particles (Bio-OSS, Geistlich-Pharma, Wolhusen, Switzerland), 0.5–1.0 mm in diameter, were implanted into a drill hole (4.5 mm in diameter and 8 mm deep) in the medial aspect of the condyles of 30 rabbits. Synthetic HA (Calcitite Calcitek, San Diego, California, USA) particles of the same size range were implanted in the contralateral medial condyle. The animals were sacrificed after 10, 20, and 40 days. Histomorphometry was performed on undecalcified ground sections to evaluate the percentage of bone within the defect site and the percentage of the surface of the particles covered by bone. While the range of particle sizes of the xenograft and synthetic HA particles were similar, the particle shape was not. The more rounded HA particle more densely packed together to provide less interstitial space (46% porosity) for new bone formation than the Bio-OSS (54%).

Within 10 days of implantation, new bone was forming directly on the surface of the Bio-OSS and HA, incorporating the particles into the host bone. New bone rapidly filled the void space within the Bio-OSS and HA particles (as expected in this fresh osseous defect) (Table 1). There was no difference in the percentage of the defects filled with bone between the two types of materials. Comparable percentages of the surface of each type of particle were covered by bone at each time period. No inflammatory response was found at the site of the synthetic or natural graft material. While osteoclasts were rarely found on the surface of the HA, they could be seen on the surface of the Bio-OSS particles with approximately the same rate of occurrence as seen on the surface of the adjacent bone trabeculae. This finding suggests that the natural bone mineral comprising the anorganic

Bone Transplantation
Eds.: M. Aebi, P. Regazzoni

Table 1. Formation of new bone with Bio-OSS and synthetic hydroxyapatite

	% SB	% VB
10 Days		
B-O	7.5 (5.3)	8.9 (6.4)
SHA	9.9 (6.9)	6.6 (4.0)
20 Days		
B-O	40 (14)	29 (12)
SHA	41 (19)	25 (11)
40 Days		
B-O	62 (14)	40 (9)
SHA	50 (11)	43 (13)

Figures are means (SD). SB, Percentage of particle covered by bone; VB, percentage of void space occupied by bone; B-O, Bio-OSS; SHA, synthetic hydroxyapatite.

xenograft undergoes physiologic remodeling while the synthetic HA remains essentially nonresorbable.

The indications for the clinical application of Bio-OSS in 12 patients were related to bone deficiencies: 5 fractures (internal fixation), 4 arthrodesis, 2 hip revision (THR), and 1 osteotomy. There were no complications and no signs of inflammation or local reactions. Radiographs generally showed incorporation of the natural bone mineral implants. Histology of biopsies was performed in three cases. Histology showed the new bone formation in the spaces between the natural bone mineral particles, but in the central part of the graft fibrous tissue was found around the natural bone mineral particles.

These results using natural bone mineral in human subjects are probably comparable to what one would expect with a synthetic HA substance, except that the Bio-OSS eventually resorbs. Additional studies are necessary to continue to show the differences in the performance of HA of natural and synthetic origin.

Bone Regeneration with Collagen-Apatite and Mineral Bone

B.-D. Katthagen and H. Mittelmeier

Orthopaedic University Hospital, Homburg, FRG

Hydroxyapatite (HA) has been proven by numerous authors to be excellently biocompatible and bioactive. Bone ingrowth into porous HA, however, depends on pore size. As we could show by own experiments, low-porosity HA exhibits perfect bone ongrowth but only marginal ingrowth. An implant with small pores acts as a barrier and hinders rather than promotes bone healing of the defect.

Utilizing the excellent bioactivity but avoiding the barrier effect of abundant material, Mittelmeier [2] developed the concept of multicentric bone regeneration around finely dispersed ceramic HA particles in a collagen web that is mouldable and styptic. This bone substitute is referred to as Collapat. A second bone substitute that we discuss is Pyrost: This is a completely deproteinized, pyrolized and sintered high-porosity mineral bone. This material consists mainly of HA. It is resistant to compression and maintains its consistency in vivo.

The effect of Collapat and Pyrost on bone regeneration was evaluated in comparison both to control defects and to other bone substitutes. The test series consisted of 96 rabbits, involving 192 tests and using a 6-mm drill hole in the distal femoral condyle. We evaluated the animals starting at week 1 in 2-week intervals for 12 weeks and then in a final assessment at 8 months. The histological and histomorphometric evaluation was performed using undecalcified sections.

The control defects showed a very limited marginal bone regeneration. Excellent bone healing of the defect was achieved rapidly and regularly using Collapat as an implant. Quantitative evaluation showed on average five times more bone regeneration with Collapat than in the control defects. This proved highly significant ($p < 0.001$) by the Wilcoxon test. No immunological or foreign body adverse reactions were observed. We can therefore conclude that Collapat promotes stimulation of the ingrowing healing tissue for intensive bone repair in orthotopic recipient beds. In addition, there is no connective tissue interface between HA particles and regenerated bone. The high-porosity mineral bone Pyrost exhibits rapid and intensive bone regeneration as well. Using an ectopic recipient bed of muscle Mittelmeier found no bone regeneration with Pyrost, but when we used Pyrost inocculated with autogenous bone marrow, bone formation occurred regularly in ectopic sites, too.

It has been shown by the experiments described in this paper that the multicentric bone regeneration obtained with Collapat and Pyrost is effective. In the meantime these results have also been confirmed in dogs.

We have used both Pyrost and Collapat in clinical trial at our University in over 700 patients. In appropriate indications they are very helpful and effective bone substitutes. In general, Collapat and Pyrost can be used in bone beds and

Bone Transplantation
Eds.: M. Aebi, P. Regazzoni

at bone surfaces with good vascularity and favourable bone replacement capability. Such a situation is found after removal of benign bone tumours and autogenous bone transplants, fractures and pseudarthroses, elongation osteotomies and spondylodeses in the case of scoliosis. These bone substitutes can be used as an augmentation of autografts as well. Implanted in soft tissues without bone contact, Collapat and Pyrost do not favour bone regeneration and can be used only in combination with autografts (bone transplants or bone marrow).

In conclusion, therefore, we can note the following:

1. Collapat and Pyrost promote bone regeneration in the orthotopic recipient bed to a statistically significant extent.
2. The mode of action is probably osteostimulation by osteoconduction.
3. Clinically, we feel these bone substitutes are very useful for bone repair.
4. However, in ectopic, poor recipient beds additional transplantation of determined osteoprogenitor cells (DOPC) is required, either by autogenous cancellous bone or bone marrow.

References

1. Katthagen B-D (1987) Bone regeneration with bone substitutes. Springer, Berlin Heidelberg New York

Demineralized Bone Matrix Induced Protein Synthesis and Bone Formation in Canine Muscle*

T. J. Albert, I. A. Guterman, C. L. Morton, J. Lank, and R. E. McLaughlin

University of Virginia Medical Center, Charlottesville, Virginia, USA

The present study was undertaken to determine the long-term consequences of transplanting demineralized bone matrix (DBM) into canine muscle pouches. Histological and biochemical analysis of specimens was carried out at various intervals between 18 and 135 days after implantation to show osteoinduction in a canine model and to determine proteins that could be used as molecular markers in relation to the observed histological changes.

Fifteen specimens were implanted into four immature (3-months-old) mongrel dogs. DBM was processed according to the methods of Oikarinen using diaphyseal cortical bone. Powder implanted was 75–140 μm in diameter and was injected into paraspinal pouches. Specimens were harvested at 18, 30, 45, 75, 100, and 135 days. A portion of each specimen was stained with hematoxylin and eosin (some specimens requiring decalcification) while the other portion was incubated in culture medium with radioactive proline. The proteins synthesized were then examined by SDS electrophoresis. Further study of protein markers was performed by selective treatment with bacterial collagenase or pepsin before electrophoresis.

Histological study showed fibrous ingrowth and large multinucleated cells increasing through the 45th day, with the 45-day specimens showing increased vascular channels and more intensely staining areas. At 75 days hypertrophic chondrocytes and osteoblasts were evident together with woven bone. The 100-day specimens resembled 75-day specimens, while the 135-day specimens lacked hypertrophic chondroblastic elements. The 18-, 45-, and 135-day specimens demonstrated incorporation of radioactivity into proteins with molecular weights of 32K, 125K, 140K, and 180K. The 125K and 140K species were suggestive of $\alpha1$ and $\alpha2$ chains of collagen. The 18-day and 45-day specimens had a 195K protein. In one of the two 135-day specimens the 32K protein exhibited proportionally more uptake than in other specimens. All specimens examined contained the 32K species, but the 30-day specimens were unique in other respects. These 30-day specimens ($n=3$) contained an 80K protein which, upon electrophoresis, migrated in the same position as chick and dog type X collagen, 120K and 130K proteins (showing less uptake and running lower than in other specimens), and a 195K protein only seen in the 135-day specimens.

Our investigation demonstrates the characteristic changes in the pattern of proteins synthesized during DBM-induced bone growth in canine muscle. With further characterization, specific protein components may serve as markers for the evaluation of successful future acceptance of grafted material. Continued studies comparing intramuscular versus intraosseus implantation as described here may provide a useful assay system for donor materials.

* Supported by National Institute of Handicapped Research.

Bone Transplantation
Eds.: M. Aebi, P. Regazzoni

Injectable Bone Graft in Rabbit Radius Defects: Influence of Demineralized Bone Matrix, Bone Marrow and Cancellous Bone

K. G. Thorngren, P. Aspenberg, and J. Wittbjer

Department of Orthopedics, University Hospital, 22185 Lund, Sweden

Injectable bone transplants would be useful in a variety of conditions requiring local stimulation of bone formation. Apart from bone defects after resection, for example in tumour surgery, conditions requiring extra stimulation to form callus, as in slow-healing fractures, could be percutaneously grafted. Apart from by a direct percutaneous approach, injectable bone grafting could be achieved using a tube, such as a cannulated rush-pin, inserted into the medullary canal of a long bone from a safe distance. An injectable bone transplant should then consist of agents previously known to stimulate the bone formation. Demineralized bone matrix has been shown to contain such factors. To allow a percutaneous application it must be particulated. Bone marrow cells have been shown to increase bone formation in connection with bone matrix both by their own bone-forming capacity and by increasing the supply of undifferentiated target cells for the inductive factors [1]. The present study compares pulverized bone matrix and autologus bone marrow with conventionally implanted whole bone matrix and marrow or cancellous bone.

A segment of the rabbit diaphysis was excised, demineralized and pulverized. These matrix particles were mixed with autologous bone marrow from the femoral canal and injected into the defect from which it had been excised [2]. On the contralateral side the demineralized bone was reimplanted without pulverization but with bone marrow. The bone yield was measured after 2 and 4 weeks by radiographic planimetry and by scintimetry using ^{99}d into standardized transverse segments. The ash-weight and ^{45}Ca content were measured. In another series, cancellous bone from the tuber ischii of the rabbit was transplanted to the radius defect and compared with a mixture of autogenous bone marrow and allogenous or autogenous bone matrix particles.

At 2 weeks the ash-weight was greater on the pulverized than on the non-pulverized matrix side. By 4 weeks, the measurements showed no difference. The other parameters determined showed no significant difference. When comparing the injectable matrix – marrow bone graft with cancellous bone, no side differences were found with ^{45}Ca, whereas the callus ash-weight of the matrix-transplanted side was around 60% of the cancellous bone side (due to the original mineral content of a cancellous bone transplant). Non-transplanted defects had very low ash-weight and ^{45}Ca values.

In summary, an injectable bone transplant consisting of pulverized demineralized bone matrix and bone marrow is quantitatively similar in bone yield both to whole matrix and marrow and to cancellous autogenous bone transplants. An optimized injectable bone graft would probably consist of three parts: firstly, addi-

Bone Transplantation
Eds.: M. Aebi, P. Regazzoni

tion of autogenous bone-forming cells provided from the bone marrow and, secondly, some kind of easily resorbable spacer giving a firmer consistency to the injectable transplant and also giving a framework for osteoconduction. We used bone matrix, as it also has the capability of osteoinduction. If, instead of bone matrix, for example, crushed tricalcium phosphate is used as framework, the third component is even more necessary. This would consist of a bone-stimulating agent such as purified bone morphogenetic protein or some other growth factors, probably in combination, when these have been further characterized and become available.

References

1. Wittbjer J, Palmer B, Rohlin M, Thorngren K-G (1983) Osteogenetic activity in composite grafts of demineralized compact bone and marrow. Clin Orthop 173:229–238
2. Aspenberg P, Wittbjer J, Thorngren K-G (1986) Pulverized bone matrix as an injectable bone graft in rabbit radius defects. Clin Orthop 206:261–269

The Role of Osteoclasts in Demineralized Bone Powder Implants During the Angiogenetic Phase of Ossicle Formation *

M. Bettex-Galland [1] and E. Burger [2]

[1] Department of Paediatric Surgery, University of Berne, Berne, Switzerland
[2] Department of Oral Cell Biology, Free University, Amsterdam, The Netherlands

Demineralized bone powder (DBP), even implanted in ectopic sites, induces the formation of bone [1]. A cytokine referred to as bone morphogenetic protein, contained in bone matrix, triggers the bone formation, which is termed bone induction or osteoneogenesis. The implant is first invaded by undifferentiated or mesemchymal cells and is enclosed in a fibroblastic capsule (days 1–7 after implantation). The mesenchymal cells then differentiate into chondrocytes, which secrete cartilage matrix. Calcification of the matrix occurs (days 8–12). As in the formation of long bone, the cartilage is then invaded by blood vessels, a phase during which bone marrow cells begin to appear as well as osteoblasts in their most active form, which secrete osteoid (days 13–17). By day 20 the cartilage has completely disappeared. The result is the formation by day 30 of a cancellous ossicle encompassing bone marrow, in which, nevertheless, DBP particles are not resorbed.

In this study we used this system as a model of enchondral bone formation, concentrating on the angiogenetic phase. DBP was prepared using the shafts of the femur, radius and humerus of male adult Wistar rats [2]. The main steps of DBP preparation are the following: The bone pieces are dehydrated and defatted in chloroform and methanol (1 : 1); they are then pulverized in a liquid nitrogen impacting mill. The powder is sieved, the fraction between 75 and 425 μm is decalcified in HCl 0.6 N, washed with water and freeze dried. On both sides of young Wistar rats weighing 250 g a quantity of 40 mg DBP was implanted into the rectus abdominis muscles. The implants were retrieved at 5, 10, 13, 15, 17, 20, 30 and 40 days after implantation. They were fixed in buffered formol, embedded without decalcification in methylmethacrylate. Groups of sections were stained after Movat, Goldner-Masson and von Kossa.

The general pattern of ossicle formation as described by many authors was also recognized in our experiments. Furthermore, by careful examination of the implants retrieved between days 13 and 17, i.e. during the invasion of cartilage by the blood vessels, we noticed a constant relation in time and localization between the blood vessels and the chondroclasts (or osteoclasts, as one generally names them). Indeed, no distinction can be made in form or reactions between these two multinucleated cells. As soon as the tiniest capillaries appear, osteoclasts can be observed in their vicinity. These at first contain few nuclei. As the capillaries grow in size, the osteoclasts seem larger and more numerous. At the end of this phase, blood vessels occupy at places almost all the space between the

* This study was supported by the Swiss National Science Foundation, grant number 3.959.-0.85.

Bone Transplantation
Eds.: M. Aebi, P. Regazzoni

DBP pieces, the osteoclasts can be observed forming rows on the sides of the blood vessels, but their protoplasm seems fluffy and their nuclei take less stain, as if they were disintegrating.

We conclude from these observations that the invasion by blood vessels is made possible by the activity of the many osteoclasts which resorb the calcified cartilage. This opinion is in accord with the observations concerning the modelling of an ossicle from calcified cartilagenous bone rudiments [3]. It recalls also the osteoclasts and blood vessel relation in the regeneration osteon after stable fixed osteotomies [4]. The regularity as well as the rapidity of these reactions during osteoneogenesis must be stressed.

References

1. Urist MR (1965) Bone: formation by autoinduction. Science 150:893
2. Bettex-Galland M (1985) Ostéonéogenèse. Etude préliminaire à l'implantation de poudre d'os décalcifiée en chirurgie humaine. Chir Pediatr 26:167–174
3. Van de Wijngaert FP, Schipper CA, Tas MC, Burger EH (1988) Role of mineralizing cartilage in osteoclasts and osteoblasts recruitment. Bone (in press)
4. Schenk R, Willenberger H (1967) Morphological findings in primary fracture healing. Symp Biol Hung 7:75–86

Evaluation of Experimental Osteoinduction in Different Animal Models

F. W. Thielemann [1] and C. Etter [2]

[1] Department of Traumatology and Reconstructive Surgery, Katharinenhospital Stuttgart, FRG
[2] Orthopaedic Department University of Bern, Bern, Switzerland

In the literature there are many contradictory results concerning osteoinductive (OI) implants in different animals. The bone formation induced by bone matrix constituents causes a biological cascade, which is still unclear in many details. Numerous experimental investigations have accumulated information which must be taken into consideration during work in the field of osteoinduction.

Demineralized bone matrix (OCG) or the so-called BMG and a dissociative extract of the matrix (similar to the crude BMP of Urist) were used as OI implants. In a first series of intramuscular implantations, the biological effect was tested in rats, sheep and dogs. Additionally using the OI OCG , the effects of storage, sterilization, addition of antibiotics and fibrin, and systemic dosage of cyclosporine were investigated. To compare the different groups the induced activity of alkaline phosphatase and histological evaluation of bone formation served as parameters. To evaluate the reliability of heterotopic osteoinduction in a more real situation a comparison was made between orthotopic and heterotopic implantation in the same animals using OI OCG. Additionally, in a small group of sheep immunosuppression with cyclosporine was used. In this series also the stability conditions were varied at the implantation site. In rats an instable intramedullary screw fixation and a rigid plate fixation were used. In dogs and sheep stable and instable plate fixations were tested.

We could confirm earlier results in rats using the three different OI implants. In dogs only the demineralized bone matrix showed a positive response. The other OI implants were not effective in osteoinduction either in dogs or in sheep. After immunosuppression we could elicit a positive response using OI OCG in sheep. The biological activity of the OI implants can be conserved by storing in a refrigerator at +4 °C over 4 months (80% of the initial activity). To sterilize the implants gamma-irradiation is the most protective procedure. Only the addition of Refobacin does not alter the activity. Treatment of the recipient with cyclosporine causes a positive response of xenogeneic implants in rats and of allogeneic implants in sheep. The value of stability is not yet clear. In rats in stable and instable situations the OI OCG seems to be superior even to fresh autogenic cancellous bone. In dogs and sheep in stable and instable situations the OI OCG does not work. In sheep only after immunosuppression with cyclosporine could a bone-forming activity of OCG be discovered.

Results obtained by heterotopic and orthotopic implantation in rats are not valuable in the same situation in dogs or sheep – or presumably in man. The biological response to OI implants depends on the immunological relation between donor and recipient; here also the results in a rat–rat system are not comparable

Bone Transplantation
Eds.: M. Aebi, P. Regazzoni

to those obtained with dogs and sheep. Additionally, the chemical preparation of a OI implant alters the immunological response of the recipient. Although stability seems to be of less importance for the biological response to OI implants in an orthotopic location, stability is an absolute necessity for valuable results not disturbed by instability-induced callus formation.

Osteoinductive Activities of Dissociative Bone Matrix Extracts

U. Holz[1], F. W. Thielemann[1], G. Herr[1], and G. Pfleiderer[2]

[1] Department of Traumatology and Reconstructive Surgery, Katharinenhospital, Stuttgart, FRG
[2] Department of Biochemistry, University of Stuttgart, Stuttgart, FRG

There are reports from Urist, Reddi and others about the extraction of osteoinductive fractions from demineralized bone matrix. The results are contradictory in terms of conditions of extracting and of biological testing. Reproducibility of the results varies widely in different test models. Therefore, a systemic investigation was performed to obtain further information about dissociative bone matrix extracts.

Using pig and rat bone matrix a dissociative extraction with solutions of GuaHCl (4 *M*), GuaSCN (4 *M*), $MgCl_2$ (3 *M*), KSCN (4 *M*). $Ca(SCN)_2$ (4 *M*), and tetramethylurea (TMU; 2 *M*) was performed. Enzyme blockers were additionally used to prevent proteolytic degradation of the extracted fractions. Reassociation of the extracted parts of the matrix was effected by dialysis against water. The matrix residues, water-insoluble fractions and water-soluble fractions were tested by intramuscular implantation in Wistar rats using gelatine capsules. A histologically observable bone formation at the implantation site served as a parameter for a osteoinductive fraction. Additionally, in the GuaHCl-extracted fraction the conditions for reassociation were varied.

The matrix residues were active in bone formation after extraction with KSCN and $Ca(SCN)_2$ and inactive in all other procedures. The results were reproducible constantly (eight of eight animals). The extracted complete fractions in the case of GuaHCl and GuaSCN extraction were inconstantly active in induced bone formation. The other fractions did not show any bone formation. After separation of the most frequently active GuaHCl-extracted fraction in a water soluble and a water-insoluble part there was an increase in the frequency of bone formation (50% positive results in GuaHCl). By lowering the protein content of the extract prior to dialysis in the GuaHCl fraction the incidence of positive implants increased to GuaHCl fraction the incidence of positive implants increase to 80%–100% depending on the source of the matrix (pig or rat). To obtain positive results in the pig-derived material, treatment of the rats with cyclosporine was always necessary.

Among dissociative extraction procedures, the extraction with GuaHCl is able to exhibit a osteoinductive activity. To obtain a high rate of positive response one must pay attention to further processing of the extracted fraction (water insolubility, reassociation). Xenogeneic GuaHCl-extracted fractions exhibit a high incidence of osteoinductive activity in rats only after immunosuppression.

Bone Transplantation
Eds.: M. Aebi, P. Regazzoni

Bone Gelatine Revisited

J. M. Rueger, R. Inglis, and A. Pannike

Department of Traumatology, Surgical Center, University Clinics of Frankfurt, Frankfurt, FRG

A protein complex of diaphyseal cortical bone that displays immunological activity and is extracted from bone gelatine is acellular bone matrix (Urist 1973). Bone gelatine proved to be osteoinductive, i.e. stimulating osteoneogenesis, after heterotopic implantation into muscle. It also is osteostimulative, i.e. it enhances bone formation and repair after orthotopic implantation in either bony drill holes or segmental defects (Rueger 1985). These effects of bone gelatine are constantly reproducible only in allogeneic implantation in rats and mice. Bone gelatine's activity is based on direct triggering of determined osteoprogenitor cells as well as on the induction, differentiation and stimulation of local pluripotent cells. Furthermore, there seems to be a chemotactically active fraction in the complex for circulating pluripotent cells (Somerman et al. 1983).

In a series of four different experiments we sought to:

1. Check the osteoinductive potency of bone gelatine compared to other bone replacement materials and their combinations.
2. Determine whether the addition of two different calcium phosphate ceramics to bone gelatine influences the time course of osteoinduction and -stimulation, reviewing the cascade theory of osteoinduction (Reddi 1982).
3. Examine differences in osteoinduction and -stimulation after the implantation of bone gelatine of five different species into one host.
4. Reduce the intensity of the immunologic reaction of a host to a xenogeneic bone gelatine.

All bone gelatine preparations, regardless of species, were produced according to Urist (1973). In the first experiment we implanted five different hydroxyapatite cermics, TCP ceramic, bovine collagen, demineralised bone powder (Glowacki 1981), bone gelatine and various combinations ($n = 16$). In the second experiment, either bone gelatine, bone gelatine with TCP ceramic or bone gelatine with hydroxyapatite ceramic was used. In the third set, sheep, dog, human, rabbit and nude rat bone gelatine was implanted into Sprague-Dawley rats. In the last experiment, human bone gelatine was implanted into T-cell-deficient, B-cell-competent nude rats. Materials were implanted between 1 and 220 days into standardised femoral drill holes and muscle pouches of the abdominal wall. After sacrifice, specimens were evaluated by, among other methods, histomorphometry of undecalcified histological sections.

In experiment 1, except for bone gelatine and its combinations with either a soluble or an insoluble calcium phosphate compound, none of the other materials or combinations was osteoinductive. In experiment 2, orthotopic implantation of the combinations resulted in an increase in bone gelatine's activity (bone yield);

Bone Transplantation
Eds.: M. Aebi, P. Regazzoni

in the heterotopic implants the osteoinductive process was accelerated by the combination of bone gelatine with TCP ceramic. In experiment 3, in only the most familiar species (nude rat) was it able to induce a measurable osteoneogenesis and to show an osteostimulative effect. And in experiment 4, in heterotopic implantation showed a poor and inconsistent activity of bone gelatine; orthotopic implantation showed on histomorphometry an activity similar to that of Spraque-Dawley bone gelatine implanted in Spraque-Dawley rats.

In conclusions, bone gelatine's activity can be increased up to five-fold by the addition of a calcium phosphate ceramic. The addition of TCP accelerates the osteoinductive process. Bone gelatine is reliably active only in allogeneic implantation. And, immunological reactions to bone gelatine in xenogeneic implantation impede on or even prevent the biological activity of the material.

References

1. Glowacki J, Altobelli D, Mulliken JB (1981) Fate of mineralized and demineralized osseous implants in cranial defects. Calcif Tissue Int 33:71–76
2. Reddi AH (1982) Regulation of local differentiation of cartilage and bone by extracellular matrix: a cascade type mechanism. Prog Clin Biol Res 110:Part B, 261–270
3. Rueger JM, Seibert HR, Pannike A (1985) Abheilung segmentaler Knochendefekte nach Auffüllung mit biologischen und synthetischen Knochenersatzmitteln im Tierexperiment. Chir Forum 1985. Langenbecks Arch Chir Suppl:13–17
4. Somerman M, Hewitt AT, Varner HH, Schiffmann E, Termine JD, Reddi AH (1983) Identification of a bone matrix derived chemotactic factor. Calcif Tissue Int 35:481–485
5. Urist MR, Iwata AH, Lecotti PA, Dorfmann RL, Boyd SD, McDowell RM, Chien C (1973) Bone morphogenesis in implants of insoluble bone gelatine. Proc Natl Acad Sci USA 70:3511–3515

Critical Factors in Successful Bone Induction

E. Munting and C. Delloye

Laboratoire d'Orthopédie, Université Catholique de Louvain, 1200 Brussels, Belgium

The aim of this paper is to highlight the factors influencing bone formation induced by demineralized bone. Denaturation of inductive proteins by proteolytic enzyme activity, physical and chemical factors such as excessive heating, freezing, sterilization and demineralizing agents were studied in 600 rats by Ca content, implant and explant weight measurements, and histology.

Regarding conservation, freezing and freeze-drying did not affect bone yield. In terms of sterilization, gluteraldehyde, formaldehyde, ethylene oxide, and 25 kGy irradiation destroyed or significantly decreased bone yield [1]. Demineralization with 0.6 *N* HCl at 4 °C or 25 °C gave a higher osteoinductive capacity than preparation according to the technique described by Urist for obtaining AAA bone [2]. Demineralization in 0.5 *N* disodium EDTA, pH 5, for 7 days at 4 °C significantly increased bone yield and prevented matrix resorption observed with HCl-demineralized implants (Fig. 1).

Inability of active matrix to induce osteogenesis may be the consequence of an inappropriate matrix morphology, the presence of bone induction inhibiting factors, immunological mismatch, or improper physiological or biomechanical environment. Regarding morphology, whereas intact demineralized diaphysis

	Final weight / initial weight		
	<1	1 – 2	>2
HCl 321	14.3 % (46)	65.7 % (211)	20.0 % (64)
EDTA 187	1.0 % (2)	29.4 % (55)	69.6 % (130)

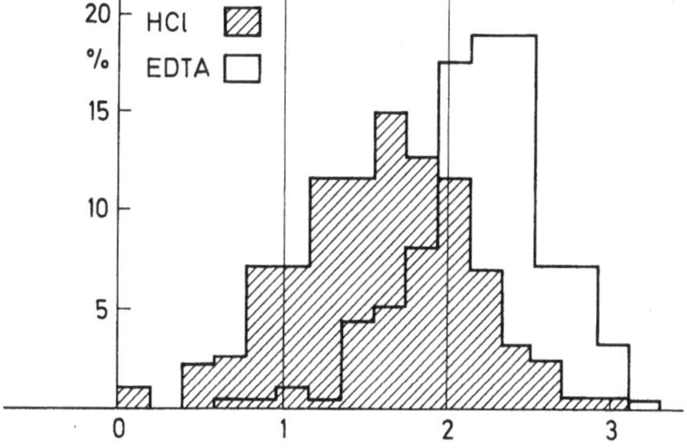

Fig. 1. Distribution in terms of implant-weight ratio

Bone Transplantation
Eds.: M. Aebi, P. Regazzoni

usually induces bone formation in rats and rabbits, ulnar defects in dogs replaced by segmental demineralized allografts almost never heal. When particulated matrix (140–800 microns) is used, induction occurs, and healing is achieved in many cases.

Other factors affecting bone induction can also be identified. Appropriate osteosynthesis is mandatory if the implant is intended to replace a load-bearing bone. Weight of implanted matrix and the resulting induced bone are directly proportional; this may explain poor results obtained with demineralized cancellous bone. Vascular supply from the host bed to the implant is essential. However, in dogs, even when using fragmented HCl-demineralized cortical bone, without exposure to sterilizing agents and used in a well-vascularized and stable environment, bone induction does not always occur. Rat experiments suggest the existence of a matrix component, extracted by EDTA, inhibiting induction. Furthermore, the effect of an immunological factor responsible for failure of bone induction is most likely in some cases.

References

1. Munting E, Wilmart J-F, Wijne A, Hennebert P, Delloye C Influence of sterilization on osteoinductive capacity of demineralized bone in the rat. Acta Orthop Scand (to be published)
2. Delloye C, Hebrant A, Munting E, Piret L, Coutelier L (1985) The osteoinductive capacity of differently HCl-decalcified bone alloimplants. Acta Orthop Scand 56:318–322

Hydroxyapatite Ceramic in a Dynamic Animal Model: Observations with the Polarizing Microscope and Biomechanical Studies

N. M. Meenen [1], J. F. Osborn [2], K. H. Jungbluth [1], and V. Wening [1]

[1] Department of Traumatology, University Hospital, Hamburg-Eppendorf, FRG
[2] Clinic for Maxillo-facial Surgery, University Hospital, Bonn, FRG

Porous hydroxyapatite ceramic (HAC) is used successfully for filling surgical and traumatic bone defects. As only little of this brittle material is replaced by bone for intervals of up to years, the integrational and remodelling processes within the ceramo-osseous regeneration complex and its mechanical properties are of great importance for the final result of the operation, especially when performed close to joint surfaces.

The aim of this study is to reveal the influence of physiological load during locomotion on the bridging of subchondral cancellous bone defects and on the remodelling with the ceramic material. As orientation is the important factor affecting the physical properties of hard tissue; we show the morphological aspect of functional adaptation of the hydroxyapatite bone compound determined by orientation of the optical axis of bone collagen fibres. By means of biomechanical methods the elastic properties of the resulting ceramo-osseous composite system is tested.

In 30 adult rabbits we drilled, with a specially designed stereotactic device, reproducible subchondral bone defects in both medial femur condyles, leaving a 0.5-mm co-planar layer of subchondral bone and cartilage (Fig. 1). The defects were filled with granules of porous HAC (Osprovit, Feldmühle Plochingen, FRG). All rabbits were allowed to move freely in their cage. For polarizing microscopy the animals were killed 2 weeks and 3, 6, and 9 months after the operation. The specimens were imbedded in methyl-methacrylate. At 18 months after the implantation we removed the femurs for testing under impressive force of up

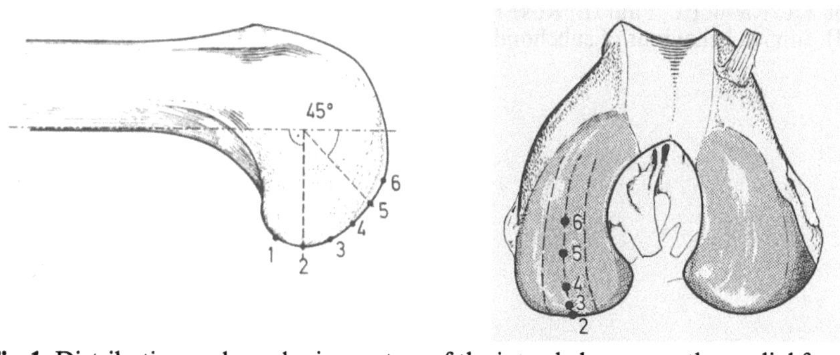

Fig. 1. Distribution and numbering system of the intended areas on the medial femur condyles. Implanted ceramic granules were located under zone 4

Bone Transplantation
Eds.: M. Aebi, P. Regazzoni

to 50 N by a plane-ended indenter of 1 mm diameter in perpendicular contact on the articular surface. We evaluated eight operated femur condyles and five non-operated ones, each on 18 reproducible measuring areas.

Using the polarizing microscope it was demonstrated that the collagen fibres have their origin in the ceramic surface and that the rate of their orientation increases continuously according to the maturation of the newly formed bone from the woven texture to the final lamellar structure. Due to their osteotropism the HAC granules become integrated into the bone, not altering the local bone physiology. No changes could be verified in the fibrillar architecture of surrounding cancellous bone and overlying subchondral bone and cartilage. Indenting the articular surface on the force-testing machine revealed no significant difference of the deformation/stress relationship over the HAC-filled defects. This means equal elastic behaviour of the ceramo-osseous regeneration complex with the overlying structures in comparison to the integrity of the non-operated femur condyles.

Our study confirmed the hypothesis that in our dynamic model adaptation to mechanical needs by the subchondral bone remodelling and scarce degradation process leads to a trabecular arrangement with the substantially integrated osteotropic ceramic material. In this state it performs physiological force-transmitting properties. This proves the good functional compatibility of HAC. When integrated by bone, it fulfils physiological demands even in large bone defects close to the articular structures, not altering their specific ability to distribute and absorb loading stress. Considering the clinical application in future, these results give further evidence to assess the biological performance of this new biomaterial.

Acknowledgement. We thank Professor Donath of University Institute of Pathology, Hamburg, FRG, for the sections.

References

1. Katz JL (1971) Hard tissue as a composite material – I bounds on the elastic behaviour. J Biomech 4:455–473
2. Meenen NM, Jungbluth KH, Donath K (1985) Besonderheiten des subchondralen Knochendefektes. Hefte zur Unfallheilkunde 185:145–153
3. Osborn JF (1985) Implantatwerkstoff Hydroxylapatit. Quintessenzverlag, Berlin
4. Simon SR, Radin EL, Paul IL, Rose RM (1972) The response of joints to impact loading. II. In vivo behaviour of subchondral bone. J Biomech 5:267–272

Experimental Spinal Fusion Using Demineralized Bone Matrix, Bone Marrow and Hydroxyapatite

T. S. Lindholm and P. Ragni

Bone Research Group, Orthopaedic Hospital of the Invalid Foundation, Helsinki, Finland

The numerous drawbacks connected with the use of autogenous bone in reconstructive surgery of the skeleton induced surgeons to look for suitable alternatives. This led to a research trend directed towards still deeper knowledge of regulative mechanisms in osteogenesis. A number of agents thought to be involved in osteogenesis have been reported, but the one best characterized to date is bone morphogenetic protein (BMP) [4]; the source of this can be demineralized bone matrix (DBM), which has been successfully used, for example, in the healing of large experimental bone defects [2]. The traditional autografting technique in spondylodesis may be a disabling procedure. There are very few reports in the literature about the use of DBM in spinal fusion [3]. This is the reason for our performing experiments on rabbits using DBM alone or combined with the osteoprogenitor cells supplier BM [1] and the synthetic bone substitute hydroxyapatite (HA).

The experiments were performed on rabbits weighing 2.5–3.5 kg. Postero-lateral spinal fusions were performed in thoracic spine, lumbar spine and interbody fusions in lumbar spine. For documentation of the results we used stability tests and radiographic and histologic measurements.

In experiment 1, DBM and BM were used. Median stability was achieved after 29 days in lumbar spine, after 49 days in thoracic spine, and after 30 days in thoraco-lumbar spine (Fig. 1 a). Radiologically, fusion was testified after 38 days in lumbar spine, after 49 days in thoracic spine and after 44 days in thoraco-lumbar

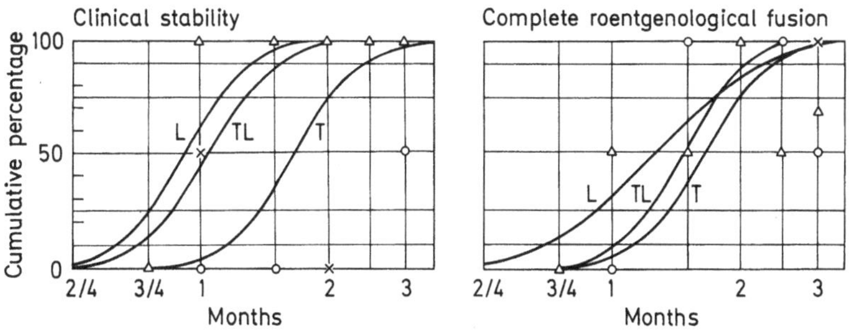

Fig. 1 a. The cumulative percentage of clinical stability in lumbar (*L*), thoraco-lumbar (*TL*) and thoracic (*T*) spine with respect to time. The most rapid, complete stability is shown after 1.5 months in the lumbar spine in a postero-lateral spondylodesis. **b** The cumulative percentage of complete roentgenologic fusion in different locations of the spine. Radiological fusion is noted after about 2.5 months on the average

Bone Transplantation
Eds.: M. Aebi, P. Regazzoni

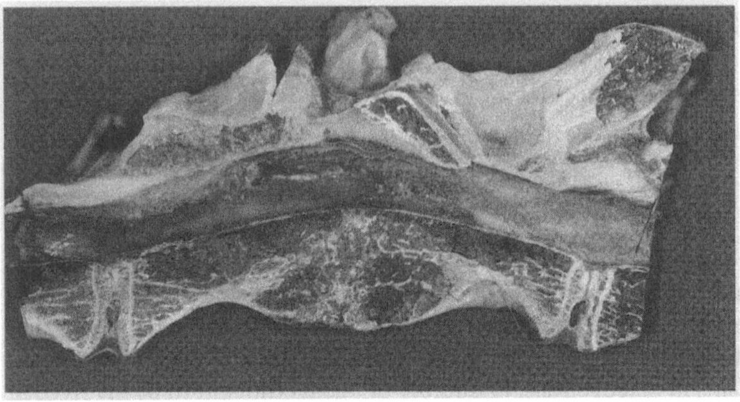

Fig. 2. Photography of an interbody spondylodesis in the lumbar spine (L4/L5) showing complete fusion after 4 months

spine (Fig. 1 b). Histologically, spondylodesis was completely remodelled after 3 months.

Experiment 2, only DBM was used in thoracic spine. In nearly all cases a spinal deformity with rotational components was achieved. The measured diameter of the spinal canal increased during the earlier stage of fusion and showed a tendency towards narrowing at a long-term follow-up.

In experiment 3, HA plus combination of DBM and BM were used. Combinations of pellets of HA and fresh autogenous BM showed the same fusion results in stability tests and X rays as did fusion with autogenous spongeous bone.

In experiment 4, interbody fusion (L4/L5 or L5/L6) was performed using DBM and blocks of HA. The fusion time was calculated to be 4 months (Fig. 2). There were no differences between the two subgroups, HA plus DBM and DBM alone. Ingrowths of new bone in HA blocks were observed after 2 months.

DBM thus confirmed its osteo-inductive potential in an experimental spinal fusion procedure, especially when combined with fresh autogenous BM. The addition of porous HA inhibited the osteo-inductive potential of DBM, whereas good results were achieved using HA and BM. The lumbar segments seemed to be the most suitable site for an experimental spondylodesis.

References

1. Lindholm TS, Urist MR (1980) A quantitative analysis of new bone formation by induction in composite grafts of bone marrow and bone matrix. Clin Orthop 150:288
2. Oikarinen J (1982) Experimental spinal fusion with decalcified bone matrix and deep-frozen allogeneic bone in rabbits. Clin Orthop 162:210
3. Takagi K, Urist MR (1982) The role of bone marrow in bone morphogenetic protein-induced repair of femoral massive diaphyseal defects. Clin Orthop 171:224
4. Urist MR (1965) Bone formation by autoinduction. Science 150:893

Bone Autografting and Allografting in Large Skeletal Resection due to Tumor Resection

R. Capanna, R. Biagini, P. Ruggieri, R. De Cristofaro, C. Martelli, A. Ferraro, P. Picci, and M. Campanacci

Istituto Ortopedico Rizzoli, Bologna, Italy

Between 1971 and 1985, 100 cases of primary bone tumors underwent resection and reconstruction with autogenous (90) or homologous (10) grafts at the Rizzoli Institute. Fifty-three resection arthrodesis with autogenous grafts were performed for tumors of the distal femur (29), proximal tibia (18), distal tibia (5), or proximal humerus (1). There were 37 benign tumors (35 giant cell tumors, 2 chondroblastoma), 7 low-grade tumours (3 parosteal osteosarcoma, 4 central chondrosarcoma) and 9 high-grade tumors (1 hemangiopericitoma, 1 periosteal osteosarcoma, 5 osteosarcoma, 2 MFH).

The surgical margins [5] were wide in 39 cases, wide but contaminated in 7, marginal in 5, intralesional in 2. We had 5 local recurrences: 2 after intralesional resection of a benign and a low-grade tumor; 1 after a marginal resection of a low-grade tumor; 2 after a wide resection of a high-grade malignant tumor. Forty-eight cases had a primary arthrodesis, while five had the grafting procedure after a temporary stabilization with Küntscher rod and cement.

Two different techniques of reconstruction were used for knee resection arthrodesis. From 1971 to 1980 the grafts consisted of anterior hemicylinders of bone taken from the ipsilateral femur and tibia turned upside-down: the osteosynthesis was performed with a Küntscher rod (Putti [16, 17] Juvara [9] Merle d'Aubigné [13] technique: 29 cases; Fig. 1). From 1980 to 1985 the grafts were taken from the ipsilateral fibula, counterlateral tibia and the ileum (corticocancellous grafts), while the osteosynthesis was performed with a Küntscher rod (13) or a condylar plate (5) (1980 techniques [4, 6, 7]: 18 cases; Fig. 2); with the 1980 protocol, if the union was incomplete on the X rays, new cancellous iliac bone was added at the diaphyseal junction of the grafts. A technique similar to the 1980 knee resection arthrodesis was used for cases of shoulder (1) or ankle resection arthrodesis (5). Among 29 patients having a Putti–Merle d'Aubigné technique, 7 developed infection (24%), which required amputation in 1 case, Küntscher rod removal and surgical debridement in 6: 2 patients achieved healing of their infection and union, 3 healing of the infection but pseudoarthrosis, and 1 achieved union with chronic osteomyelitis. Nine patients (31%) had a mechanical failure: 5 fracture of the rod or plate with nonunion, 2 bending of the rod and nonunion, 2 telescopage of bone grafts with union and shortening. Among 9 patients with nonunion, 2 had amputation for concomitant local recurrence, while 7 achieved union after introduction of a new Küntscher rod and repeated bone grafting. Minor complications were nerve palsy (3) and stress fracture of the bone grafts (5); all regressed without surgical treatment.

Bone Transplantation
Eds.: M. Aebi, P. Regazzoni

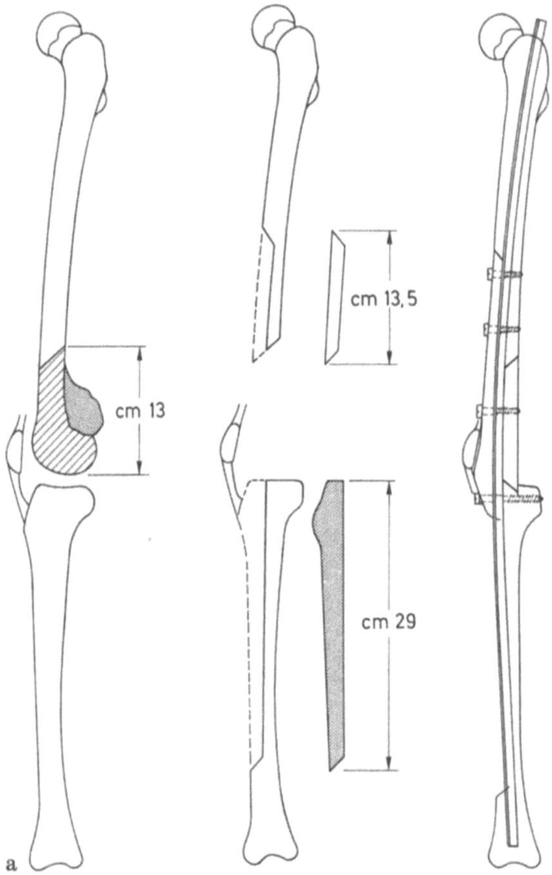

Fig. 1 a and b. Knee resection arthrodesis according to Putti–Juvara–Merle d'Aubigné technique for the distal femur **a** or proximal tibia **b**. (From [4])

On the other hand, with the 1980 technique in knee resection arthrodesis we had only 1 infection (5%; treated by amputation), 1 rupture of a plate with non-union (successfully treated by a new plate and autogenous grafts) and 3 transient stress fractures of the grafts; only 4 patients (22%) required supplementary bone grafts at 6 months. Except for 1 case of infection with consequent delayed fusion, no complications were noted in 6 patients with shoulder or ankle resection arthrodesis. The advantages of the 1980 technique in respect to the original Putti Juvara one, are [1, 3]:

1. Decreased surgery on the same limb, with reduced exposure and surgical time.
2. Increased stability: the diaphyses residual to the resection are intact; the contact between the grafts and the host bone is end-to-end instead of side-to-side.
3. The blood supply of the host bone is better preserved, especially if a condylar plate is used instead of Küntscher rod. However, to ensure sufficient stability,

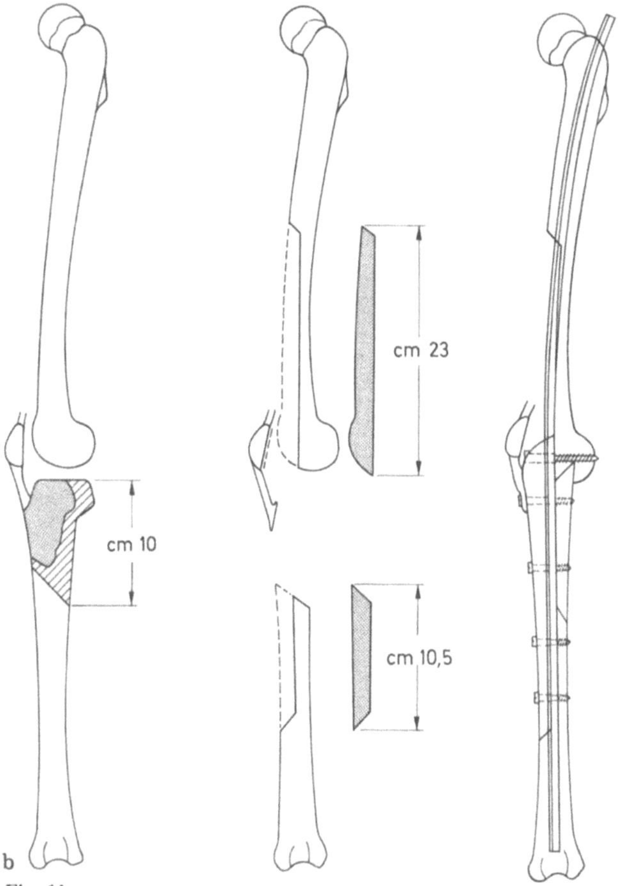

Fig. 1b

the use of a condylar plate is recommended only in short resections, especially of the proximal tibia and in absence of osteoporosis.

4. An improvement of the technique is represented by the systematic use of supplementary cancellous autogenous grafts if, at 6 months, a delayed union is suspected.

In our opinion resection arthrodesis with autogenous grafts is indicated: (a) in young and active people who desire an unrestricted weight-bearing activity; (b) in benign stage III and malignant stages I and II tumors, where an en bloc resection with the surrounding muscular compartments is indicated; and (c) when the resection length is less than 20 cm.

In high-grade tumors a two-stage procedure (temporary stabilization with rod and cement followed after several years by reconstruction with autogenous grafts) is recommended for the following reasons: the technique allows immediate ambulatory status without external supports; reducing the amount of the surgery during chemotherapy, it reduces the immunodepression; chemotherapy does not in-

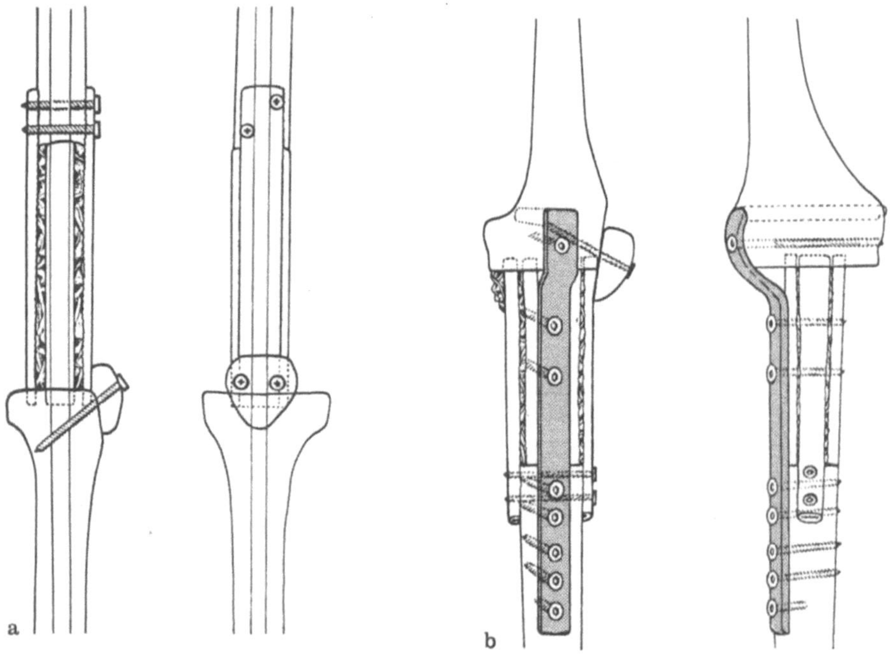

Fig. 2 a and b. Knee resection arthrodesis according to the 1980 technique. A Küntscher rod is used as osteosynthesis for reconstruction of the distal femur **a** while a condylar plate for reconstruction of the proximal tibia **b**. (From [4])

terfere with the incorporation of the grafts; grafting may be avoided in patients who have uncontrolled metastasis, local infection, or recurrence.

Between 1971 and 1985, 30 diaphyseal resection and reconstruction with grafts were done at the Rizzoli Institute. There were 6 benign (2 ABC, 1 osteoblastoma, 1 GCT, 2 desmoid tumors) and 24 malignant tumors (parosteal Ogs 3; periosteal Ogs 5; central chondrosarcoma 5; periosteal chondrosarcoma 1; Ewing's sarcoma 4; adamantinoma 1 MFH; usual Ogs 3). The resection diaphysis were: femur (12 cases), humerus (9), tibia (5), radius (1), unal (1), fibula (1) metatarsus (1).

The average resection length was 11 cm (range 4–19); a plate (20), a Küntscher rod (4), or other methods (6) of osteosynthesis were used. Twenty patients had reconstruction with autogenous grafts taken from the ipsilateral tibia (11), ipsilateral tibia and iliac crest (7), ipsilateral tibia counterlateral fibula and iliac crest (2). Ten patients had an intercalary homograft. Among 30 resections, we experienced only two local recurrences.

We had 2 osteosyntheses failures (requiring surgical treatment), 4 delayed fusions (3 requiring additional bone grafts), 6 infections (all complicated by pseudoarthrosis), and 7 stress fracture of the grafts (1 complicated by pseudoarthrosis). Twenty-three patients achieved fusion.

Between 1971 and 1985, 17 distal radius resections and reconstructions with autogenous proximal fibula were done at the Rizzoli Institute (Fig. 3) [2, 8, 10, 11, 14, 15, 18]. There were 15 giant cell tumors, 1 central chondrosarcoma, and

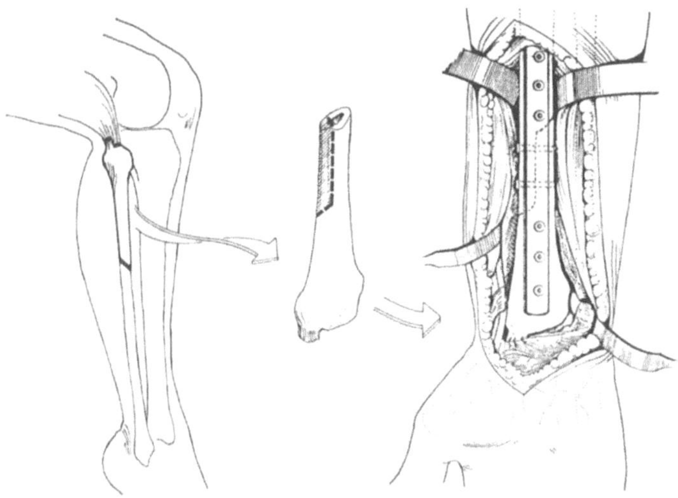

Fig. 3. Resection of the distal radius and reconstruction done with the proximal fibula. (From [12])

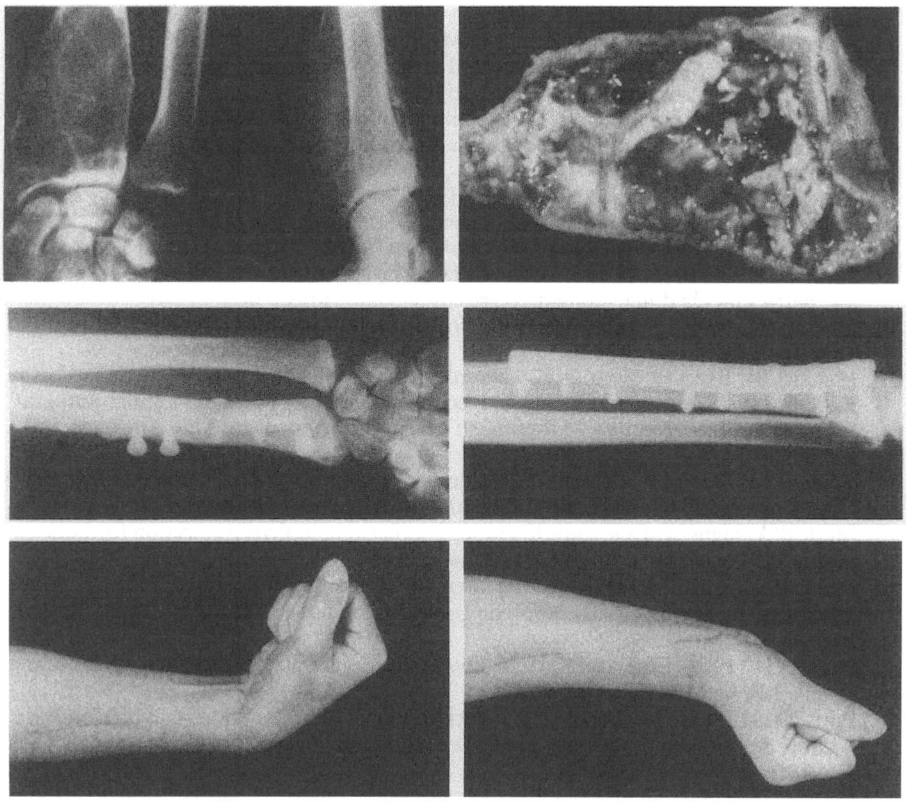

Fig. 4 a–f. Giant cell tumor of the distal radius (**a**) treated by resection (**b**) and reconstruction by fibular autograft; 41 months after resection the graft has healed completely (**c, d**), and the motion of the wrist is almost normal (**e, f**)

1 osteosarcoma. The resection length ranged from 5 to 12 cm. (average 6.5); a plate (16) or screws (1) were used as ostheosynthesis. The surgical margins were wide in 14 cases, wide but contaminated in 2, marginal in 1. We had no local recurrence.

We had 1 infection, 1 fracture of the graft below the plate and 7 subluxations of the wrist joint. All patients achieved proximal fusion of the grafts except one case with an infected pseudoarthrosis; a satisfactory joint motion of the wrist was conserved in 45% of the cases (Fig. 4). Only 2 patients referred a minimal lateral instability of the knee joint.

References

1. Campanacci M, Costa P (1979) Total resection of distal femur or proximal tibia for bone tumors. Autogenous bone grafts and arthrodesis in twenty-six cases. J Bone Joint Surg [Br] 61:455
2. Campanacci M, Laus M, Boriani S (1979) Resezione dell'estremità distale del radio. Ital J Orthop Traumatol 5:153
3. Capanna R, Ruggieri P, Casadei R, Ferraro A, Campanacci M (1986) Arthrodesis in limb saving surgery. Abstracts of international congress: bone and cancer, 9–10 Oct 1986 Helsinki
4. Enneking WF (ed) (1987) Limb salvage in musculoskeletal oncology. Churchill Livingstone, New York, Edinburgh, London, Melbourne
5. Enneking WF, Spanier SS, Goodman M (1980) A system for the surgical staging of musculoskeletal sarcoma. Clin Orthop 153:106
6. Enneking WF, Shirley PD (1977) Resection-arthrodesis for malignant and potentially malignant lesions about the knee using an intramedullary rod and local bone grafts. J Bone Surg [Am] 59:223
7. Enneking WF, Eady JL, Burchardt H (1980) Autogenous cortical bone grafts in the reconstruction of segmental skeletal defects. J Bone Joint Surg [Am] 62:1039
8. Gilbert A (1979) Vascularized of the fibular shaft. Int J Microsurg 1:100
9. Juvara E (1921) Procédé de résection de la partie superieure du tibia avec substitution, à la partie enlevée d'une greffe prélevée sur le fémur. Presse Med 29:241
10. Lawson TL (1952) Fibular transplant for osteoclastoma of the radius. J Bone Joint Surg [Br] 34B:74
11. Mercuri M, Bacci G, Bertoni F, Calderoni P, Capanna R, Cervellati C, Gherlinzoni F, Giunti A, Guernelli N, Guerra A, Picci P, Campanacci M (1982) Fibular autograft for distal radius resection. Attualità in chirurgia ortopedica. Aulo Gaggi Editore, Bologna
12. Mercuri M, Biagini R, Ferruzzi A, Calderoni P, Gamberini G, Campanacci M (1987) Perone pro radio. Chirurgia degli Organi di Movimento 72:63–68
13. Merle d'Aubigné R, Dejouany JP (1958) Diaphyso-ephiphysial resection for bone tumor at the knee. J Bone Joint Surg [Br] 40:305
14. Merle d'Aubigné R (1974) Résection large de l'extremité inférieure de radius. In: Merle d'Aubigné R, Mazas F (eds) Nouveau traité de technique chursurgical, vol 8. Masson, Paris, p 521
15. Pho RVH (1979) Free vascularized fibular transplant for replacement of the lower radius. J Bone Joint Surg [Br] 61:362
16. Putti V (1912) Eine Methode, um die Verkürzung der Extremität bei Ausgedehnter Resektion des Oberen Endes des Schienbeines zu verringern. Zbl Chir Mech Orthop 4(5):181
17. Putti V (1928) A study of two cases of tumor of the femur. The Robert Jones Birthday Volume. Oxford University Press, London, p 35
18. Yoshimura M, Shimamura K, Iwai Y, Yamauchi S, Ueno T (1983) Free vascularized fibular transplant. J Bone Joint Surg [Am] 65:1295

Clinical Aspects I:
Vascularized and Non-Vascularized Autografts

Free Vascularized Fibular Graft

J. Brennwald

Kantonsspital Basel, Departement für Chirurgie, Spitalstr. 21, CH-4031 Basel

Microsurgery opened a completely new field in bone transplantation with the free vascularized bone transfer. Oestrup and Fredrickson (1974) stressed that successful transplantation of bone is dependent on both the endosteal blood supply, i.e., the nutrient blood supply, and the periosteal blood supply. Using microsurgical techniques both blood supplies can be reestablished by anastomosing the donor vessels, artery and vein, to the recipient vessels (Berggren et al. 1982). After restoration of the blood supply the bony segment should be as well vascularized as a living bone, and therefore incorporation of the bone graft should be similar to fracture healing. Non-vascularized bone grafts will undergo complete remodeling until the periosteal and endosteal blood supply is reestablished. However, it is questionable whether, for example in free iliac crest grafts, the endosteal blood supply remains as effective as it was in the original site, since the medulla is no longer supplied by the original nutrient artery and vein.

Clinically, however, it seems that the blood supply is less important than the minimal donor morbidity and the ability of the bone graft to satisfy the various requirements of the recipient site. Over the years only a few free vascularized bone grafts have been shown to be of use: the rib, the fibula, the iliac crest, the second metatarsal, the radius, and the ulna. All these bone grafts can be harvested in combination with soft tissue such as muscle and skin.

In the following the free vascularized fibula graft is taken as an example of a free vascularized bone graft; there is minimal donor site morbidity , endosteal and periosteal blood supply can be maintained and the bone is stronger than the rib and iliac crest.

The fibula is vascularized by the peroneal artery, the vessels entering the fibula posterior and slightly proximal to the middle of the shaft, and by segmental periosteal vessels. When larger defects in long bones are to be filled, the lateral half of the soleus muscle can be included (Baudet 1981), a small longitudinal lateral skin strip used (Chen and Wang 1983), or a smaller skin island added as a graft survival monitor (Yoshimura et al. 1983).

No significant morbidity resulting from harvesting the fibula is known, although in children bowing of the tibia has been reported (Gilbert 1979), as well as a valgus ankle deformity caused by uneven growth in the lower tibial epiphysis (Tamai 1984).

Bone Transplantation
Eds.: M. Aebi, P. Regazzoni

Dissection

Preoperative angiography is helpful in showing the vascularization of the fibula and in determining the blood supply to the foot that will remain when the fibula is transferred. Two approaches are possible, a posterior (Taylor 1977) and a lateral one (Gilbert 1979). With the lateral approach the patient can be placed in a supine position, whereas the posterior approach requires a more or less prone po-

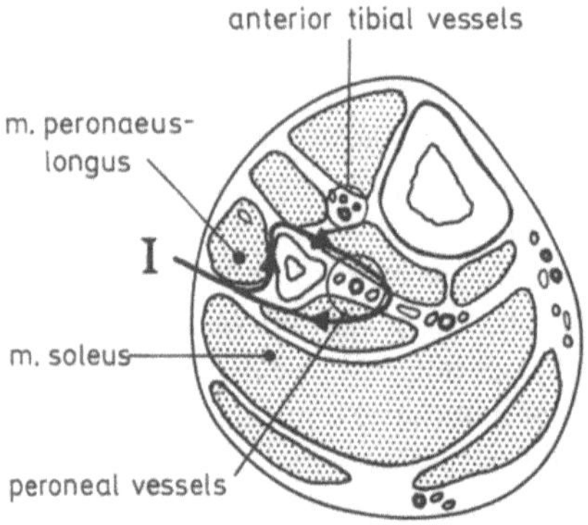

Fig. 1. Midshaft section of the lower leg: the dissection for a purely fibular graft (method I)

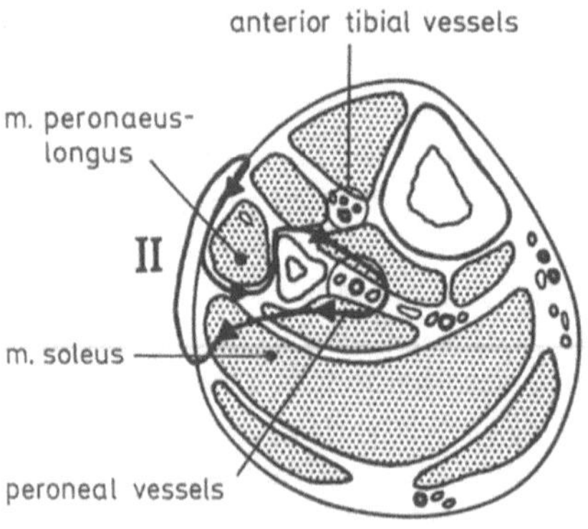

Fig. 2. The plan of dissecting if an overlaying skin flap is required (method II)

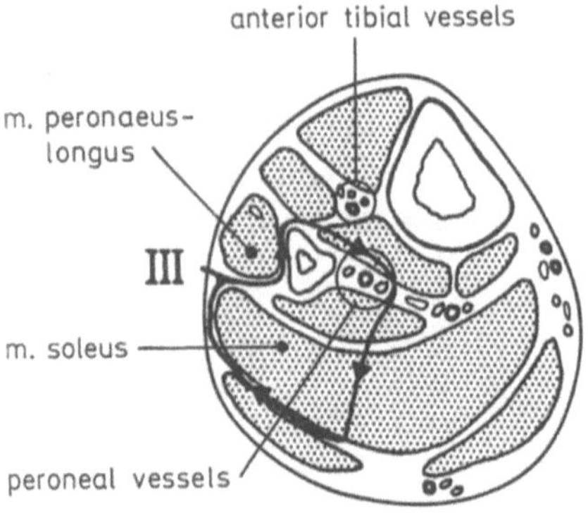

Fig. 3. The plan of dissection if an additional muscle graft is included (method III)

sition. Each approach therefore offers different advantages and disadvantages and the approach must be selected according to the reconstructive procedure.

After applying a tourniquet, the dissection for a free vascularized fibula graft is carried out as shown in Fig. 1 (method I). For a fibular graft with a skin island flap part of the lateral solus muscle must be removed because of the cutaneous branch which can emerge out of the solus muscle, so method II is used (Fig. 2). For a fibular graft with muscle the lateral part of the soleus muscle can be included, and method III used (Fig. 3).

The bone length varies from patient to patient. On average, roughly three-quarters of the total fibula length can be used: the fibula head should be left in place for knee stability, and the distal quarter of the fibula for ankle stability.

If a particularly high functional load on the transplanted fibula graft is expected, the graft can easily be doubled by osteotomizing the fibula in the middle and folding it parallel so that the same vessel pedicle supplies each half (Jones et al. 1988).

Fixation of the Fibular Graft

Fixation of the transplanted graft is important for ensuring union between the bones in the recipient area. Rigid, stable fixation between graft and host bones must be achieved and the whole graft area must be stabilized either by external fixation or by internal fixation using plates and screws. Asymmetric functional loading of the graft or implant will lead to fatigue fractures. Therefore, a cancellous bone graft placed in a second operation can be used to provide the stability necessary in long bone reconstructions.

As a final step, when the graft is already securely fixed the vessel anastomoses, preferably end-to-side, should be carried out. An effective drainage system should be installed because of the possibility of hematomas resulting from the open bone cavities.

Aftertreatment

Regular X-ray examinations show whether the bone union takes place without disturbance. It is to be expected that the bone will heal more slowly than in an uncomplicated fracture without tissue damage. Therefore, full functional load can only be allowed when complete bony union has occurred.

References

Baudet (1981) Presentation Internat. Soc. of Reconstr. Microsurgery, Meeting Melbourne Australia 1981 Jan

Berggren A, Weiland AJ, Dorfman H (1982) Free vascularized bone grafts: factors affecting their survival and ability to heal to recipient bone defects. Plast Reconstr Surg 69:19–29

Chen-Zong-Wei, Wang Yan (1983) The study and clinical application of the osteocutaneous flap of the fibular. Microsurgery 1:11–16

Gilbert A (1979) Vascularized transfer of the fibula shaft. Int J Microsurg 1:100–102

Jones NF, Swartz WM, Mears DC, Jupiter JB, Grossman A (1988) The "double barrel" free vascularized fibular bone graft. Plast Reconstr Surg 81:378–385

Oestrup L, Fredrickson J (1974) Distant transfer of a free living bone graft by microvascular anastomoses. An experimental study. Plast Reconstr Surg 54:274–285

Tamai S (1984) Vascularized fibula transplantation for congenital pseudoarthrosis and radial club hand. In: Buncke H, Furnas D (eds) Symposium on clinical frontiers in reconstructive microsurgery. Mosby, St. Louis, ch 31

Taylor GI (1977) Microvascular free bone transfer. Orthop Clin North Am 8:425–447

Yoshimura M, Shimarrura K, Yoshinobu I, Yamauchi S, Uena T (1983) Free vascularized fibular transplant. J Bone Joint Surg 65A:1295–1301

Pedicled Autograft and Osteotomy in Revascularization of the Femoral Head

R. Ganz

Department of Orthopaedic Surgery, University of Berne, Inselspital, CH-3010 Berne

The incidence of idiopathic femoral head necrosis in general is increasing. This entity is found much more frequently in men than in women with the peak age between 20 and 40 years. Quite often both hips are involved. The pathophysiology is rather clear in posttraumatic conditions, but a more complex picture is involved in the idiopathic group. The currently favored etiology is that of a bone marrow fibrosis causing increased perivascular pressure [11]. There is a resultant necrotic segment which lies in the anterosuperior quadrant of the femoral head, an area which is supplied by terminal vessels and is exposed to the maximum mechanical load.

In the treatment of idiopathic femoral head necrosis there is no general agreement as to the preferred treatment modality. In the preradiologic stage (stage I) core decompression seems to give good results, but besides Ficat and Arlet [5] and Hungerford [10] no one has published results of a large series demonstrating this. For stage II and III lesions, various osteotomies, either alone or in combination with free bone grafting procedures, have been used [2, 4, 14, 16, 19, 20]. In our own series with combined flexion osteotomy and free cancellous bone-grafting of the necrotic segment, the long-term success rate was no better than 65% [7].

Attempts at improving the circulation in the femoral head date back to the early 1960s [6]. Several types of muscle pedicle grafts have been described [13, 15, 18]. In 1965 Boyd and Ault [3] published preliminary results on the implantation of an artery into the femoral head. In 1973 Hori [9] tried to revitalize the femoral head by vascular bundle transplantation. A technically demanding procedure has been described by H. Judet et al. [12] in which a microvascular fibular graft is used for revascularization and stabilization of the femoral head. However, none of these techniques combined a revascularization procedure with an osteotomy to decrease the mechanical load on the involved segment and increase the blood supply to the femoral head.

Our attempts at revascularization of the femoral head necrosis date back to 1978 when we used an arteriovenous vessel loop. In 1979 we adopted the method of Hori, but the preparation of the vascular bundle was sometimes difficult and, in cases of previous surgery, impossible. Since 1979 we have used a vascularized bone block harvested from the lateral iliac crest. Its vascular pedicle is from the deep circumflex iliac vessels and it has a length of up to 16 cm, sufficient for rerouting of the graft to the femoral head [8]. Our technique of flexion osteotomy has been modified since our previous presentation [7]. Currently we routinely perform a trochanteric osteotomy which allows more flexion and decreases static load, during the flexion, on the anterior joint area.

Bone Transplantation
Eds.: M. Aebi, P. Regazzoni

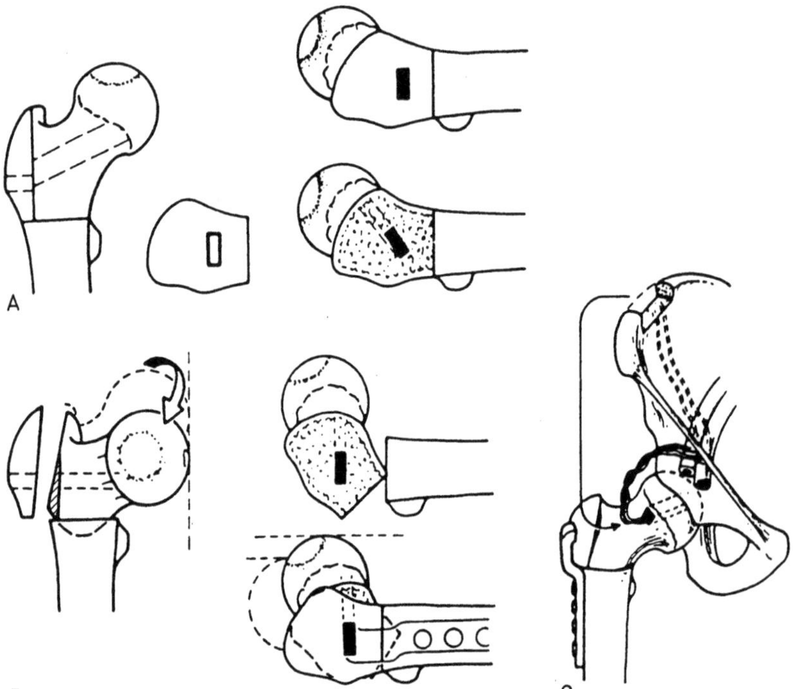

Fig. 1 A–C. Technique of flexion osteotomy and revascularization in femoral head necrosis. **A** Blade channel in the greater trochanter and the neck-head fragment. **B** Wedge resection of the neck (hatched), no intertrochanteric wedge. Insertion of the plate's blade into the greater trochanter and the neck. **C** Implantation of the pedicled iliac bone graft into the head

By avoiding the removal of a bone wedge the dorsal displacement of the femoral shaft is minimal and a standard osteotomy plate (90°/15 mm offset, 60 mm blade length) can be attached easily to the distal fragment. The desired correction includes 50° of flexion and 10°–15° of adduction. After fixation of the osteotomy plate the previously harvested pedicle bone graft is rerouted anterior to the rectus femoris to the femoral neck where it is inserted through a canal of about 12 mm in diameter into the necrotic area (Fig. 1). Postoperatively, special emphasis is placed on extension exercises of the hip. Partial weight bearing of 10–15 kg is also required for 4–6 months.

Our experience with the described technique of an osteotomy combined with the pedicle bone block consists of 60 hips. The long-term results, with a mean follow-up of 32 months (11–84 months), are available for 45 hips. Of these, only 12 could be classified as Ficat stage II, with all the others being stage III. The clinical evaluation (Merle d'Aubignié system [17]) showed a very good or good result in 68.3%, an acceptable result in 14.6% and a bad result in 17.1%. The average value increased from 11.23 preoperatively to 14.94. The subjective results were even better: 85% of the patients classified their result as optimal or markedly improved compared to before operation, 2.5% had minimal improvement, 5% had no improvement, and 7.5% said that their hip was worse than before surgery. The walking ability improved in general from 3.56 to 5.0. Preoperatively, nine hips allowed a normal gait compared to 21 after surgery. The radiographic improvement was less dramatic. All cases showed an improvement of congruency in the weight-bearing area. None of our stage II cases showed further flattening of the contour. In none of the cases did the size of the necrotic segment increase. Scintigraphy and computed tomography (CT) have been used to examine 26 cases. CT was especially helpful and allowed good observation of graft incorporation. Signs of incorporation of the graft were seen in 17 cases, but only two cases that were stage II showed perfect reintegration of the necrotic segment and the pedicle bone graft. Increased sclerosis around the necrotic segment indicated less reincorporation of the graft in the necrotic sector. The worst radiological and clinical results were seen in cases with a completely loose osteochondral fragment.

Compared to our previous series the improvement in results was not significant, but we can say that the new series includes more advanced cases and cases with a greater extension of the necrosis. We will continue with this technique but will include some modifications. Any avascular necrosis of the femoral head that is stage III will get CT scan preoperatively. This is not only necessary to make a tridimensional reconstruction with a better picture of the necrosis, but also helps to exclude cases with completely loose osteochondral fragments. In our opinion, this rather complex surgery is contraindicated in such patients.

For stage II lesions, the combined procedure of an osteotomy and a pedicle graft will be used. The stage III cases will only receive the osteotomy without revascularization because this does not seem to aid very much in this advanced stage. In cases where osteotomy is not indicated we perform a total hip replacement.

There is limited experience with total hip replacement after failed flexion osteotomy; however, it does not appear to represent major technical difficulties. The negative aspect of this second procedure is the increased risk of infection. There is, however, also a positive argument, namely, that the sclerotic wall of the osteotomy will help to narrow the upper part of the medullary cavity and therefore increase the osseous press-fit contact of the prosthesis.

References

1. Baksi DP (1983) Treatment of post-traumatic avascular necrosis of the femoral head by multiple drilling and muscle-pedicle bone grafting. J Bone Joint Surg 65-B:268
2. Bonfiglio M, Basdenstium MB (1958) Treatment by bone grafting of aseptic necrosis of the femoral neck and nonunion of the femoral neck. J Bone Joint Surg 40-A:1329
3. Boyd RJ, Ault LL (1965) An experimental study of vascular implantation into the femoral head. Surg Gynecol Obstet 121:1009
4. Camera U (1954) Die biologische Haloplastik. Verh Dtsch Orthop Ges 42:341
5. Ficat P, Arlet J (1977) Ischémie et nécrose osseouse. Masson, Paris
6. Frankel CJ, Derian PS (1962) The induction of subcapital femoral circulation by means of an autogenous muscle pedicle. Surg Gynecol Obstet 115:473
7. Ganz R, Jakob RP (1980) Partielle avasculäre Hüftkopfnekrose: Flexionsosteotomie und Spongiosaplastik. Orthopäde 9:265

8. Ganz R, Büchler U (1983) Overview of attempts to revitalize the dead head in aseptic necrosis of the femoral head – osteotomy and revascularisation. In: Hungerford DS (ed) The hip: proceedings of the eleventh open scientific meeting of The Hip Society. Mosby, St. Louis, p 296
9. Hori Y (1980) Revitalisierung des osteonekrotischen Hüftkopfes durch Gefässbündel-Transplantation. Orthopäde 9:255
10. Hungerford DS (1979) Bone marrow pressure, venography and core decompression in ischemic necrosis of the femoral head. In: Hungerford DS (ed) The hip: proceedings of the seventh open scientific meeting of The Hip Society. Mosby, St. Louis, p 218
11. Hungerford DS, Zizic TM (1983) Pathogenesis of ischemic necrosis of the femoral head. In: Hungerford DS (ed) The hip: proceedings of the eleventh open scientific meeting of The Hip Society. Mosby, St. Louis, p 249
12. Judet H, Judet J, Gilbert A (1981) Vascular microsurgery in orthopaedics. Int Orthop 5:61
13. Judet R, Judet J, Lamois B, Gubler JP (1966) Essaie de révascularisation expérimentale de la tête fémorale. Rev Chir Orthop 52:277
14. Kerboull M (1973) L'ostéotomie intertrochantérienne dans le traitement de la nécrose idiopathique de la tête fémorale. Rev Chir Orthop (suppl 1) 59:52
15. Lee CK, Rehmatullah N (1981) Muscle-pedicle bone graft and cancellous bone graft for the "silent hip" of idiopathic ischemic necrosis of the femoral head in adults. Clin Orthop 158:185
16. Merle d' Aubigné R, Postel M, Mazabraud A, Massias P, Guegneu J (1965) Idiopathic necrosis of the femoral head in adults. J Bone Joint Surg 47-B:612
17. Merle d'Aubigné R (1970) Cotation chiffré de la fonction de la hanche. Rev Chir Orthop 56:481
18. Palazzi C, Xicoy J (1975) The pediculate bone grafts as treatment for the aseptic necrosis of the femoral head. Arch Orthop Unfall Chir 83:115
19. Patterson RJ, Bickel WH, Dahlin DC (1964) Idiopathic avascular necrosis of the head of the femur. J Bone Joint Surg 46-A:267
20. Wagner H (1967) Aetiologie, Pathogenese, Klinik und Therapie der idiopathischen Hüftkopfnekrose. Verh Dtsch Orthop Ges 54:224

Autologous Bone-Grafts: Problems at the Donor Site

D. Grob

Klinik Wilhelm Schulthess, Neumünsterallee 3, 8008 Zurich, Switzerland

Contrary to most other publications about autologous bone grafting, the discussion in this paper does not concern the biologic reaction and the ingrowth of the graft but the problems that arise at the donor site. Even if cancellous bone of all parts of the skeleton may act as grafts, the quantity and quality of the pelvic bone favor the iliac crest, either anteriorly or posteriorly. Corresponding to the need of the mechanical properties of the graft, the pelvis offers both the pure cancellous bone and the corticocancellous bone in a sufficient amount. However the price of taking bone from the iliac crest is paid by a fairly high complication rate: up to 21% of operations with autologous corticocancellous bone grafts caused more or less severe complications. Only 16 out of 50 nonselected patients who underwent autologous bone grafting from the pelvis for anterior spondylodesis were without any complaints concerning the donor site. In four patients, reintervention at the iliac crest were necessary.

To reduce this rate of complications, we suggest respecting the following points: (a) The risk of complication increases with the taken amount of bone graft. If at all possible, take just cancellous bone. (b) A defect in the cortical part of the iliac wing should be replaced by a homologous graft. (c) An atraumatic operative technique and a careful hemostasis has to be strictly respected, as well as the particular anatomy of the nerves near the iliac crest. (d) The long bones of the extremities are not suitable for donor sites. They should be used only in unexpected situations where intraoperatively the need for autologous bone graft arises.

Bone Transplantation
Eds.: M. Aebi, P. Regazzoni

Technique for Harvesting Autogenic Bone Paste

W. Dick, P. Regazzoni, and B. Gerber

Orthopaedic Clinic, Department of Surgery, University of Basel, Basel, Switzerland

In comparison with solid bone grafts, the particulate form of autogenic grafts as a paste-like material offers several advantages:

- The surface of the graft is multiplied, and vascularisation and remodelling of bone are thereby facilitated.
- The healing that occurs in the bone graft area is a field phenomenon, occurring simultaneously throughout the entire defect.
- Ingrowth of capillaries is quick, as clefts give access everywhere.
- Irregularly shaped defects can be filled more completely. The contact between host site and graft is closer and more extensive than with solid bone chips.

The position of two bone fragments to be united can still be corrected after graft insertion without extrusion of the graft.

Only a small access is necessary to fill a large defect cavity.

From a curved incision underneath the posterior iliac crest the posterior iliac wing and iliac spine are prepared subpriostally. The gluteus muscles are reflected with two Hohmann retractors (Fig. 1). A normal alcetabular reamer, as is used for total hip replacements with 44–48 mm diameter, is then used to procure the graft and to transform it simultaneously into a paste-like material. Some milliliters of blood from the donor site are added. To procure a better initial grip for the reamer, a small window is chiselled into the cortical layer. The outer wing of the ilium and the cancellous table are reamed; the inner wing is preserved. By pulling the reamer sideways in all directions a large amount of bone can be gained. Bleeding at the donor site is controlled by a collagen haemostatic felt.

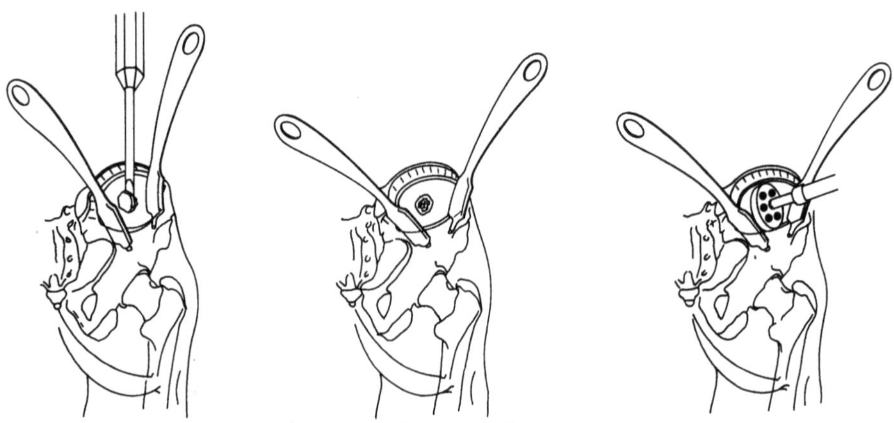

Fig. 1. Harvesting autogenic bone paste by acetabular reamer

Bone Transplantation
Eds.: M. Aebi, P. Regazzoni

The method presented here for collecting a homogeneous mixture of ground cortical and cancellous autogenic bone has proven in over 100 cases of spine surgery to be very simple, time-saving and productive. The acetabular reamer is much quicker and cheaper than a bone mill.

References

Dick W (1986) Use of the acetabular reamer to harvest autogenic bone graft material: a simple method for producing bone paste. Arch Orthop Trauma Surg 105:235–238

Dick W (1987) Innere Fixation von Brust- und Lendenwirbelbrüchen, 2nd edn., Huber, Bern

The Use of Autogenic Bone Paste in Anterior Interbody Spine Fusion

W. Dick and H. Bereiter

Orthopaedic Clinic, Department of Surgery, University of Basel, Basel, Switzerland

The rate of pseudarthrosis in conventional interbody fusions by insertion of solid autogeneic or homogeneic strut grafts in the disc space is high and may reach 30%. This is due to several factors. (a) Vascularisation and ingrowth start only from the ends of the graft, coming from the opposite end plates of the vertebrae only. (b) Remodelling of the graft takes very long, not rarely leading to a fatigue fracture and consecutive pseudarthrosis in the middle of the graft (being not yet revitalised), whereas both ends are firmly consolidated with the neighbouring vertebrae. (c) The position of the graft very near to the instantaneous axis of rotation, causing a short lever arm and thereby high forces acting on the graft, makes the necessary protection from movements in the zone of ossification difficult.

Changing the technique of operation and of graft preparation can avoid these disadvantages. In addition to the usual preparation of the disc space, two-thirds of the anterior and lateral walls of the adjacent vertebral bodies is stripped subperiosteally, and the anulus fibrosus is removed completely on the anterior and lateral aspect. The anterior rim of the vertebra is nibbled down to the open cancellous bone. The autograft, a mixture of ground cortical and cancellous bone (see abstract Dick et al.; this volume), is then inserted in a paste-like consistency around the outer surfaces of the vertebrae and into the disc interspace. Thus an imitation of the spontaneous callus formation in fractures is reached (Fig. 1). If distraction is needed, an additonal strutt graft may be inserted as a spacer between the end plates of the vertebrae.

This technique and the graft healing process has been demonstrated radiologically in 12 cases of lumbosacral spondylolisthesis and degenerative lumbar spine

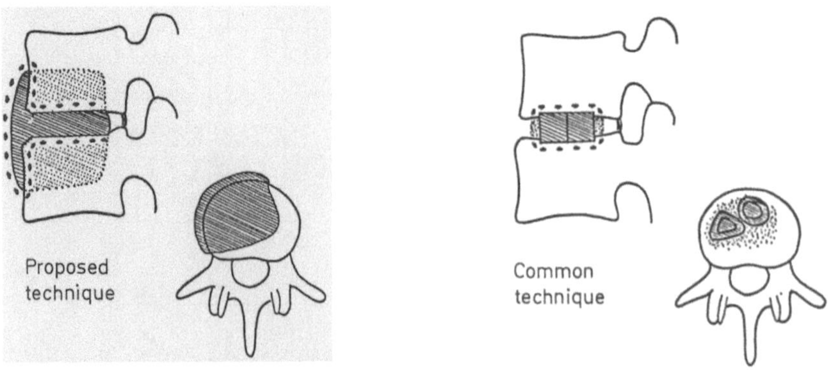

Fig. 1. Proposed grafting technique for anterior spine fusions

Bone Transplantation
Eds.: M. Aebi, P. Regazzoni

instability. It has proven to lead to solid bridging of the vertebrae in all cases within 12 weeks and to a mature fusion within 6–9 months. The advantages are: (a) multiplication of graft surface and contact area; (b) vascularisation of the graft, starting from both the well-vascularised retroperitoneal layer and the vertebral bone; (c) healing occurring as a field phenomenon simultaneously over the whole graft area; and (d) position of the graft far away from the centre of rotation in an eggshell-like semicircle shape – thus the biomechanically favourable position of the bridge formation helps to control interbody movements in all directions.

References

Dick W (1987) Innere Fixation von Brust- und Lendenwirbelfrakturen, 2nd edn. Huber, Bern

Production of Autologised Cancellous Bone with the Use of Homologous Cancellous Bone

A. Sárváry and G. Berentey

Semmelweis University of Medical Sciences, Department of Traumatology, Péterfy Hospital, Budapest, Hungary

The free transplantation of cancellous bone is often used for the stimulation of osteogenesis, for the replacement of traumatic or pathologic bone defects and for the curing of nonunions. The effectiveness of transplantation depends not only upon the blood supply of the recipient bed but also upon the quantity and activity of cancellous bone. Of the donor sites used, the margin of the iliac crest and the lateral mass of the sacrum are the most advantageous because (a) the greatest quantity of cancellous bone can be gained from these sites; (b) in these regions there is a certain haemopoiesis, even in adults; and (c) removal of the cancellous bone from these regions has no marked detrimental effect on the statics of the bone. The donor sites of the iliac crest and the sacrum do not regenerate spontaneously; thus, in case of repeated transplantations the sources of cancellous bone might become exhausted.

After the removal of the cancellous bone, the iliac crest is filled with large quantities of homologous spongiosa. In 6–10 weeks the implanted cancellous frame displays an osteo-inductive effect and becomes filled with antologous tissue suitable for further transplantation (Figs. 1–3). The advantages of this method are as follows:

1. After an adequate incubation period the implanted homologous cancellous bone has the same osteo-inductive effect as the autologous spongiosa.

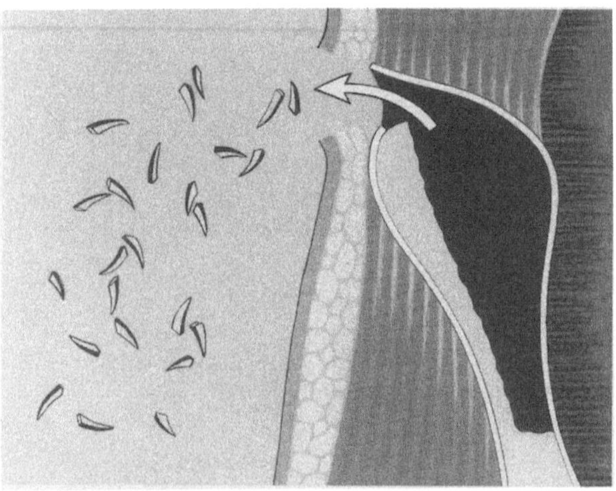

Fig. 1. The autologous cortical and cancellous bone removed from the internal surface of the crista iliaca

Bone Transplantation
Eds.: M. Aebi, P. Regazzoni

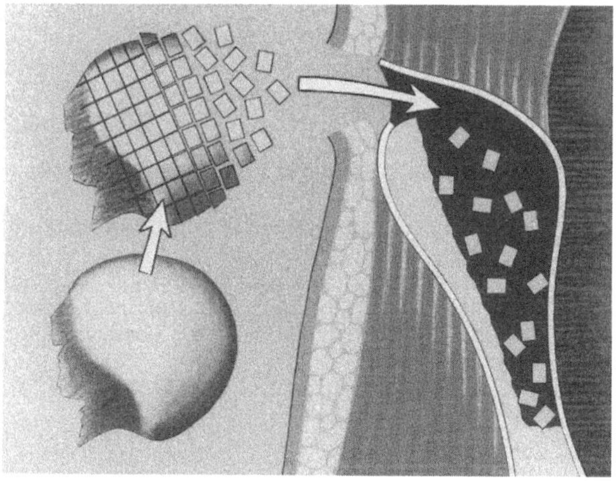

Fig. 3. The filled area is covered with the fascio-periosteal flap

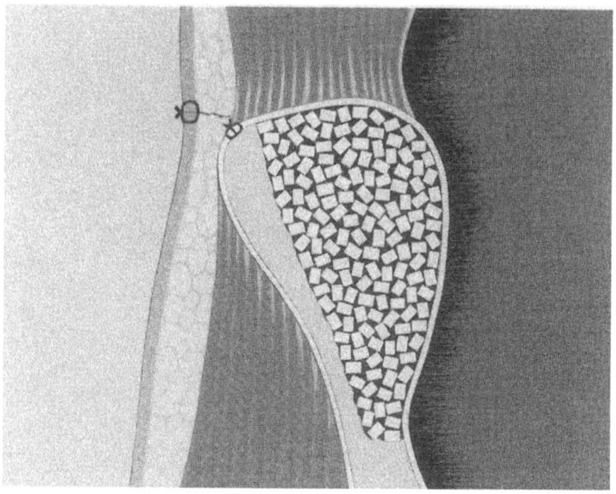

Fig. 2. The donor bed is filled with about $0.5 \times 0.5 \times 0.5$ cm homologous cancellous bone cubes from the bone bank in a quantity two to three times that of the original volume

2. The expulsion reaction against the T-antigen does not take place at the final recipient site.
3. An autologous material twice or three times the volume of the original quantity can be produced.
4. A known quantity of autologous material is at disposal for further transplantations.
5. The procedure can be repeated as often as necessary.
6. The surgical technique is simple, and its costs are low.

The case of an 11-year-old girl is presented, in whom, because of Ewing's sarcoma, a 12-cm long resection was performed and the bone defect filled once with autologous and twice with autologised homologous cancellous bone. In 31 weeks the bone defect was bridged.

References

1. Holz U, Weller S, Borell-Kost S (1982) Indikation, Technik und Ergebnisse der autologen Knochentransplantation. Chirurg 53:219–224
2. Sárváry A (1981) Uj typusu autolog spongiosa elo 'llitása dezantigenizált heterolog spongiosából. Magy Traumatol Orthop Helyreallito Sebesz 24:65–71
3. Schweiberer L (1970) Experimentelle Untersuchungen von Knochentransplantaten mit unveränderter und mit denaturierter Knochengrundsubstanz. Hefte Unfallheilkd 103:
4. Urist MR, Silvermann R, Buring K, Dubuc FL, Rosenberg JM (1967) The bone induction principle. Clin Orthop 53:243–283

Skeletal Reconstruction by Vascularized Fibular Transfer: Indications and Results

H. H. de Boer and M. B. Wood

Department of Orthopaedics, Mayo Clinic, Rochester, Minnesota, USA

Although the value of vascularized bone transfer is implied in terms of reconstruction and massive defects, there are still relatively few scientific reports in the literature regarding the results of vascularized fibular transfer in a large series of patients. Herein we review our experience with 62 patients who underwent this procedure.

The records of all patients treated at the Mayo Clinic who underwent a vascularized fibular transfer for reconstruction of a bony defect, and who had at least 1 year follow-up were reviewed. Unequivocal X-ray evidence of bone healing at both ends of the graft was required to declare the bone segment united. All major complications and required secondary procedures were recorded. The results were analyzed chiefly in relation to the indication of the procedure and the recipient bone site.

The range of follow-up time of the 62 patients in this study was 12–87 months (mean, 31 months). Twenty-five (40%) patients had a reconstruction after bone tumor resection, 20 (32%) had a skeletal reconstruction after traumatic bone loss or established nonunion with bony defects, and another 17 (28%) after radical débridement of chronic osteomyelitis.

There were 22 (36%) patients who had their femur reconstructed, 20 (32%) their tibia, and 20 (32%) with reconstruction performed in the upper extremity. Forty-three (69%) had primary union of the bone graft; in addition, nine patients had union of the graft after further surgical intervention. Therefore, the overall eventual rate of union was 84%.

We achieved the best results with limb reconstruction after tumor resection and with recipient sites that involved the upper extremity. In contrast, our results were least favorable with reconstruction after resection for chronic osteomyelitis.

The overall results suggest that a vascularized fibular transfer seems to be a valuable reconstructive technique for the management of clinical problems that involve massive skeletal defects.

References

Wood MB, Cooney WP (1984) Vascularized bone segment for management of chronic osteomyelitis. Orthop Clin North Am 15

Wood MB, Cooney WP, Irons GB (1984) Post-traumatic lower extremity reconstruction by vascularized bone graft transfer. Orthopaedics 7:255

Bone Transplantation
Eds.: M. Aebi, P. Regazzoni

Vascularized Pedicular Rib Grafts in Operative Treatment

Z. Milinkovich, B. Bojanich, B. Radojevich, M. Zlatich, C. Abaidoo, N. Stankovich, and V. Brusich

Special Orthopedic Surgical Hospital Banjica, Belgrade, Yugoslavia

In large bone defects of traumatic, infectious, or tumoral process or after spinal decompression in congenital deformities, there is a significant risk of graft resorption and nonunion of bone grafts due to poor, insufficient, or damaged vascularization of the recipient bed in the spine. Experimental studies and clinical practice confirm that in such conditions priority is given to vascular pedicular grafts of ribs. These grafts, with well-preserved blood supply, provide vitality, direct union without cell substitution, and revascularization. As live grafts they retain biomechanical strength after transplantation.

Our experience since 1982 with pedicular rib grafts in 28 patients confirms this. The analysis is related to the first 19 patients, with follow-up periods of 18 months or more. Among these, 10 cases were of specific TBC spondylitis, 2 cases of nonspecific spondylitis, 2 after decompression in congenital anomalies, and 5 were considered failures. In this group of 5 patients, after twisting of the grafts, tests of vitality and vascularization were negative in 3, and in 2 which we did after tumoral resection they united fast and became well incorporated in spite of tumoral process. In 14 cases all grafts united 12–16 weeks after the operation. These were confirmed both clinically and radiologically. In spondylitis these grafts proved effective, and this allowed us to reduce the postoperative immobilization in cast to 4 months (with further protection with plastic orthosis for up to 1 year after the operation).

The operative technique involved careful planning of the surgical approach regarding the level of decompression: in the thoracic region one or two ribs above the level of decompression or below in the upper thoracic region. In lumbar region it is limited to the L2 vertebrae. After skin incision, dissection is made through the muscle attachment 2 mm above the desired rib. After thoracotomy we dissect the rib together with periosteum and vessels to the costochondral junction, divide it by osteotome and ligate vessels, and continue careful dissection proximally to the vertebrocostal junction. After dislocation in this junction, the desired length of rib is measured and osteotomized in the proximal or distal part, leaving a long pedicle for further insertion. After vertebrectomy and decompression, the rib graft is inserted in the recipient bed. Before insertion, ligature is taken out, and we perform the test of vitality. A small incision of the periosteum can confirm the presence of vascularization.

Our experience is encouraging and points up the necessity for wider application of such bone transplants. Surgical application of vascular rib grafts does not require a microsurgical team, and it is accessible to all spinal surgeons.

Bone Transplantation
Eds.: M. Aebi, P. Regazzoni

The Pedicle Bone Graft: An Indication for Superselective Angiography

V. Klingmüller [1] and G. Schwetlick [2]

[1] Department of Pediatric Radiology, [2] Orthopedic Clinic, Justus Liebig University, Giessen, FRG

Therapy of idiopathic necrosis of the femoral head by transplantation of a pedicle bone graft should provide good arterial supply. This operation is based on the idea that ischemic processes play an important role in the origin of this necrosis [2, 3]. The pedicle bone graft is taken from the ipsilateral iliac crest together with the deep circumflex iliac artery (ACIP), and vein where their main branches run into the bone [1, 4]. The advantage of the pedicle bone graft is, that the transplanted bone is perfused by its original vessels. The success of the operative therapy depends on the state of the vessels. Therefore, the operation should be accompanied by angiographies. Only the superselective method using the Seldinger technique provides angiograms of the relevant vessel without superposition of other vessels [3].

Preoperative angiographies were performed in 45 patients aged 32–56 years with idiopathic necrosis of the femoral head (except one who had a medial fracture of the femoral neck). The medial circumflex artery of the thigh (ACFM), the

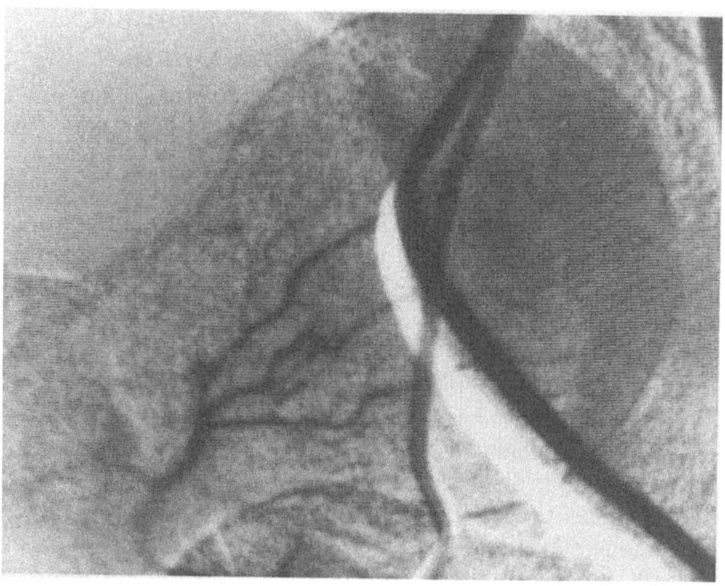

Fig. 1. Preoperative angiogram of the arteria circumflexa femoris medialis. Only three tiny rami nutritii are still open

Bone Transplantation
Eds.: M. Aebi, P. Regazzoni

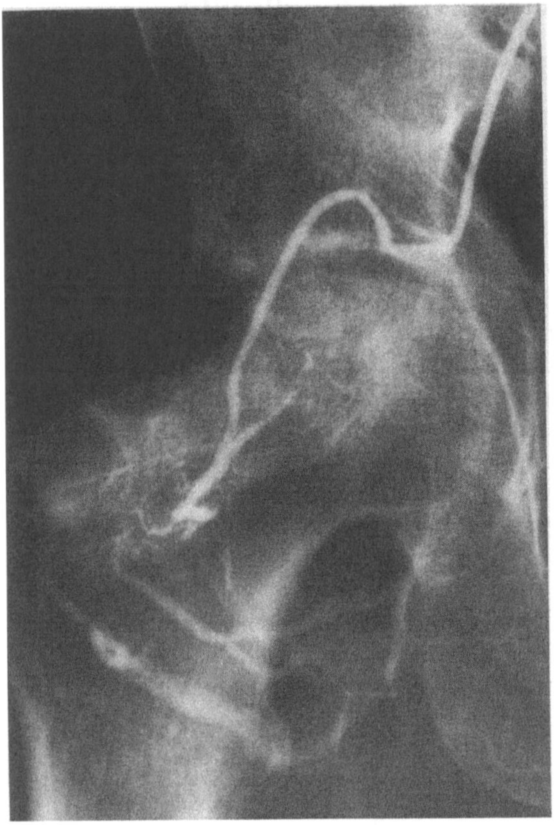

Fig. 2. Postoperative angiogram of the reset arteria circumflexa ilium profunda demonstrates good perfusion to the transplanted bone

main supplying artery of the femoral head, showed pathological findings in 28 cases with idiopathic necrosis and obstruction, rarefaction, or dilatation of the rami nutritii (Fig. 1).

The superselective imaging of the ACIP is very helpful in preoperative planning. Among the 36 angiograms of the ACIP, 27 showed an origin distal to, 5 a projection on, and 4 proximal to the slit of the joint. In the distal group, 10 arteries had no branches, but the remaining 17 had maximally 4 branches or subbranches. Collaterals to the lumbar artery were a common finding.

The pedicle bone graft has already been transplanted in 24 cases. The postoperative angiographies of the reset ACIP were performed 3 months after the operation (Fig. 2). To date, 19 patients have been examined. In two cases the ACIP could not be demonstrated, and in two other cases only a short part of the artery could be seen. In the case of medial fracture the artery was well perfused.

Angiographies of the reset ACIP in different positions of the leg became very important. These demonstrated that the reset ACIP can be obstructed in some positions, especially with extreme rotations. These positions need not be painful, but the patient must to be adequately informed to avoid them.

Pre- and postoperative superselective angiography provides important and interesting information to improve therapy with the pedicle bone graft. The preoperative examination of the ACFM is a useful diagnostic tool in cases of the necrosis of the femoral head. The preoperative angiogram of the ACIP is helpful in planning the operation. The postoperative angiography is a direct demonstration of the state of the vessels, not an indirect scintigraphy. Examinations in different positions of the leg help to avoid harmful gymnastic exercises.

References

1. Ganz R et al. (1983) In: Hungerford DS (ed) The hip. Mosby, St. Louis
2. Klingmueller V et al. (1987) Fortschr Roentgenstr 146:196–200
3. Schwetlick G et al. (1987) Orthopaede 125 (in press)
4. Xunyuan D et al. (1986) Chirurg 57:340–343

Treatment of Idiopathic Osteonecrosis of the Femoral Head by Free Vascularized Peroneal Graft

H. Judet, J. Judet, and A. Gilbert

Clinique Jouvenet, 6 Square Jouvenet, 75016 Paris, France

We have used the technique of free vascularized peroneal graft for idiopathic necrosis of the femoral head since 1978. A total of 72 hips have been operated, of which 68 have been reviewed during the last 6 months. The average follow-up is 3 years. The oldest cases have been followed up for 7 years, and all the cases have at least 1 year follow-up.

Technic

The femoral head is anteriorly dislocated. The necrosed bone is totally removed. The cavity is filled with autogenous spongious bone surrounding a segment of the opposite fibula vascularized by microanastomosis between its pedicle and the anterior circonflex pedicle. The articular cartilage is carefully elevated and replaced over the graft. There is no weight bearing for 6 months.

Results

Of the 68 hips reviewed, 8 were bilateral. Ages ranged from 20 to 60 the average being 35. Postoperative complications were one case of deep sepsis and two of thrombo-phlebitis. The result for these cases were:

- 18 immediately unsuccessful (25%), with persistance of evolution of the necrosis, all reoperated by total hip replacement
- 35 very good and good according to Merle d'Aubigné, Postel scale
- 9 fair
- 6 bad

Correlation between clinical results and pre-operative X-ray stage according to the Marcus and Enneking classification gives:

Stage II and III	78% and 75% good results
Stage IV	60% good results
Stage V	less than 50%

Conclusions

This procedure is indicated in our experience when the sphericity of the femoral head has been preserved and there is still a safe amount of cartilage. In this condition, whatever the extent of the necrosis, the results are good in two-thirds of the cases. This is encouraging considering the fact that most of the patients are young and the results of other possible treatments are disappointing.

Bone Transplantation
Eds.: M. Aebi, P. Regazzoni

Vascularized Periosteal Grafts *

A. C. Masquelet [1], C. Romana [1], and C. V. Penteado [2]

[1] Service de Chirurgie Orthopédique et Réparatrice, Hôpital Trousseau, 26, avenue du Docteur A. Netter, 75012 Paris, France
[2] Anatomy Department, Institute of Biology, State University of Campinas, São Paulo, Brazil

The idea of employing vascularized periosteal grafts (VPG) in orthopaedic and reconstructive surgery is not new, but until now the experimental results concerning their osteogenic capacity have been conflicting [1–3]. Clinically, few cases have been reported [4]. In order to justify VPG in bone healing and reconstruction, we have undertaken anatomical, experimental and clinical studies.

The goal was to determine systematically the possible VPG donor sites on fresh injected specimens. Blood supply of the periosteum of the limbs was studied. The bones investigated were the ilium, femur, tibia, humerus, radius, and ulna.

We tested on 20 rats the association of a VPG with a cancellous bone graft (CBG) in compact bone formation. A musculo-periosteal flap (MPF) was raised from the lower third of the femur and isolated on the descending genicular vascular pedicle. Cancellous bone was harvested from the proximal tibia. We compared bone formation in three situations: (a) a MPF alone, closed up on itself; (b) a CBG buried in a well-vascularized muscular bed; and (c) a composite graft formed by a vascularized MPF wrapped around a CBG. Examinations included X rays, bone scanning, tomodensitometry, verifications of the inclusions after killing the rats, and histology of new bone formation.

We applied our concept of the association between VPG and CBG in five clinical cases of long bone reconstruction or non-united fractures (Table 1). Three patients had previously undergone conventional bone grafting without success.

We discovered many reliable VPG donor sites. These grafts can be employed as free revascularized or as vascularized, pedicled flap. Most of them can include a muscle. Results are summarized in Table 2. This experimental work has shown regular and undoubted results in all cases after 6 weeks. Cancellous bone buried in muscles practically disappeared. Vascularized MPF alone revealed a fine-fibered compact bone formation. And CBG buried into a vascularized MPF produced a fast densification and a significant amount of compact bone.

Our first case was a reconstruction of the ulnar shaft in a 16-year-old boy, 3 years after a post-traumatic osteomyelitis. The free periosteal transplant, 10 cm × 4 cm, was wrapped around the two segments of the ulna to constitute a tubular structure and to restore the continuity of the shaft. Autologous cancellous bone chips were put inside the tube before suturing it, and vessels were anastomosed. Bone healing was acquired 2 months and 3 weeks later (Fig. 1). In all cases, we applied the association of VPG and CBG. In cases 1, 2 and 5, healing was obtained in 3 months or less. In case 4, the lower part of the reconstruction

* Study Grant CNPq Proc. no. = 20.2848/85-BM

Bone Transplantation
Eds.: M. Aebi, P. Regazzoni

Table 1. Clinical case report

	Case	Previous bone grafting	Flaps employed	Healing duration
1	Reconstruction of the ulna	0	Free periosteal flap from the lower third of the femur	2 months, 3 weeks
2	Non-united arthrodesis of the hip	8	Pedicled musculo-periosteal flap from the ilium	3 months
3	Non-united fracture of the midshaft of the femur	2	Pedicled musculo-periosteal flap from the lower third of the femur	4 months
4	Reconstruction of the upper part of the femur	1	Pedicled musculo-periosteal flap from the ilium	5 months (at the upper extremity)
5	Non-united fracture of the proximal humerus	0	Pedicled periosteal flap from the lower third of humerus	2 months

Table 2. Vascularized periosteal grafts donor sites

Donor site	Vascular supply	Pedicled graft	Free graft	Periosteal graft	Musculo-periosteal graft
Upper limb					
Lower third of the humerus	Posterior branch of the deep brachial artery	+	+	+	0
Ulnar shaft, radius shaft	Anterior interosseous artery	+	0	+	0
Lower limb					
Inner aspect of the ilium	Deep circonflex iliac artery	+	+	0	+ (Iliac muscle)
Upper third of the femur	Deep branch of the lateral circumflex artery	+	0	+	
Lower third of the femur	Descending genicular artery	+	+	+	+ (articular muscle of the knee)
	Perforating branch of the deep femoral artery				
Tibial shaft	Tibialis posterior artery (huge branch from)	+ (On the main branch)		+	0
	Tibialis anterior artery (segmental vascular supply)	+ (On the TAA)	+	+	0

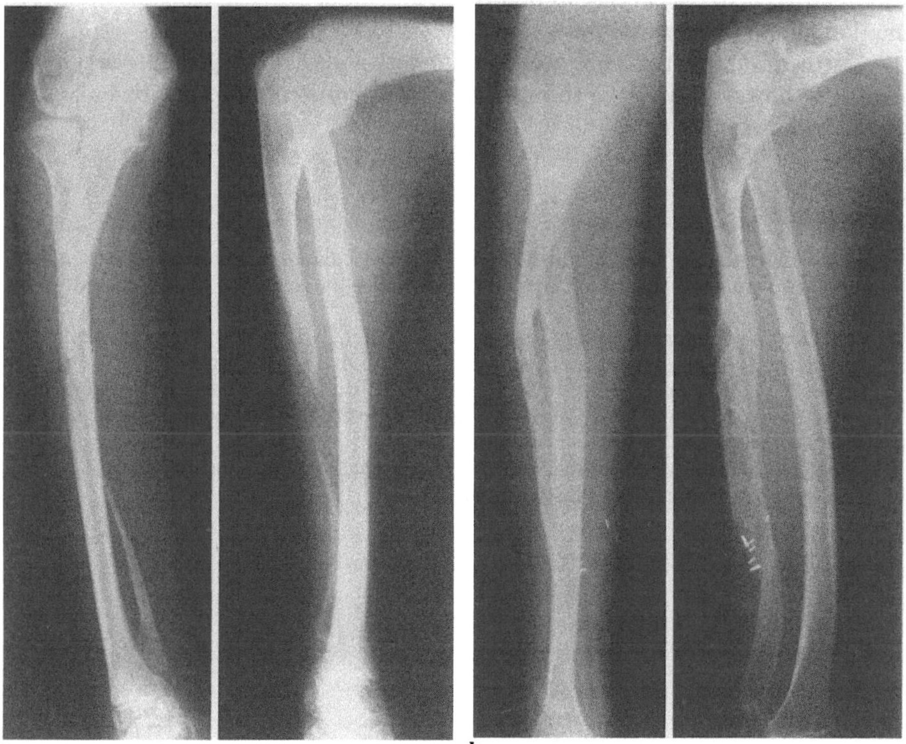

a b

Fig. 1 a and b. Reconstruction of the ulna in a 16-year-old boy. **a** Bone defect of the ulna 3 years (*3Y*) after a post-traumatic osteomyelitis. A free periosteal flap was planned to restore the continuity of the shaft. The periosteal tube was filled up with cancellous bone chips. **b** New compact bone formation was fastly obtained and healing acquired 2 months and 3 weeks (*2M 3W*) after the operative procedure

was not solid at 5 months, but the pedicle of the MPF had been too short to cover this area.

Undoubtedly, there is a relation between the revascularization of a periosteal graft and bone formation, but in the experimental studies reported, the OCP seem to vary with the donor site, and tibial periosteum gives more bone formation than rib periosteum [2]. Prerequisites of stress to bone formation was asserted 10 years ago [1]. Japanese authors have recently shown [3] that VPG produces a significant amount of bone even if not subjected to stress or weight. Moreover, OCP seems to depend on blood circulation, and a vascularized MPF is better than a simple VPG.

In all these previous studies, bone formation from periosteal grafts was effective, but slow and not massive. According to our experimental work and clinical results, it would seem that association of a VPG (or MPF) with cancellous bone gives a fast, compact bone formation. In orthopaedic surgery, clinical experience shows that conventional bone grafting to reconstruct bone defects may fail even in a well-vascularized bed. We think that a vascularized MPF provides a well vascularized bed to a cancellous bone graft and induces a fast, compact bone formation due to the periosteum.

Further investigations are needed to understand the biological process. Nevertheless, however, we have shown that many periosteal flaps can be harvested in the human body.

References

1. Finley JM, Acland RD, Wood MB (1978) Revascularized periosteal grafts: a new method to produce functional new bone without bone grafting. Plast Reconstr Surg 61:1
2. Van Den Wildenberg FAJM, Goris RJA, Tutein MBJE (1984) Free revascularized periosteum transplantation: an experimental study. Br J Plast Surg 37:226
3. Tsuyoshi T, Kiyonori H, Takashi M, Kazuki U, Tohru O (1986) Vascularized periosteal grafts: an experimental study using two different forms of tibial periosteum in rabbits. Plast Reconstr Surg 78:489
4. Satoh T, Tsuchiya M, Harii K (1983) A vascularized iliac musculo-periosteal free flap transfer: a case report. Br J Plast Surg 36:109

Clinical Aspects II: Bone Allografts and Alternatives

Allograft Reconstruction in Revision Total Hip Surgery

R. D. Oakeshott, J. P. McAuley, A. E. Gross, D. A. F. Morgan, D. J. Zukor, J. F. Rudan, and P. J. Brooks

Division of Orthopaedic Surgery, University of Toronto, Toronto, Canada

Introduction

Orthopedic surgeons are encountering increasing numbers of patients with aseptic, time-related loosening of total hip arthroplasties. Compounding the problem is the well-documented loss of bone stock associated with prosthetic loosening and wear particles [1–9]. Conventional methods of reconstruction may be inadequate for such situations [10–13]. Even the option of excision arthroplasty may be lost due to severe bone deficiency.

Allograft bone can be used to reconstruct such severe deficiencies of bone stock and restore some semblance of normal bony architecture. The aim of this prospective study was to determine the clinical results of allograft bone in such reconstructions and to determine the most appropriate use of the various allograft reconstructive modalities.

Materials and Methods

Procurement and Preparation of Allograft Bone. Under sterile operating room conditions, bone is procured from cadaveric donors who conform to the guidelines of the American Association of Tissue Banks [14]. Sterility is assured by (a) cultures of bone surface, marrow, and donor blood; and (b) later irradiation with 2.5 Mrad [15]. From the time of procurement until irradiation, the bone is stored at −20 °C. Once irradiated, it is maintained at −70 °C until utilized. Once selected for use, the allograft is again cultured and then thawed by immersion in half-strength betadine in normal saline.

The Recipient Population. Of the 85 patients who underwent allograft reconstruction of total hip revisions, 72 were available for clinical and radiographic evaluation. Ages ranged from 28 to 88 years, with an average of 58 years; 68% were female. Seven patients required bilateral reconstructions. An average of 2.5 hip procedures were performed on each patient.

The commonest underlying etiology was osteoarthritis (29 patients), followed by hip dysplasia (11 patients). The sequelae of femoral neck fractures resulted in the primary arthroplasty in 9 patients. Numerous other etiologies were encountered, including Legg-Perthes disease, hemophilia, epiphyseal dysplasia, primary bone tumors, infantile sepsis, villonodular synovitis, tuberculosis, achondroplasia, and fibrous dysplasia.

All patients were prospectively followed using a modified Harris Hip Rating Protocol [16]. A failure constituted an increase of less than 20 points in the hip

Bone Transplantation
Eds.: M. Aebi, P. Regazzoni

score or a complication related to the allograft resulting in reoperation. Anteroposterior and lateral radiographs were obtained preoperatively and sequentially postoperatively. The radiographs were evaluated following the techniques of DeLee and Charnley (acetabulum) [17] and Gruen et al. (Femoral) [18]. Evidence was sought of union of host bone to allograft for intact allografts (as evidenced by bridging trabeculae) and consolidation of morsellized allograft (the development of similar radiodensity as the surrounding host bone). Migration of allografts and implants was also assessed. Because of the inevitable variations in projections and positioning in sequential radiographs, a positional change of up to 3 mm was not considered significant. Femoral and acetabular lucencies were felt to be significant if greater than 2 mm or progressive.

Both acetabular and femoral deficiencies were encountered, and 32 patients required reconstruction of both levels of deficiency. Acetabular deficiencies were frequent, resulting in 69 reconstructions, of which 31 were performed for protrusio, 18 for shelf defects (coverage), and 20 for major defects (column deficiencies or total acetabular insufficiency). Femoral reconstruction was required in 43 cases, predominantly for calcar deficiencies (26 grafts) or complete proximal femoral insufficiency (12 grafts). The remaining 5 grafts were cortical struts for reconstitution of a lateral femoral cortical defect.

Surgical Techniques

Preoperative planning was performed in all cases using routine radiographs and, if needed to clarify the deficiency, various combinations of Judet views, inlet and outlet views, and computerized axial tomography. A modification of the lateral transgluteal approach was used, with additional femoral or acetabular exposure as required. Trochanteric osteotomy was used if required in a difficult exposure.

Several principles were carefully followed in fixation of the allografts. Solid acetabular allografts were fixed to host bone with 6.5-mm cancellous screws with washers. The metallic femoral component was cemented to the allograft prior to insertion. Either this alloimplant was impacted into the host bone, or the host bone was longitudinally osteotomized and used to envelope the allograft. In the latter case fixation was obtained with cerclage wires. Rotational stability was frequently achieved by producing a step-cut osteotomy at the junction of allograft and host bone. Rarely was an antirotation plate utilized. All host–recipient bone interfaces were autogenously grafted to promote union, and extreme care was taken to avoid the interposition of cement between allograft and host bone. Cementing into host bone was similarly avoided.

Clinical Results

Improvements in hip scores averaged 41 points. Wide ranges of both preoperative scores (6–61 points) and postoperative scores (21–95) were encountered. Twelve cases were considered as failures. Seven failed to improve their scores by the requisite 20 points. Seven patients required reoperation for complications related to the allograft and were thus failures. However, five went on to become clinical successes. Three of the seven sustained fractures of calcar grafts, which were revised with good results. Two suffered acetabular component dislocations: one from excessive medial morsellized grafting which was successfully salvaged and the second with a shelf reconstruction and calcar allograft which because of persistent instability resulted in excision arthroplasty and clinical failure (improvement of 15 points).

There were also complications not directly related to the allograft, as expected in any group of revision arthroplasty patients [20–23]. Three patients developed radiographically confirmed deep vein thromboses, with two resulting in nonfatal pulmonary emboli. One patient with a history of deep vein thrombosis developed another postoperatively despite anticoagulant prophylaxis. Two patients sustained culture-proven superficial wound infections which were treated successfully with antibiotics and did not recur. Two deep infections resulted in excision arthroplasty. Both these patients had undergone anterior approaches, with subsequent wound dehiscence and positive cultures for *Streptococcus* (*viridans* and *faecalis*). One went on to an excellent functional result with the excision arthroplasty; however, the second improved by only 4 points from the original score. It should be noted that both patients had undergone four previous operations prior to the initial allograft reconstruction.

Reoperation was required in one patient for evacuation of a hematoma, and in a second for removal of a retained plastic drain. Intraoperative fractures were produced in four patients. Three femoral fractures were appropriately treated by internal fixation. The fourth, an extremely osteoporotic female, sustained a proximal tibial fracture while the limb was being prepped and draped for surgery.

One mortality occurred. This patient was 70-year-old woman who dislocated the total hip 1 month after surgery and succumbed to a pneumonia that developed after open reduction and further reconstruction.

Radiographic Analysis

Acetabular Allograft Reconstructions

Reconstruction in Protrusio Acetabulae. Medial defects were reconstituted with 31 allografts, usually morsellized femoral head (24 cases). Femoral head slices were used in 5 cases and in isolated cases morsellized tibia and rib. Polymethylmethacrylate (PMMA) was utilized to augment fixation of the acetabular component in 14 grafts and metal ring or mesh in 14. Cementless acetabular components were used in 17 cases. Of the 31 grafts, 30 were consolidated radiographically. Prosthetic migration was detected in 11 grafts. Notably, 8 of the 9 bipolar cementless prostheses migrated, in contrast to only 2 of the 14 cemented prostheses and 1 of the 6 cementless acetabular components. Radiolucencies exceeding 2 mm were found in 4 cemented acetabulae, without clinical symptoms.

Acetabular Shelf Reconstructions. In the 18 shelf allografts, appropriately shaped segments of femoral heads were fixed to host bone with 6.5-mm cancellous screws, with cancellous autografting of host–donor interfaces (Fig. 1). All 12 cases with a follow-up period longer than 8 months clearly demonstrated radiographic

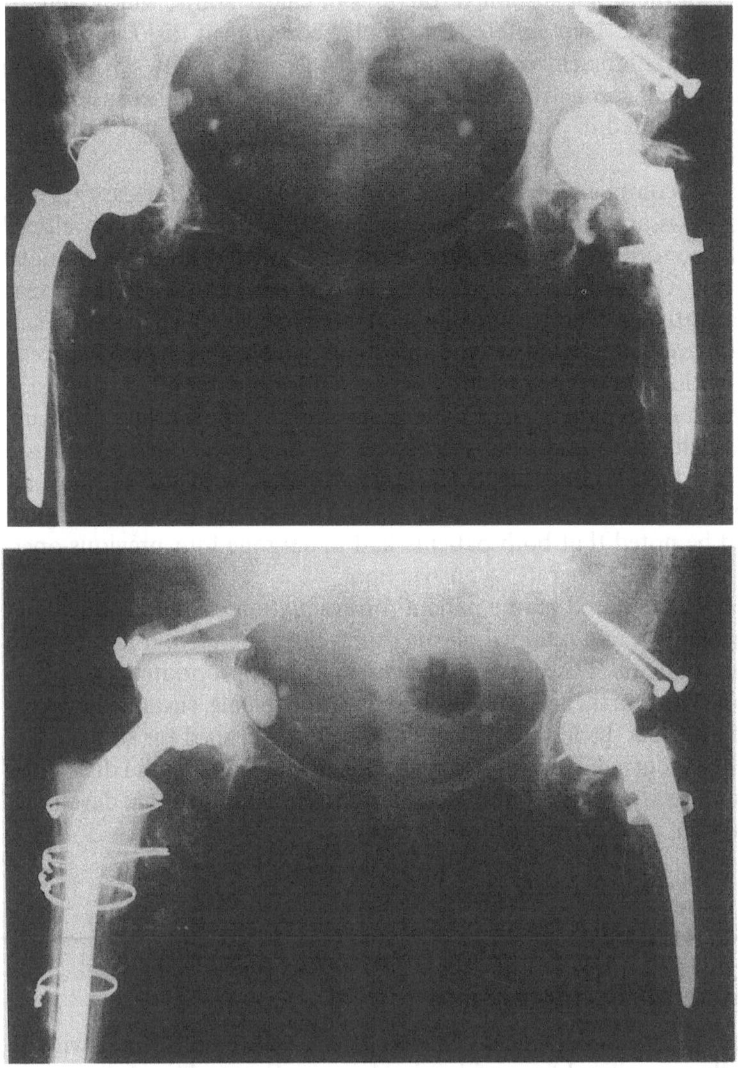

a

b

Fig. 1 a and b. Preoperative **a** and postoperative **b** radiographs of a 67-year-old woman who had previously undergone bilateral total hip arthroplasties for congenital hip dysplasia and presented with severe right hip pain. She was reconstructed with a large-fragment femoral allograft and acetabular shelf allograft. Her postoperative radiograph demonstrates the acetabular shelf allograft fixed to host bone by 6.5-mm cancellous screws, with a fixed acetabular component. Her femoral deficiency was reconstructed with a large fragment femoral allograft, step-cut osteotomy at the host allograft junction, and retention of the host proximal femur as an envelope

union. No fractures were detected. However, one graft completely resorbed. Localized bone resorption was found in 5 cases, confined only to areas of the graft not involved in stress transfer. The two bipolar prostheses in this group again migrated (4 mm and 1 mm), in contrast to the absence of migration in the remaining 16 cases. No significant radiolucencies were encountered.

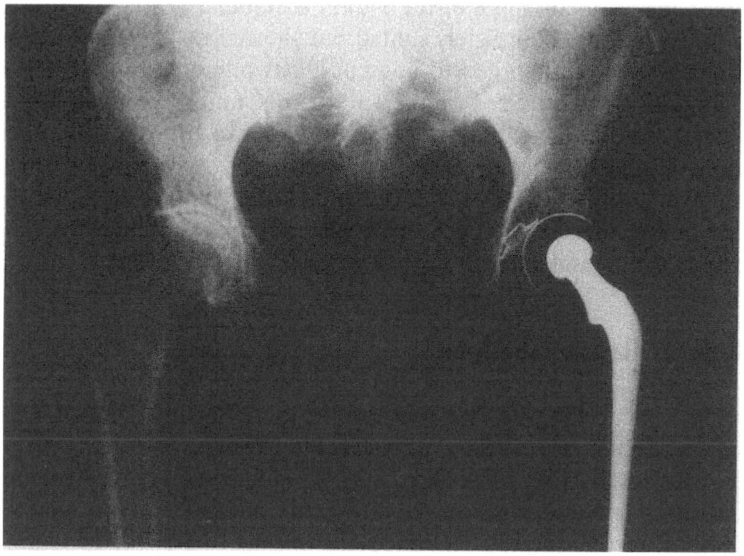

a

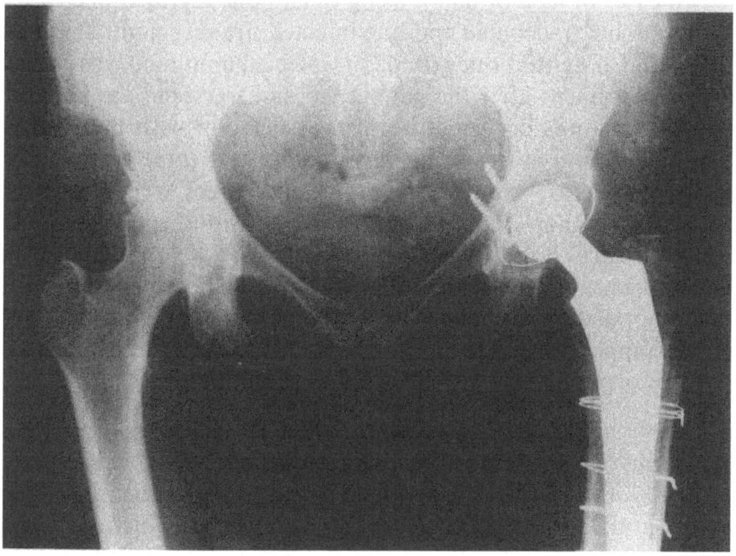

b

Fig. 2 a and b. Preoperative **a** and postoperative **b** radiographs of a 69-year-old woman with osteoarthritis. Her failed left total hip had obvious calcar and lateral femoral cortical deficiencies which were reconstructed. The 1-year postoperative radiograph reveals union of the lateral cortical strut graft and partial resorption of the calcar graft with an excellent clinical result

Column and Total Acetabular Reconstruction. Eleven femoral head segments were used to reconstruct acetabular column deficiencies, and 9 had extensive deficiencies necessitating reconstruction with total acetabular allografts. Naturally, all required some internal fixation [24]. Cement augmentation was required in only 6 cases, 5 of which also had a modular support ring [16, 25]. Radiological union was evident in 15 grafts, including 8 of the 9 total acetabular grafts. Two of the femoral head grafts had not completely united but showed no evidence of component loosening. Three grafts failed to unite at all, two femoral head and one total acetabular graft. One required excision for sepsis, and the remaining two continued to be asymptomatic with no signs of failure of fixation or component loosening. Implant migration occurred in four cases, again, all with bipolar prostheses. The infected graft exhibited partial resorption and component loosening. One cementless acetabular component demonstrated radiographic loosening, confirmed at reoperation and correction with a cemented component.

Femoral Allograft Reconstructions

Calcar Allografts. Calcar allografts were defined as those having a medial longitudinal axis of less than 5 cm, used to reconstruct defects above the level of the inferior edge of the lesser trochanter (Fig. 2, 3). In all, 26 such reconstructions were performed using femoral calcar and tibial metadiaphyseal allograft bone. Of the 7 tibial allograft reconstructions, 5 united, in contrast to 8 of the 19 femoral allografts. The two cases of lack of union using tibial bone revealed one case of questionable radiographic tracebulae and one infected, frankly nonunited case. Similarly in the femoral allograft bone group, one infected nonunion was excised. Another required replacement after the patient fell and fractured the allograft. Two other allograft fractures occurred, both in association with non unions. Femoral graft subsidence into host bone 1–2 cm occurred in three cases of nonunions. Resorption of the graft was observed in varying degrees in eight cases. Six of these were in grafts less than 2 cm in length, and the two others were in 3-cm grafts compromised by drill holes. There were 12 instances of subsidence of the metal femoral component; 11 migrated more than 1 cm and occurred in cases reconstructed with femoral allograft bone. The subsidence was evident between the allograft/cemented component and the host. In cementless cases, it resulted from proximal allograft resorption and a subsidence into the allograft.

Large-Fragment Femoral Reconstructions. Eight allograft femora and four allograft tibial meta/diaphyseal segments were utilized to reconstruct deficient proximal femora (see Fig. 1). Two-thirds had component-to-allograft cementing. Three of the four tibial allografts united; the fourth was the only one in which a dynamic compression plate was used for stability, and it did not unite. Four of the eight femoral reconstructions united radiologically, with three others clinically stable in the surrounding envelope of host femur. Graft absorption was not observed. Migration occurred in only two cases, both in uncemented femoral allograft reconstructions. In one case the metal component subsided within the allograft. The second case demonstrated host bone fracture, with subsidence into the host bone by the alloimplant.

Lateral Femoral Cortical Reconstructions. For deficiencies in the lateral cortex of the host femur, tibial or femoral diaphyseal bone was cerclaged over the defect in five cases. Three united completely, and one at a single end. The fifth resorbed completely in the absence of sepsis.

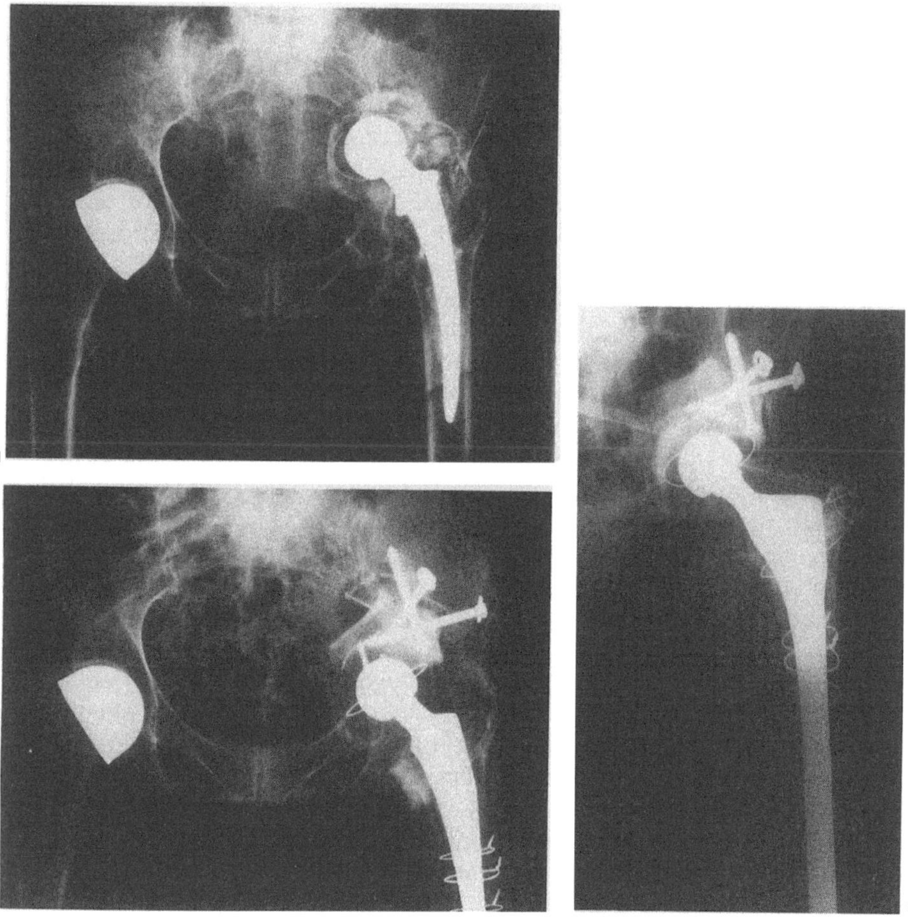

a b c

Fig. 3 a–c. Preoperative **a** and postoperative **b** radiographs of a 55-year-old rheumatoid arthritic who presented with a failed left total hip severe protrusio. Her 9-month postoperative film demonstrates the total acetabular and femoral calcar allografts. She subsequently fell and fractured the calcar allograft, resulting in painful loosening of the femoral component. She was successfully revised **c** to a long-stem femoral component with a new calcar graft. Her acetabular component was loose at operation, but excellent acetabular allograft union and integrity were present. This allowed relatively easy revision of the acetabular and femoral components because of the increased bone stock and lack of cement in host bone

Discussion

The results of allografting are appearing increasingly as experience in this relatively new modality develops [12, 13, 26–30]. The greatest advantage of these techniques over conventional reconstruction is the restoration of bony architecture. Likely due to very slow revascularization and remodeling, the allografts are able to maintain structural integrity under physiologic loading [31]. Naturally, rates of union comparable to those obtained with autografts will not be obtained. However, with autogenous bone augmentation the great majority of allografts obtain bony continuity with host bone. The use of allograft bone does not appear to increase complications or the risk of postoperative sepsis when compared with other revision series [21, 22, 32].

In cases of reconstructions of protrusio acetabulae the greatest problem was recurrence of the deformity, with loss of allograft and host bone with time. Bipolar prostheses were particularly problematic and were responsible for 8 of the 11 cases of recurrence. No migration occurred if femoral head slices or segments were used to reconstruct the defect, even in the absence of protrusio ring supplementation.

The technique of shelf reconstructions has proven successful, particularly when appropriate graft shaping and fixation are performed. Bipolar prosthetic use again resulted in migration into the graft, but both cemented and cementless fixed acetabular components gave comparable good results.

The success with acetabular reconstructions was particularly encouraging. Despite the larger deficiencies encountered in the use of this technique, union rates and clinical success are comparable to those with the femoral shelf grafts. Technically the surgery utilizing total acetabular grafts is no more exacting than that in femoral head grafts and has the advantage of easier component placement and bicortical structural integrity.

Concerning calcar allograft reconstruction, regardless of the type of allograft bone (tibia or femur) small size and compromise with drill holes resulted in increased graft resorption. Cementing of the allograft to metal implant resulted in an absence of fractures and decreased graft resorption. The use of tibial bone seems to be superior to femoral allograft bone in the reconstruction of calcar defects; the reasons for this are not clear. The numbers are small, and the difference may simply relate to the relative ease of shaping tibial meta/diaphysis to fit host and prosthesis. The cement/allograft composite seems to function well. The allograft acts as a biological collar transmitting forces to host bone and allowing union to it.

In large femoral reconstruction stability is obviously essential for clinical performance and union of the allograft to host. This is optimally obtained with a minimum of metallic fixation, using rather a step-cut junction between allograft and host healthy diaphyseal bone. Host bone is not sacrificed. The deficient proximal femur is retained for use as a surrounding vascularized envelope for the allograft; this provided additional stability in 25% of cases. Again, cement fixation of the metallic implant to allograft provides additional stability and protection from subsidence and fracture.

In lateral femoral cortical reconstruction the technically undemanding technique of the use of diaphyseal allograft bone to reconstruct host lateral cortical deficiency has proven very successful.

Summary

Despite the obvious difficulties encountered in total hip revisions with deficient bone stock, an 85% overall success rate was obtained in the 72 patients reviewed.

Adherence to the following principles optimizes chances for the lasting success in allograft reconstructions in total hip revisions:

1. A fixed acetabular component is the most appropriate implant for use with morsellized protrusio allografts.
2. Femoral head segments used in protrusio and shelf reconstructions give excellent results.
3. Major acetabular defects are more easily corrected with total acetabular allografts rather than multiple femoral head segments, with comparably good results.
4. The optimum use of calcar allografts requires allografts which are longer than 2 cm and are cemented to the implant but not host bone.
5. Stability of large femoral grafts should be achieved by a step-cut junction between allograft and healthy host diaphyseal bone, augmented by retention of the host proximal femur to function as an envelope, stabilized with cerclage wires.
6. Long-stem femoral components should be cemented to the allograft but not to host bone and provide additional stability to the host allograft junction.
7. The violation of femoral allografts by drill holes should be avoided to decrease resorption and fracture.
8. All host allograft junctions should be kept clear of cement and autogenously bone-grafted to facilitate union.
9. A fully equipped bone bank is a necessity for undertaking these modalities of reconstruction.

References

1. Freeman MAR, Bradley GW, Revell PA (1982) Observations upon the interface between bone and polymethylmethacrylate cement. J Bone Joint Surg [Br] 64:489
2. Goldring SR, Jasty M, Roelke MS, Rourke CM, Bringhurst FR, Harris WH (1986) Formation of a synovial-like membrane at the bone-cement interface. Arthritis Rheum 29:836
3. Goldring SR, Schiller AL, Roelke M, Rourke Cm, O'Neill DA, Harris WH (1983) The synovial-like membrane at the bone-cement interface in loose total hip replacements and its proposed role in bone lysis. J Bone Joint Surg [Am] 65:575
4. Goodman SB, Schatzker J, Sumner-Smith G, Fornasier VL, Geften N, Hunt C (1985) The effect of polymethylmethacrylate on bone: an experimental study. Arch Orthop Trauma Surg 104:150
5. Howie D, Oakeshott R, Manthy B, Vernon-Roberts B (1987) Bone resorption in the presence of polyethylene wear particles. J Bone Joint Surg [Br] 69:165
6. Jasty MJ, Floyd WE, Schiller AL, Goldring SR, Harris WH (1986) Localized osteolysis in stable, non septic total hip replacement. J Bone Joint Surg [Am] 68:912
7. Linder L, Lindberg L, Carlsson A (1983) Aseptic loosening of hip prostheses. Clin Orthop 175:93
8. Pazzaglia UE, Ceciliani L, Wilkinson MJ, Dell'Orbo C (1985) Involvement of metal particles in loosening of metal plastic total hip prostheses. Arch Orthop Trauma Surg 104:164
9. Revell PA, Weightman B, Freeman MAR, Vernon-Roberts B (1978) The production and biology of polyethylene wear debris. Arch Orthop Trauma Surg 91:167
10. Harris WH (1982) Allografting in total hip arthroplasty. Clin Orthop 162:150
11. McGann W, Mankin HJ, Harris WH (1986) Massive allografting for severe failed total hip replacement. J Bone Joint Surg [Am] 68:4

12. Mnaymneh W, Malinin T, Yead W, Borja F, Burkhalter W, Ballard W, Zych G, Reyes F (1986) Massive osseus and osteoarticular allograft in nontumorous disorders. Contemp Orthop 13(3):13
13. Trancik TM, Stulberg BN, Wilde AH, Feiglin DH (1986) Allograft reconstruction of the acetabulum during revision total hip arthroplasty. J Bone Joint Surg [Am] 68:527
14. American Association of Tissue Banks (1979) Guidelines for the banking of musculoskeletal tissue. Am Assoc Tissue Banks Newsletter 3:2
15. Freidlander GE, Mankin HJ, Sell KW (eds) (1983) Osteochondral allografts, biology, banking and clinical applications. Little Brown, Boston, p 223
16. Gross AE, Lavoie MV, McDermott AGP, Marks P (1985) The use of allograft bone in revision of total hip arthroplasty. Clin Orthop 197:115
17. De Lee JG, Charnley J (1976) Radiological demarcation of cemented sockets in total hip replacement. Clin Orthop 121:20
18. Gruen TA, McNeice GM, Amstutz HC (1979) Modes of failure of cemented stem type femoral components. Clin Orthop 141:17
19. Hardinge K (1982) The direct lateral approach to the hip. J Bone Joint Surg [Br] 64:17
20. Ejsted R, Olsen NJ (1987) Revision of failed total hip arthroplasty. J Bone Joint Surg [Br] 69:57
21. Weber FA, Lautenbach EEG (1986) Revision of infected total hip arthroplasty. Clin Orthop 211:108
22. Wroblewski BM (1986) One stage revision of infected cemented total hip arthroplasty. Clin Orthop 211:103
23. Eftekhar NS, Tzitzikalakis GI (1986) Failures and re-operations following low friction arthroplasty of the hip. Clin Orthop 211:65
24. Harris WH, Crothers O, Oh I (1977) Total hip replacement and femoral head bone grafting for severe acetabular deficiency in adults. J Bone Joint Surg [Am] 59:752
25. Oh I, Harris WH (1982) Design concepts, indications, and surgical techniques for use of the protrusio shell. Clin Orthop 162:174
26. Borja FJ, Mnaymneh W (1985) Bone allografts in salvage of difficult hip arthroplasties. Clin Orthop 197:123
27. Gross AE, McKee N, Farine I, Czitrom A, Langer F (1984) Reconstruction of skeletal defects following en bloc excision of bone tumors. In: Uhthoff HK, Stahl E (eds) Current concepts of diagnosis and treatment of bone and soft tissue tumors. Springer, Berlin Heidelberg New York, p 163
28. Mankin HJ, Doppelt SH, Sullivan TR, Tomford WW (1982) Osteoarticular and intercalary allograft transplantation in the management of malignant tumors of bone. Cancer 50(4):613
29. Parrish FF (1973) Allograft replacement of all or part of the end of a long bone following excision of a tumor. J Bone Joint Surg [Am] 55:1
30. Scott RD (1984) Use of a bipolar prosthesis with bone grafting in acetabular reconstruction. Contemp Orthop 9(3):35
31. Kandel RA, Gross AE, Ganel A, McDermott AGP, Langer F, Pritzker KPH (1985) Histophatology of failed osteoarticular shell allografts. Clin Orthop 197:103
32. Tomford WW, Starkweather RJ, Goldman MH (1981) A study of the clinical incidence of infection in the use of banked allograft bone. J Bone Joint Surg [Am] 63:244

Long-Term Results of Osteoarticular Allografts in Weight-Bearing Joints

B. A. Waber, W. W. Tomford, H. J. Mankin, and L. A. Butterfield

Massachusetts General Hospital, Department of Orthopaedics,
Boston, Massachusetts, 02114, USA

Introduction

The long-term results of osteoarticular allografts used in weight-bearing joints are not well documented due to a lack of a sufficient number and follow-up of patients in most series. Lexer (1925) reported a 50% failure rate of such grafts [1] with follow-up of approximately 2.5 years. Parrish reported good results in 68% of his 16 patients with an average follow-up of 5 years [2]. We have reviewed a group of 104 patients who had an osteoarticular transplant at the hip or knee with a minimum 3-year follow-up and maximum 16-year follow-up. This study was performed in an attempt to document more clearly the results after transplantation of these grafts and to determine what factors most affected results.

Materials and Methods

From a series of 218 patients who had transplants of massive allografts between 1971 and 1983, we reviewed 115 consecutive patients who had large osteoarticular allografts involving part or all of the articular surface of one side of a major weight-bearing joint. Eleven patients who died of metastatic disease early in the course of their treatment were eliminated from the series to provide 104 patients (112 allografts) that had a minimum follow-up time of 3 years. Allografts studied included hemipelvises (3), proximal femurs (9), distal femurs (65), and proximal tibias (35). The average of the patients was 31 years with a range from 11 to 67 years. Average follow-up was 6 years, with a maximum of 16 years. There were 45 men and 59 women. The original diagnosis was a primary bone tumor in 91 patients and a nontumor condition in 13 patients. Nontumor conditions included traumatic defects (7), osteonecrosis (5), and pigmented villonodular synovitis (1). Six of the patients with tumors had a second allograft, and two of these patients had a third allograft. Giant cell tumor was the most frequent tumor diagnosis, accounting for 63% of the tumor patients. Osteosarcoma (parosteal and central) accounted for 18% and chondrosarcoma accounted for 10%. The knee was involved in 92 patients and the proximal femur or hemipelvis in 12 patients. All grafts were procured from cadavers according to guidelines promulgated by the American Association of Tissue Banks.

Proximal femoral grafts had approximately 1 in. of abductor tendon and capsule attached to the graft, and distal femoral grafts had approximately one-half the length of the medial collateral and lateral collateral ligaments attached to the graft along with 2–3 in. of the posterior capsule which was sewn to the host cap-

Bone Transplantation
Eds.: M. Aebi, P. Regazzoni

Table 1. Transplant grading system

Excellent:	Pain-free, with no recurrence of disease, normal limb function and able to return to normal activities with minimal limitations.
Good:	Restoration to limited but functional range of motion and strength, and without pain. Patients returned to most activities without brace or support, excluding active sports.
Fair:	A functional deficit which required brace or support. Patients were unable to return to preoperative activities or work.
Failure:	Any patient requiring an amputation or removal of the graft for infection, fracture, or recurrence of the tumor.

sule. Cruciate ligaments when excised for tumor control were not reconstructed. Proximal tibial grafts had one-half of the medial collateral ligament (superficial) attached and the entire length of the patella tendon from the tibial tubercle to just distal to the patella. All cartilage surfaces were cryoprotected with 10% dimethysulfoxide (DMSO).

Two methods of assessment were used to rate the results of the transplants. In the first method, patients were assessed at each office visit by the operating surgeon with the use of a grading system previously developed and described [3]. Patients were rated either excellent, good, fair, or failure depending on recurrence of their disease, use of their limb, and return to normal activities with varying limitations (Table 1). The second method of assessment was based on radiographic examinations which included the graft, the osteosynthesis site, and the joint at two different postoperative intervals: (a) immediately after implantation and (b) the most recent office visit. If subsequent surgery, including joint replacement, was necessary, X-rays used were thosen taken just before the second procedure. Analysis of the roentgenograms was performed by using scoring systems for both the immediately postoperative (Table 2) and follow-up assessments (Table 3). Radiographs of 20 fracture/nonunion cases and all 11 joint replacement cases were compared with a control group of 33 patients who had excellent or good results with no complications.

The immediate postoperative X-ray assessment first evaluated the osteosynthesis site (junction between the host bone and the allograft). A gap of less than a 1 mm received 3 points, a gap of 1.0–1.5 mm received 2 points, a gap of 1.5–2.0 mm received 1 point, and a gap greater than 2 mm received 0 points. Second, the osteosynthesis technique was evaluated on the basis of AO recommended procedures [4] in accord with the number of cortices fixed by screws, contouring of the plate to the bone, and alignment of the bones at the osteosynthesis site. Third, an evaluation of the joint space between the allograft and the host bone was performed. An anatomic fit was given 3 points, a minor mismatch with less than 2 mm overlap at either side of the joint on an anteroposterior X-ray was given 2 points, a mismatch equal to or greater than 2 mm but less than 4 mm was given 1 point, and a mismatch where the total was considered to be greater than or equal to 4 mm was given 0 points.

Table 2. Osteoarticular allografts: initial radiological evaluation score

	Points
Appearance of osteosynthesis site	
Gap <1 mm	3
Gap <1.0–1.5 mm	2
Gap <1.5–2.0 mm	1
Gap >2.0 mm	0
Fixation evaluation (AO protocol)	
Optimal	3
Minor modification	2
Major modification	1
Unstable	0
Joint space	
Anatomic (0)	3
Minor mismatch (<2 mm)	2
Moderate mismatch (2–4 mm)	1
Major mismatch (>4 mm)	0

Table 3. Osteoarticular allografts: final radiological evaluation score

	Points
Time to healing of osteosynthesis site	
Less than 1 year	3
1–2 years	2
More than 2 years	1
No healing	0
Bone resorption	
Allograft more dense than host	4
Allograft equal to host	3
Slight allograft resorption compared to host	2
Moderate allograft resorption	1
Fracture	0
Fixation evaluation	
No complication	3
Minor complication	2
Major complication	1
Failure (removal)	0
Joint space	
No change	3
Mild narrowing/small osteophytes	2
Narrowed/osteophyte	1
Collapsed (Charcot-like)	0

For the follow-up X-ray analysis, the time of healing of the osteosynthesis site was scored first. Three points were given if healing occurred at less than 1 year, 2 points if healing occurred between 1 and 2 years, 1 point if healing took more than 2 years, and no points if there had been no healing by 3 years. Second, a category of bone resorption compared the X-ray appearance of the allograft with the contiguous host bone. In this evaluation, 4 points were given if an allograft appeared more dense than the host bone, 3 points if it appeared the same as the host bone, 2 points if it appeared to have minimal resorption compared to the host bone, 1 point if the allograft appeared to have moderate resorption compared to the host bone, and complete resorption (fracture) was given 0 points. Third, the osteosynthesis site was evaluated for evidence of complications. Three points were given for no complications. Minor complications such as screw or plate loosening without change in the alignment of the bones at the osteosynthesis site was given 2 points. Any major complication such as hardware failure and subluxation or dislocation of the joint received 1 point. Either failure which necessitated removal of the allograft or another operation such as an arthrodesis, received 0 points. Fourth, the joint space was assessed. A joint space assessed as no change from the original received 3 points, mild narrowing with small osteophytes received 2 points, narrowing with large osteophytes received 1 point, and a collapse or Charcot-like joint received 0 points.

Clinical Results

Of the 112 allografts followed for a minimum of 3 years, 56 had an excellent, 25 had a good, 10 had a fair end result and 21 allograft procedures were failures. Excellent and good results were distributed evenly among women and men. Results for anatomic areas were essentially the same: 73% excellent and good results in allograft procedures around the knee compared to 67% similar results for procedures involving the hemipelvis or hip. Of the allograft procedures performed for tumors, 19% (17/91) failed, and the same percent (19%, 4/21) of procedures performed for nontumor problems failed.

Complications following allograft surgery occurred in 46 patients (44%) (Table 4, 4a). These complications included local tumor recurrence, fractures, delayed union or nonunion, and infection. Seventeen of these 46 patients had more than one complication.

Six local tumor recurrences were noted. Four patients had a giant cell tumor which recurred, and two patients had a parosteal osteosarcoma which recurred. The treatment was wide excision in two patients, wide excision and reallograft in three patients, and amputation in one patient.

Of the four major complications encountered, fracture was the most frequent, occurring in 22% (25/112) of cases. Five of the fractures occurred in allografts of the hemipelvis or proximal femur, and 20 occurred in allografts around the knee (distal femur or proximal tibia, with the split being approximately 50% on each side). Mean time from initial surgery to allograft fracture was 23 months. Following treatment, which consisted of autograft with or without replating (17 cases), total joint replacement (5 cases), or reallograft (3 cases), the result was good in 9 cases (36%). The remaining 16 were rated as fair or failure requiring a second or third revision, but no amputations were performed for fracture problems.

Table 4. Complications

Local tumor recurrence	6/91 patients (7%)
Giant cell tumor	4/57
Parosteal osteosarcoma	2/12
Fracture	25/112 allographs (22%)
Hemipelvis/proximal femur	5/12
Distal femur	11/65
Proximal tibia	9/35
Nonunion	13/112 allographs (12%)
Hemipelvis/proximal femur	1/12
Distal femur	10/65
Proximal tibia	2/35
Infection	15/104 patients (14%)
Hemipelvis/proximal femur	2/12
Distal femur	9/59
Proximal tibia	4/33
Total number of complications	46/104 patients (44%)

Table 4a. Complication rate vs. diagnosis

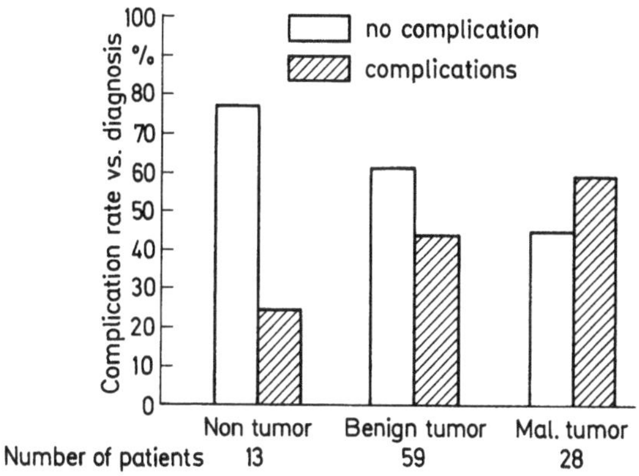

Nonunion occurred in 12% of cases (13/112). Treatment consisted of autograft and replating (6), reallograft (5) and joint replacement (2). All nonunion cases in which reallograft or joint replacement was necessary had a second complication of either fracture or infection. End results were excellent or good in seven of these cases (54%).

In the ratings based on radiographic examinations, patients who had a fracture or nonunion showed no differences in compression at the osteosynthesis site or fixation when compared to the ratings of patients in the control group who had a good or excellent result and no complications. There was a difference in time to healing of the osteosynthesis site of the fracture/nonunion group, which was delayed about 1 year compared to the control group. Slight resorption was noted in the fracture/nonunion group, compared to no resorption in the uncomplicated allografts. No difference between the two groups was noted in the final assessment of fixation.

Fifteen patients developed an infection (Table 5), five of these almost immediately postoperatively (within 1 month). Organisms cultured in these cases included *Staphylococcus aureus* (2), *Escherichia coli* (1), enterococcus (1), and *Bacteroides* (1). Ten patients developed an infection several weeks to several months postoperatively. Organisms cultured in these cases included *S. epidermidis* (8), *S. aureus* (1), and *Pseudomonas* (1).

Of the five early infections, one of these patients had an extensive skin slough shortly after surgery which may have been related to the infection. Of the remaining ten infections, all of which were considered late infections, eight followed additional procedures such as autogenous graft for a nonunion, muscle flaps, or skin grafts for wound healing problems, or excision of soft tissue tumor recurrence.

In this group of 15 infections, one healed with débirdement and antibiotics, and one developed chronic drainage. Six allografts were removed, but replaced with new allograft. Seven patients had an amputation. Two of the 15 patients with infection ultimately had an excellent result and three patients had a good result. The remaining ten cases were rated as failures.

Table 5. Infections in weight-bearing allografts

Patient	Time to infection	Prior procedures	Organism	Treatment and result	Rating
C.H.	1 month	–	*Enterococcus*	Allo. removal/ reallograft	E
R.L.	1 month	Skin slough	*Bacteroides*	Graft removal/ reallograft	P
R.M.	1.5 months	–	*E. coli/pseudomonas*	Débridement/ amputation	P
C.M.	1 month	–	*S. aureus*	Allo. removal/ amputation	P
S.M.	1 month	–	*S. aureus*	Allo. removal/ reallograft	E
C.B.	17 months	Graft + replate	*S. epidermidis*	Allo. removal/ new allo.	P
C.C.	36 months	–	*S. epidermidis*	Débridement/ healed	G
B.D.	12 months	Full-thickness loss	*S. epidermidis*	Débridement/ amputation	P
N.F.	10 months	Full-thickness loss	*Enterobacter/ S. aureus*	Débridement/ amputation	P
G.H.	22 months	Autograft for nonunion	*S. epidermidis*	Débridement/persistent drainage	G
R.M.	3 months	Open fixation	*Pseudomonas*	Débridement/ amputation	P
M.N.	17 months	p̄ Third allo. for fixation/nonunion	*S. epidermidis*	Débridement/ amputation	P
A.P.	22 months	–	*S. epidermidis*	Graft removal/ joint replacement	P
S.R.	7 months	p̄ Autograft for fracture	*S. epidermidis*	Débridement/allo. arthrodesis	G
L.T.	6 months	p̄ Excision of local recurrence	*S. epidermidis*	Débridement/ amputation	P

Joint deterioration resulting in joint replacement was not considered a complication, but the incidence was analyzed for this study. Eleven patients (Table 6) had a joint replacement of the joint in which an allograft was used (11%). Four of these had joint fragmentation, and five had allograft fractures. The replacements were performed in 1 of 3 hemipelvis, 2 of 9 proximal femoral, 7 of 65 distal femoral, and 1 of 35 proximal tibial allografts. Eight of the 11 arthroplasties were performed within 3 years of the original allograft transplant, and ten were performed within 5 years.

Cemented total hip replacements were performed for the failed hemipelvis and two proximal femoral allografts. One of the femoral allografts lasted for 4 years, and the other for 9 years before replacement was necessary. The hemipelvis allograft included a proximal femoral allograft from the same donor; nonetheless, this "anatomic" joint failed at 3.5 years.

Cemented total knee replacements were performed for failed distal femoral and proximal tibial allografts. Six of the seven femoral allografts that necessitated

Table 6. Failed allografts resulting in joint replacement

Patient	Diagnosis	Type of graft	Time to joint replacement	Type of joint replacement
K.P.	GCT	Hemipelvis/ proximal femur	2.5 years	THR
E.F.	CHSA	Proximal femur	9 years	THR
R.M.	GCT	Proximal femur	4 years	THR
L.B.	GCT	Distal femur	5 years	TKR
J.C.	Trauma	Distal femur	3.5 years	TKR
L.O.	PAROSA	Distal femur	3 years	TKR
F.O.	GCT	Distal femur	2 years	TKR
K.P.	GCT	Distal femur	3 years	TKR
P.S.	GCT	Distal femur	3 years	TKR
L.S.	PAROSA	Distal femur	2 years	TKR
V.F.	GCT	Proximal tibia	1.5 years	TKR

joint replacement lasted 3 years or less; the seventh lasted 5 years. The proximal tibial allograft failed at 1.5 years. The arthroplasty rate for the distal femoral allografts (7/65, 11%) was much higher than the rate of replacement for proximal tibial allografts (1/35, 3%). Five of the seven distal femoral allografts that needed arthroplasties were judged to have an unstable joint following the implantation of the allograft originally.

X-ray analysis for the joints that failed showed that in the initial X-ray, the osteosynthesis site had a gap of between 1.0–1.5 mm, fixation was performed according to AO recommendations with minor modifications, but the joint was frequently mismatched due to a discrepancy in size of the allograft compared to the size of the host bone (Figs. 1, 2). Six of the 11 grafts had a mismatch of greater than 4 mm at the time of implantation of the allograft, and the average mismatch in size was 2–4 mm. In the control group of uncomplicated cases (none of which required joint replacement), the average mismatch was less than 2 mm.

Average time to healing at the osteosynthesis site of the failed joints was 1–2 years. The allografts showed minimal resorption, fixation showed no or minor complications, but all of the joints showed collapse or a Charcot-like appearance on X ray. In comparison, the average time to healing of the osteosynthesis site of the joint in the control group was 1–2 years. The control group showed no bone resorption, similar minor complications in fixation, and in analysis of the joint space, showed mild narrowing.

Follow-up of the total joint replacements after failed allografts was not sufficiently long to determine the end result of such a procedure. Of the 11 joints replaced by prostheses, two have been revised. The first, a constrained knee prosthesis inserted in 1977, 3 years after insertion of a distal femoral allograft, had the tibial component recemented in 1982 and the femoral component revised in 1984. The second, an unconstrained prosthesis inserted in 1982, 1.5 years after insertion of a proximal tibial allograft, failed in 1986, necessitating revision of the tibial component.

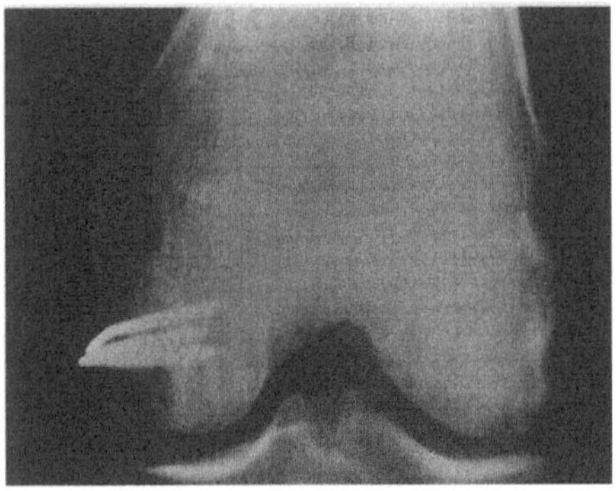

Fig. 1. This joint is well matched with no discernible size discrepancy on X-ray. It has lasted for 16 years

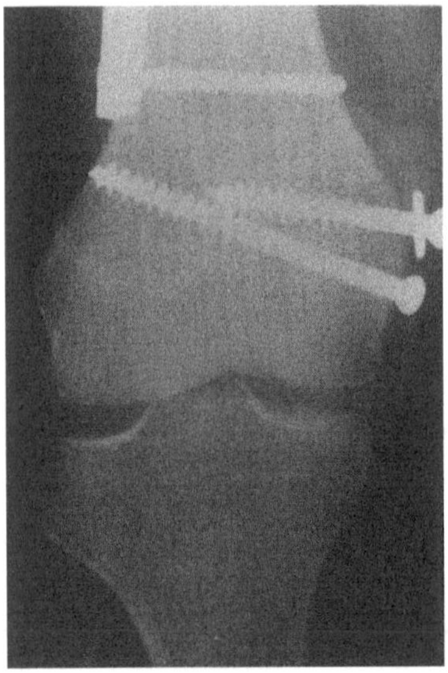

Fig. 2. This joint is mismatched approximately 3 mm and necessitated replacement within 2 years

Discussion and Conclusion

This study attempted to answer two questions: (a) What happens to weight-bearing joints in which osteoarticular allografts are used? and (b) What common factors were found in patients who developed complications? The study examined two joints (the hip and the knee), and four types of allografts (hemipelvis, proximal femur, distal femur, and proximal tibia).

The results of osteoarticular allografts were not hard to determine from this study because many patients have been followed for long periods. Fractures and nonunions present formidable but not limb-threatening problems. Many of the infections that occurred in this series followed a second operation on the allograft; *S. epidermidis* was the predominant organism in these infections. About 10% of the transplanted joints in this series deteriorated within 3 years, suggesting a moderately rapid rate of cartilage deterioration in these failed joints. The study suggests that most weight-bearing joints with allografts appear to hold up satisfactorily.

The overall proportion of good and excellent results was 72%. This figure is not different from results (75.3% good and excellent) recently published by Mankin et al. [3] in a study including both weight-bearing and non-weight-bearing joints, suggesting that weight bearing may not be a major factor in complications of osteoarticular allografts.

Our attempt to determine factors which led to complications in the allografts in this series was more difficult. For fracture/nonunion, the appearance on X ray of increased resorption compared to the host bone suggests that a metabolic response to allografts, perhaps on an immune basis, may be partially responsible for failure of incorporation and eventually fracture. For infection, an allograft is particularly susceptible at a second operation, and therefore special precautions such as laminar flow rooms may be helpful in reducing the incidence of this complication. Finally, accurate sizing and matching appears to be important to the longevity of a joint which includes an osteoarticular allograft. Further follow-up of these patients should result in valuable information on these factors affecting allografts.

References

1. Lexer E (1925) Joint transplantation and arthroplasty. Surg Gynecol Obstet 40:782–809
2. Parrish FF (1973) Allograft replacement of all or part of the end of a long bone following excision of a tumor. J Bone Joint Surg [Am] 55:1–22
3. Mankin HJ, Gebhardt MC, Tomford WW (1987) The use of frozen cadaveric allografts in the management of patients with bone tumors of the extremities. Orthop Clin North Am 18:275–299
4. Rittmann WW, Perren SM (1974) Cortical bone healing after internal fixation and infection. Springer, Berlin Heidelberg New York

The Combination of Bone and Bone Substitutes in Tumor Surgery of the Pelvis and Hip

W. Mutschler and C. Burri

Department of Trauma and Reconstructive Surgery, University of Ulm, 7900 Ulm, FRG

The treatment of bone tumors of the pelvis and hip joint is still one of the most challenging problems in orthopedic surgery. Any therapeutic concept has to take into account the histological characteristics of the tumor, its anatomic setting with respect to compartmental barriers and involvement of vessels and nerves and the presence of metastases, as well as the potential benefits of adjuvant chemotherapy, irradiation and surgical reconstruction [3]. Thus, the adequate surgical procedure for a tumor-like lesion or a high-grade malignant sarcoma might be intracapsular excision or hemipelvectomy respectively.

The use of bone and bone substitutes is generally indicated when performing limb-saving tumor resections in the pelvic region and hip joint in order to maintain the stability of the pelvic ring and the function of the hip joint and lower limb. Pelvic resections are divided into three major types according to Enneking and Dunham [6]: type I iliac ring resections; type II, periacetabular resections; type III, anterior arch resections. On the basis of the extent of the resection, the type I and type III procedures can each be subdivided into three classes: IA, wedge resection of the iliac wing without interruption of the pelvic ring; IB, resection of the iliac wing with interruption of the pelvic ring; IC, complete resection of the iliac wing with the sacroiliac joint; IIIA, resection of the anterior arch including the inferomedial part of the acetabulum; IIIB, monolateral resection of the anterior arch; IIIC, bilateral resection of the anterior arch [3].

Our experience with tumors of the pelvis and proximal femur includes the following methods for reconstruction: bone cement plug with secondary autograft; autogenous/allogenous bone grafts plus bone cement plus osteosynthesis; autogenous/allogenous bone grafts; prosthetic replacement of the hemipelvis and hip plus autogenous/allogenous bone grafts; prosthetic replacement of the hip and proximal femur with different types of prosthesis. The indication, technique, advantages, disadvantages and results of these procedures will now be described with regard to the types of resection mentioned above.

Reconstruction after resection of bone metastases of the pelvis and hip will also be discussed.

Reconstruction After Type I Resections

Bone lesions involving the wing of the ilium can almost always be removed by means of a local procedure. In type IA resections without interruption of the pelvic ring reconstruction is not necessary from a biomechanical point of view. However, after biopsies of tumors with uncertain categorization and after curet-

Bone Transplantation
Eds.: M. Aebi, P. Regazzoni

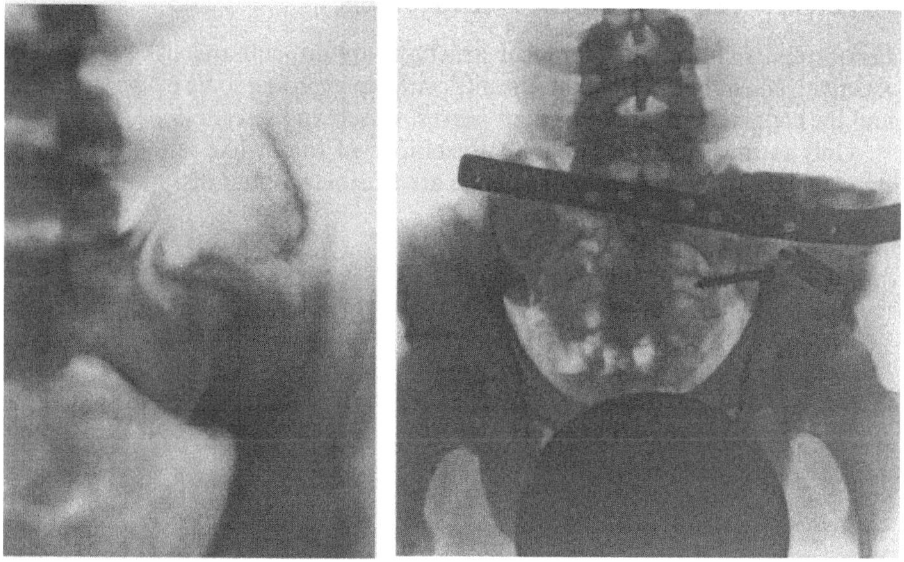

a b

Fig. 1 a and b. Male, 21 years: chondrosarcoma type I of the sacroiliac joint. **a** Preoperative X-ray. **b** X-ray after reconstruction using autogenous grafts, AO plate and bone cement.

tage of benign lesions we favor *bone cement plugging*. This procedure prevents bleeding and allows carefully oncologic follow-up. As a second step, removal of the cement plug and filling of the remaining defect with autogenous bone chips can be done simultaneously with a repeat biopsy.

Type IB resections with interruption of the pelvic ring require adequate restoration of the ring. Frequent indications are bone metastases and primary low-grade malignant bone tumors. In metastases a combination of *bone cement and internal rigid fixation* is suitable for immediate stability and weight bearing. In primary bone tumors large bone defects from the paracetabular region to the sacrum have to be bridged. Bridging is best achieved with large *autogenous corticocancellous grafts* which are harvested from the contralateral iliac crest and fitted into the defect, secured by screws and small plates. The grafts should be placed near the inner border of the pelvis.

If the sacroiliac joint is involved and parts of the sacrum have to be removed (type IC), anchorage of grafts and implants is difficult. In this case, a long plate fixed at the contralateral sacrum and/or ilium of the other side is effective. Again, additional bone cement embedded above the grafts and included in the internal rigid fixation (Fig. 1) will give immediate stability. This method of securing grafts also seems suitable in cases where subsequent postoperative adjuvant chemotherapy and irradiation are indicated. From the literature it is clear that chemotherapy and irradiation cause partial graft necrosis [1, 5]. The bone cement and the metal implants are removed 1–2 years later. If necessary, autografts or allografts are then used for reinforcement of the pelvic ring and reattachment of the gluteal muscles.

Reconstruction After Type II Resections

Periacetabular resections and reconstructions are difficult and risky because of the involvement of the hip joint, the difficulties in exposing some pelvic structures and the connections with important nerves, vessels and viscera [3, 4].

Only intracapsular and marginal excisions of tumor-like lesions or benign bone tumors of the paracetabular bone are feasible without disrupting the con-

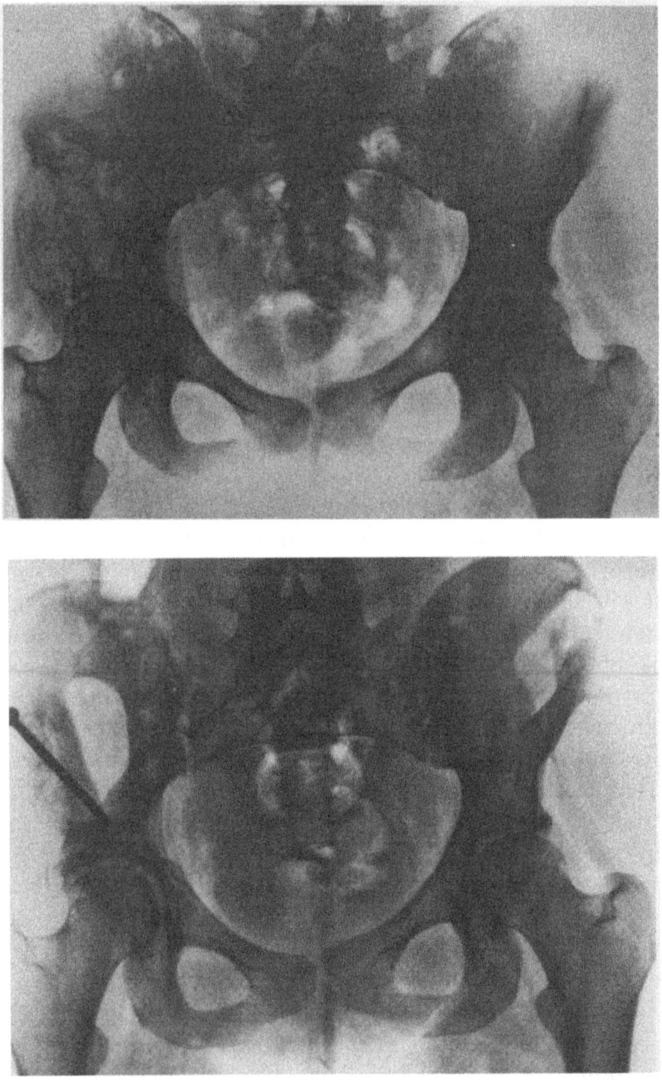

a b

Fig. 2a and b. Female, 17 years: aneurysmal bone cyst fibroma of the ilium involving the acetabulum. **a** Preoperative X-ray. **b** X-ray after two-step operation. First step: reconstruction of the inner pelvic ring and acetabulum with an autogenous corticocancellous graft and bone chips taken from the contralateral side. Second step: Metal removal and remodeling of the ilium column by an allogenous graft, fixed with a screw

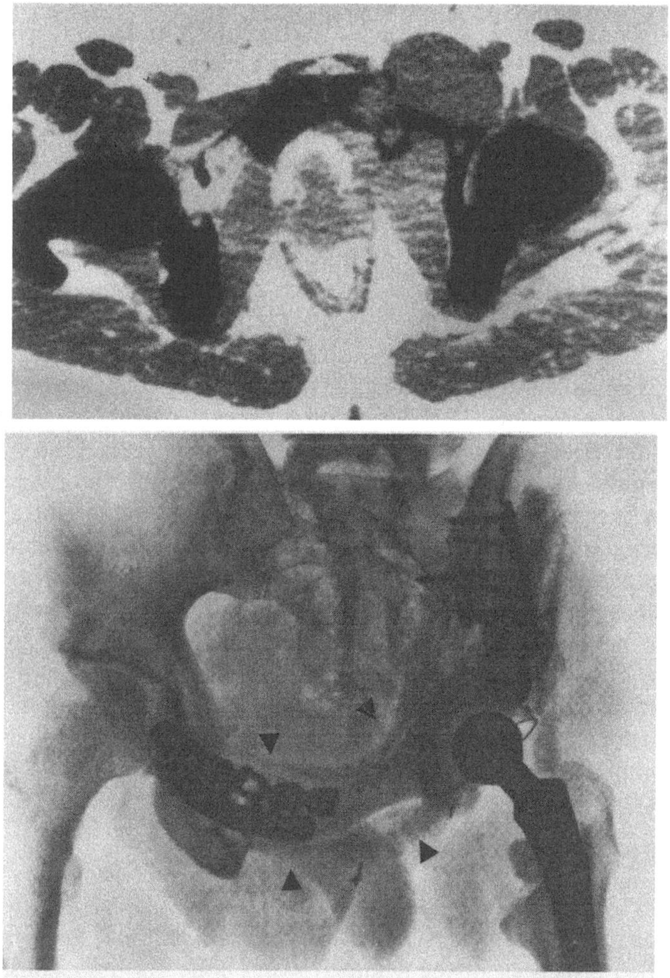

Fig. 3 a and b. Male, 37 years: malignant fibrous histiocytoma of the pubis and acetabulum. **a** Preoperative CT. **b** X-ray after reconstruction using a polyacetate hemipelvis. *Arrowheads* indicate pulverized autografts and allografts

gruity of the hip joint. If the margin of excision extends to the subchondral plate or if up to one-third of the acetabulum has to be removed, *autogenous/allogenous grafting* is sufficient for support. Spontaneous healing of the grafts provides stability without causing a significant functional defect. Sometimes the grafts may be anchored by screws (Fig. 2).

When the lesion involves the entire acetabulum and total acetabular resection is necessary, fusion or creation of a pseudarthrosis – either medially in relation to the pubis or laterally in relation to the ilium or sacrum – has been claimed to be the best type of reconstruction [1, 3, 6, 11, 12]. However, most patients exhibit marked pelvic tilt and leg length discrepancy after such operations [10]. Acceptable cosmetic and functional results are best achieved if the normal local anatomy is recreated as accurately as possible. To this end, Burri et al. [2] and also Karpf and Wang [8] performed *total internal hemipelvectomy with complete prosthetic replacement*.

Our technique for this operation is as follows: The skin incision begins at the level of the sacroiliac joint, follows the pelvic rim upward and then downward to continue to the inguinal ligament, ending at the public symphysis. After separation of subcutaneous tissue and fascia the anterior spines are chiseled for subsequent reinsertion if no tumor is present. Careful dissection of the femoral artery, vein and nerve is carried out in the inguinal region and the symphysis is visualized. Then the pelvic shell is mobilized on both sides, removing the gluteal and iliac muscles by respectively raising them subperiosteally up to the sacroiliac joint. The hip joint capsule is approached below the gluteal muscles and an osteotomy of the neck of the femur is performed. The dissection is continued, detaching the muscles from the ischial tuberosity.

Osteotomies of the pubis, the ischium and the ilium are performed, taking care not to injure the obturator nerves and vessels, the sciatic nerve or the gluteal vessels. The hemipelvis can now be carefully extracted. The polyacetate hemipelvic prosthesis is implanted. Sacroiliac fixation is achieved with screws or plates. The symphyseal end is secured by one or two plates placed contralaterally. For replacement of the hip joint an acetabular cup and its femoral component are cemented. Autogenous bone grafts taken from the femoral head and allogenous grafts pulverized in a bone mill are used for additional "biological stabilization". This is a means of attaching muscles to the implant via a pseudotendinous attachment and preventing implant loosening (Fig. 3).

Reconstruction After Type III Resections

In patients with high-grade malignant tumors of the anterior arch involving the acetabulum and the surrounding soft tissues, adequate reconstruction may be achieved with a modified prosthesis of the hemipelvis and bone grafting. Thus, type IIIA procedures follow the same principles as mentioned above. Tumor-like lesions, benign bone tumors and small low-grade malignant tumors limited to the anterior arch may be cured by resection without reconstruction, as the anterior ring is thought not to be a prerequisite for pelvic stability [7]. In type IIIC procedures bone autografts/allografts combined with bone cement and plates for internal rigid fixation are the preferred method of reconstruction.

Reconstruction After Resection of Bone Metastases of the Hip and Proximal Femur

The combination of bone and bone substitutes for reconstruction in patients with bone metastases is seldom indicated. The operative treatment of bone metastases is palliative; the great majority of patients develop multiple metastases and die on average 10.8 months after any bone operation. In view of this poor prognosis and considering the patient's age, short operations with low morbidity and maximum

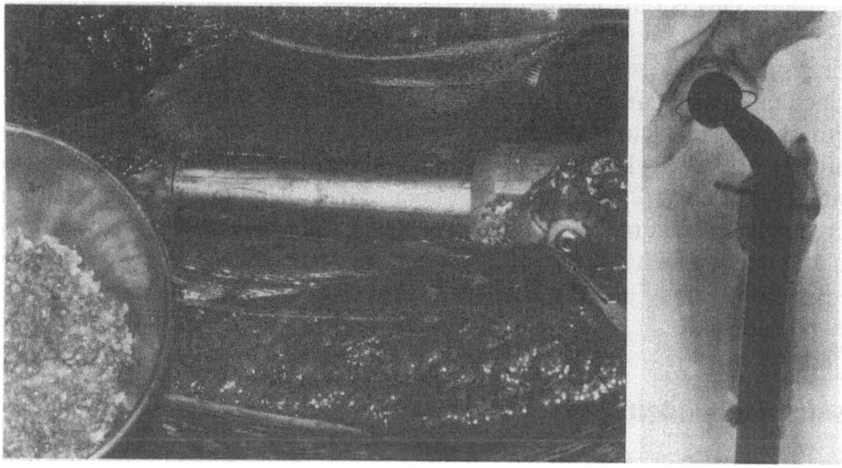

a b

Fig. 4a and b. Female, 68 years: solitary breast cancer metastasis of the proximal femur. **a** Intraoperative site after tumor resection and implantation of a tumor prosthesis. The prosthesis is covered by a Dexon net which is filled with milled allograft. **b** Postoperative X-ray

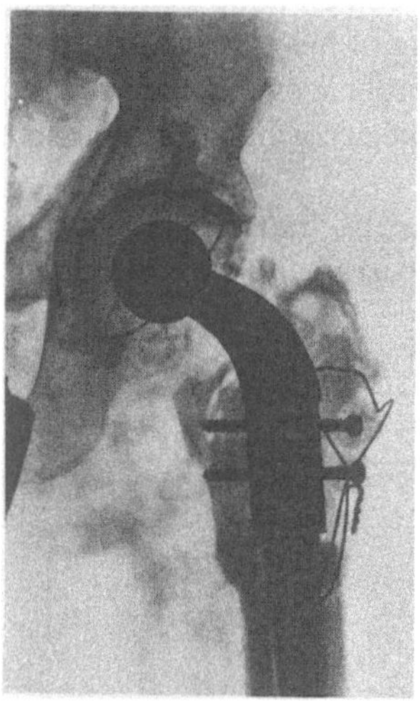

Fig. 5. Male, 43 years: chondrosarcoma type I of the proximal femur treated by resection and implantation of a Cane prosthesis reinforced by autologous grafts. X-ray 20 months after operation

benefit regarding function and stability should be chosen [9]. As most metastases are located in the neck of the femur, all types of cemented total hip prostheses can be used for reconstruction. When the acetabulum is involved an extended approach is sometimes necessary to resect part of the acetabulum and build it up, e.g., by means of a metallic reinforcement ring anchored in bone cement or in bone grafts.

In patients suffering from so-called solitary (isolated) bone metastases, we try to follow the rules of primary bone tumor surgery. That means no-touch isolation of the tumor and reconstruction by means of extended *tumor prostheses* (Cane prostheses). This is only justifiable if solid anchorage of the artificial socket as well as of the femoral stem can be accomplished. Therefore, "biological repair" of the paracetabular region in such cases demands corticocancellous autografts in which the socket can be fixed. To avoid loosening of the femoral component and to obtain satisfactory soft tissue attachment to the implant, modified Cane prostheses are used which permit the anchorage of the greater and lesser trochanters to the stem (2). An additional long-term protection against mechanical failure might be a net made out of resorbable Dexon which totally surrounds the stem and is filled with milled frozen allogenous bone graft. As shown in Figs. 4 and 5, a bony "coat" develops which is able to protect the stem against non-physiological load.

Results and Conclusions

Seventy-one patients with primary tumors of the pelvis and 123 patients with bone metastases of the hip and pelvis were treated at our department between July 1, 1978 and February 1, 1987. Twenty-three of the patients with primary tumors underwent biopsy, curettage, tumor resection and hemipelvectomy without any reconstruction. The treatment of the remaining 48 patients is summarized in Table 1.

Complications were rare in tumor-like lesions and benign bone tumors. Only one infection occurred, and was curable. No loosening of metal implants or significant resorption of grafts was observed. Of the 14 patients evaluated, the functional results were graded excellent in 13 and fair in one according to Enneking's system [5].

The results of 34 patients suffering from malignant tumors are listed in Tables 2 and 3. No complication was observed due to graft failure and implant

Table 1. Reconstruction in 48 patients with primary tumors of the pelvis

Type of resection	Reconstruction	Benign	Malignant	Total
Curettage	Bone cement	3	–	3
Curettage	Bone graft	4	–	4
IA	Bone graft + internal fixation	2	2	4
IB	Bone graft + internal fixation	2	2	4
IC	Bone cement + plate	–	4	4
	Bone graft + internal fixation	3	4	7
II	Bone graft + internal fixation	–	2	2
III	Bone graft + internal fixation	–	2	2
Internal hemipelvectomy	Polyacetate hemipelvis	–	18	18
		14	34	48

Table 2. Complications, recurrences, and metastases after treatment of 34 primary malignant tumors of the pelvis (as at March 1, 1987)

Type of resection	Local complications	General complications	Recurrence	Metastases
I (*n*=12)	2	–	2	–
II (*n*= 2)	1	–	1	–
III (*n*= 2)	–	1	–	–
Internal hemipelvectomy (*n*=18)	11	1	7	8
34	14	2	10	8

Table 3. Functional and oncological outcome after treatment of 34 primary malignant tumors of the pelvis (as at March 1, 1987)

Type of resection	Function					Oncological outcome			
	Excellent	Good	Fair	Poor	?	NED	AD	DD	?
I (*n*=12)	9	2	1	–	–	10	–	2	–
II (*n*= 2)	–	–	–	1	1	–	–	1	1
III (*n*= 2)	1	1	–	–	–	2	–	–	–
Internal hemipelvectomy (*n*=18)	2	3	1	6	6[a]	5	1	11	1

NED, No evidence of disease; AD, alive with disease; DD, died with disease.
[a] No functional evaluation possible before death.

loosening in type I, II and II resections. Internal hemipelvectomy and hemipelvic replacement was followed by loosening of plates in two cases and luxation of the prosthesis in another three cases. The functional and oncological results were mainly influenced by the type and extent of the tumor, as almost all recurrences, metastases and major complications were observed in patients with high-grade malignancies.

A total of 131 operations were performed in 123 patients with metastases of the hip and pelvis. Thirty-two underwent internal rigid fixation and bone cementing for reconstruction, 19 received conventional total hip prostheses, 17 had additional acetabular reconstruction, 31 received Cane prostheses and nine were given extended tumor prostheses. In two patients internal hemipelvectomy and replacement by polyacetate hemipelvis was performed. Overall, 84.5% of the patients were able to walk with or without crutches. A total of 21 complications occurred, of which 12 were luxations of the prosthesis. Two loose prostheses were replaced by new ones. The low rate of mechanical failure is probably related to the short survival time (average 10.8 months).

The following conclusions were derived from the findings of this study:

1. The functional results in patients with primary bone tumors of the pelvis are improved by some form of reconstruction.

2. Different combinations of bone and bone substitutes have been demonstrated to work well for reconstruction of the pelvis including the hip joint. According to the site and extent of the lesion, combinations of bone autografts and frozen bone allografts with internal fixation, bone cement and prosthetic replacement are used with success.
3. The surgical technique is demanding, the complication rate is high, and the results depend mainly upon the stage of the tumor.
4. In bone metastases all types of prostheses for total hip replacement are considered suitable for use in reconstruction. Solitary bone metastases require an additional biological repair.

References

1. Abstracts of International Symposium of Limb Salvage in Musculoskeletal Oncology. Orlando, Florida, 1985
2. Burri C, Claes L, Gerngross H, Mathys R (1979) Total internal hemipelvectomy. Arch Orthop Trauma Surg 94:219
3. Campanacci M, Capanna R (1984) Pelvic malignancies – resections of the pelvic bones. In: Uhthoff H (ed) Current concepts of diagnosis and treatment of bone and soft tissue tumors. Springer, Berlin Heidelberg New York, p 359
4. Capanna R, Van Horn J, Guernelli N, Briccoli A, Ruggieri P, Biagini R, Bettellin G, Campanacci M (1987) Complications of pelvic resections. Arch Orthop Trauma Surg 106:71
5. Enneking WF (1983) Musculoskeletal tumor surgery. Churchill Livingstone, New York
6. Enneking WF, Dunham WK (1978) Resection and reconstruction for primary neoplasms involving the innominate bone. J Bone Joint Surg [Am] 60A:731
7. Karaharju E, Korkola O (1985) Resection of large tumors of the anterior pelvic ring while preserving functional stability of the hip. Clin Orthop 195:270
8. Karpf PM, Mang W (1978) Das Retikulumzellsarkom des Beckens. Fortschr Med 31:1559
9. Mutschler W, Burri C (1984) Treatment of tumors of the pelvis and proximal femur. In: Weller S (ed) Late results after osteosynthesis. Seventy-fifth meeting of German section of AO International. Köhler, Tübingen
10. Nilsone U, Kreiebergs A, Olsson E, Stark A (1982) Function after pelvic tumor resection involving the acetabular ring. Int Orthop 6:27
11. Sim FH, Bowman WE (1984) Limb salvage in pelvic tumors. In: Uhthoff H (ed) Current concepts of diagnosis and treatment of bone and soft tissue tumors. Springer, Berlin Heidelberg New York, p 367
12. Steel HH (1978) Partial or complete resection of the hemipelvis. J Bone Joint Surg [Am] 60A:719

Reconstruction of Post-Traumatic Articular Surface Defects Using Fresh Small-Fragment Osteochondral Allografts

D.J. Zukor, B. Paitich, R.D. Oakeshott, P.J. Brooks, J.P. McAuley, J.F. Rudan, F. Langer and A.E. Gross

Combined Orthopaedic Unit, Mount Sinai Hospital and Toronto General Hospital; Division of Orthopaedic Surgery, University of Toronto, Toronto, Canada

Introduction

The late reconstruction of articular surface defects following trauma involving joints continues to be a challenge for the orthopaedic surgeon. Prosthetic replacement or arthrodesis, while viable options, are often undesirable or inappropriate treatments in young, high-demand patients. Since 1972, as part of the comprehensive bone transplantation programme at the Combined Orthopaedic Unit of Mount Sinai and Toronto General Hospitals, University of Toronto, fresh small-fragment osteochondral allografts have been used to replace damaged joint surfaces following trauma. Other aspects of the programme have previously been reported [10, 15–19, 34].

Initially, small-fragment grafts were used for a variety of other indications, including primary osteoarthritis, osteonecrosis and osteochondritis dissecans. Long-term follow-up of the first 100 cases showed the most favourable results when the aetiology of joint loss was trauma [31]. Since that study most grafts have been performed for traumatic defects. Grafts are now rarely performed for osteoarthritis or steroid-induced osteonecrosis. However, osteochondritis continues to be a relative indication.

This paper reports the experience and long-term clinical and radiographic results of 59 fresh small-fragment allografts for post-traumatic joint defects studied prospectively over the past 14 years.

Materials and Methods

Since 1972, 85 fresh osteocartilaginous allografts have been performed in 79 patients for post-traumatic joint defects. Of these, 59 grafts in 55 patients had a follow-up longer than 1 year and were included in this study. All patients were prospectively followed both clinically and radiographically. For knee patients a strict point protocol was used. This includes both subjective and objective data and was previously reported by McDermott [31] (Table 1].

Radiographs were carefully scrutinized. Factors examined included joint alignment, fit and fixation of graft, bony union, graft collapse and fragmentation, preservation of cartilage space, and development of osteoarthritis. Pre- and post-operative anteroposterior, lateral, oblique and skyline views and weight-bearing films were utilized for this analysis.

Bone Transplantation
Eds.: M. Aebi, P. Regazzoni

Table 1. Knee rating score

Subjective factors (60 points)
- Pain intensity (0–35)
  - None = 35
  - Mild = 28
  - Moderate = 21 (occasional analgesics)
  - Severe = 14 (regular analgesics)
  - At rest = 0
- Instability (0–10)
  - None = 10
  - Occasionally = 7
  - Moderate with decreased activity = 4
  - Severe, using braces = 0
- Walking aids (0–5)
  - None = 5
  - Cane = 3
  - Crutches, two canes = 1
  - Walker = 0
- Walking distance (0–10)
  - One mile or more = 10
  - One to five blocks = 6
  - One block = 3
  - Inside the house = 1
  - Confined to bed = 0

Objective factors (40 points)
- Extension (0–10)
  - No deformity = 10
  - Less than 5° = 7
  - 5°–10° = 4
  - 10°–20° = 2
  - Greater than 20° = 0
- Flexion (0–20)
  - Greater than 120° = 20
  - 90°–120° = 15
  - 45°–90° = 8
  - Less than 45° = 0
- Effusion (0–10)
  - None = 10
  - Moderate = 5
  - Severe = 0

Total (normal knee) = 100

The average age was 37.8 years (range, 10–70) with an average follow-up of 4.3 years (range, 1–13.7). Among the patients were 34 men and 21 women. The average interval from injury to graft was 3.9 years (range, 2 months to 27 years). Of the 59 grafts, 55 involved the knee, two the talus, and one each the lateral humeral condyle and the middle phalanx of a finger (Fig. 1). Among the knee allo-

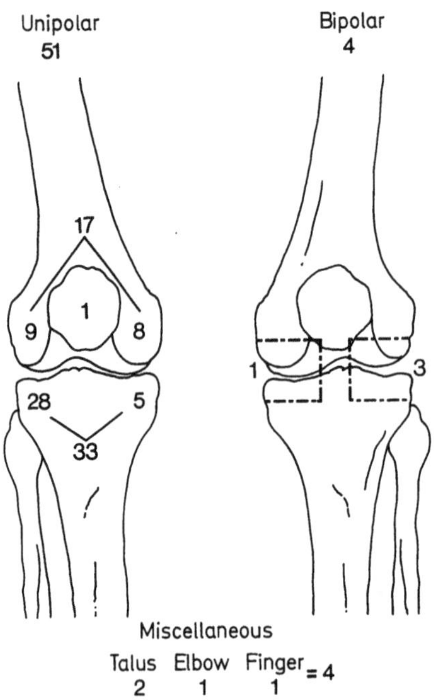

Fig. 1. Distribution of grafts

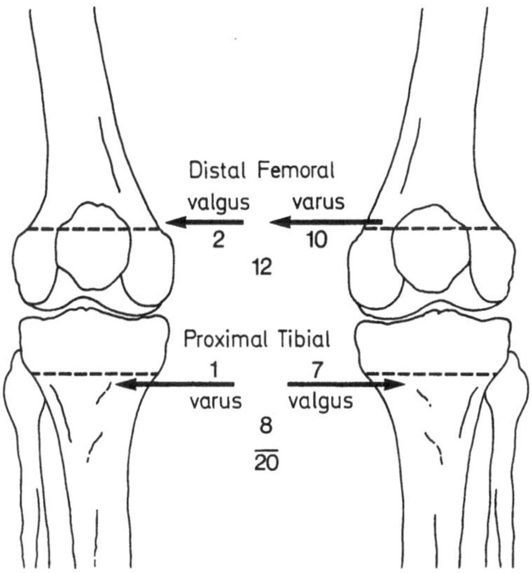

Fig. 2. Osteotomies

grafts, 33 were of the tibial plateau (5 medial and 28 lateral); 17 involved the femoral condyle (8 medial and 9 lateral), 4 involved both femoral condyle and tibial plateau of the same compartment and were termed unicompartmental bipolar grafts (1 medial and 3 lateral), and one graft was used to resurface the patella.

Twenty realignment osteotomies were carried out in 19 patients who received transplants involving their knees (Fig. 2). Distal femoral ostetomies were performed in 10 patients to achieve varus and in 2 to achieve valgus alignment. High tibial valgus osteotomies were performed in 7 patients and varus tibial osteotomy in 1. Of the 20 osteotomies, 9 were carried out prior to or simultaneously with allograft implantation. This practice increased in frequency towards the end of the series.

Menisci were included with 28 of the grafts. Of these, 21 were left attached to their corresponding lateral tibial plateau allograft at time of implantation and 5 to the medial plateau. Two were actual free-meniscal allografts at the time of replacement of the lateral femoral condyle.

The medial aspect of the talus was replaced in two patients. One patient had allograft replacement of the humeral capitellum. The final patient had an osteoarticular replacement of the distal half of the middle phalanx of her long finger.

Graft Procurement, Handling and Operative Technique

Donors are located by the Multiple Organ Retrieval and Exchange programme of Toronto, and to be suitable they must meet the criteria outlined by the American Association of Tissue Banks [12]. They must also be under 30 years old (and preferably younger) to provide healthy, viable cartilage. Graft procurement ist carried out within 24 h of death under strict aseptic conditions with the specimen consisting of the entire joint with the capsule intact. After taking appropriate cultures the graft is stored in 1 l sterile Ringers's lactate at 4 °C with added cefazolin (1 g), bacitracin (50000 U) and gentamicin (80 mg). Tissue typing is no longer performed, and no attempt is made to match donor and recepient other than on the basis of size. No immunosuppression is used.

The recipient patient is notified as soon as a donor has been located and immediately makes his or her way to the hospital as pre-arranged. Implantation is usually achieved within 12 h and always within 24 h. This schedule can be adhered to despite the fact that many of the patients come from diverse parts of the United States and Canada.

The transplantation procedure is usually performed in a clean-air room, with the operating team waring body exhaust suits. The patients routinely receive pre- and post-operative prophylactic antibiotics (cefazolin if no allergy exists). The favoured surgical approach is direct midline, which allows easy access for both the transplant and either proximal tibial or distal femoral osteotomy. Should later salvage procedures be necessary, the same approach is used with little risk of skin complications. Following arthrotomy the involved damaged articular surface is resected to a good bleeding cancellous bone surface. The donor tissue is then cut to appropriate size and implanted aiming for a tight fit with accurate reproduction of normal anatomy. Fixation is augmented by cancellous screws. If the meniscus is irreparably damaged or has previously been excised, it is replaced by an allograft meniscus which is sutured to the capsule of the recipient.

Some changes in technique have evolved since this procedure was last reported. The graft itself is no longer used to correct alignment. This is achieved by osteotomy either prior to or at the time of allograft implantation. This decision depends on whether the graft involves the same side of the joint as the osteotomy or not. For example, a lateral tibial plateau graft can be done simultaneously with a distal femoral varus osteotomy, and a medial femoral condyle graft can be accompanied by a high tibial valgus osteotomy.

The preference is to perform either distal femoral varus or proximal tibial valgus osteotomies. If the realignment procedure involves the same side of the joint as the graft, it should be carried out well prior to transplantation to allow sufficient time for revascularization of host bone. This also obviates the technical difficulties of performing these two procedures simultaneously at the same site.

Post-operatively, the limbs are no longer immobilized but started immediately in the recovery room on continuous passive motion (CPM) in order to maximize cartilage nutrition and prevent stiffness. The machines have been specially modified to allow positioning in either varus or valgus alignment.

Patients are protected from full weight bearing for approximately 1 year by a long leg brace with an ischial ring.

Results

Clinical Analysis. Cases were rated either as successes or as failures. A successful result required improvement of the rating score by at least 10 points or maintenance of a score of 75 points or higher. Cases were rated as failures if there was any decrease in the rating score, or if subsequent salvage surgery was necessary.

Overall, 45 of the 59 grafts (76%) were successful. Of the 55 knees 42 were successful. These had an average pre-operative score of 66.5 (range, 31–93) and an average post-operative score of 91 (range, 68–100).

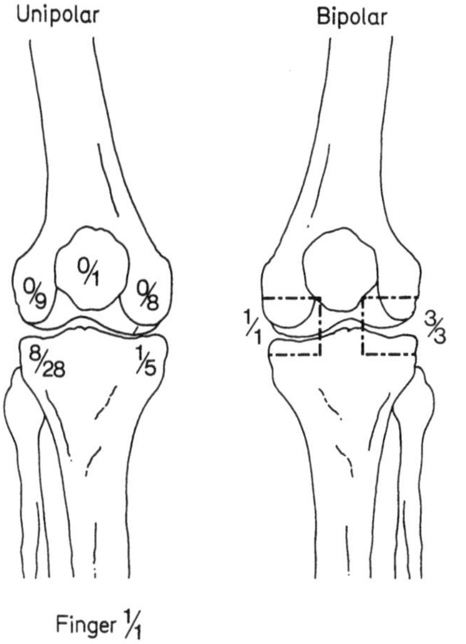

Fig. 3. Distribution of failures

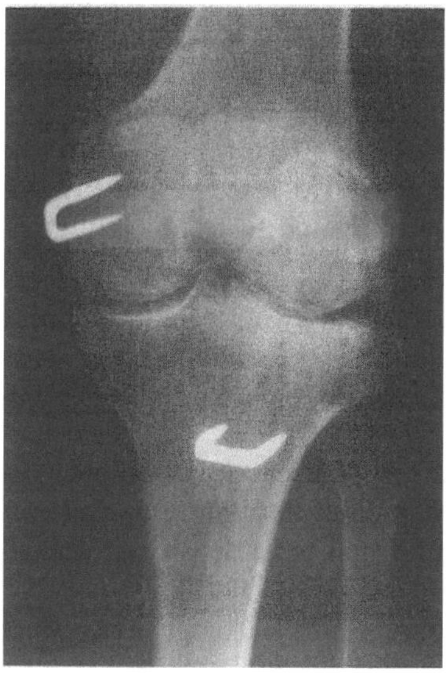

Fig. 4. Anterioposterior X ray showing failed lateral compartment bipolar graft in 28-year-old man 7 years after transplantation

Of the 13 failures at the knee, 4 were unicompartmental bipolar grafts, 8 were lateral plateau replacements and 1 a medial plateau graft (Fig. 3). Of these one underwent arthrodesis at 8 years, and three have undergone total knee replacement at 2, 4 and 6 years. The others were still functioning but were considered failures because of varying degrees of pain of stiffness. Of the 13 failures, 7 were Workers̀ Compensation Board (WCB) patients.

The 17 femoral condyle replacements and single patellar graft were successful, as were 4 of the 5 medial plateau grafts and 20 of the 28 lateral plateau replacements. All 4 bipolar grafts failed (Fig. 4). Of the 19 patients who had osteotomies

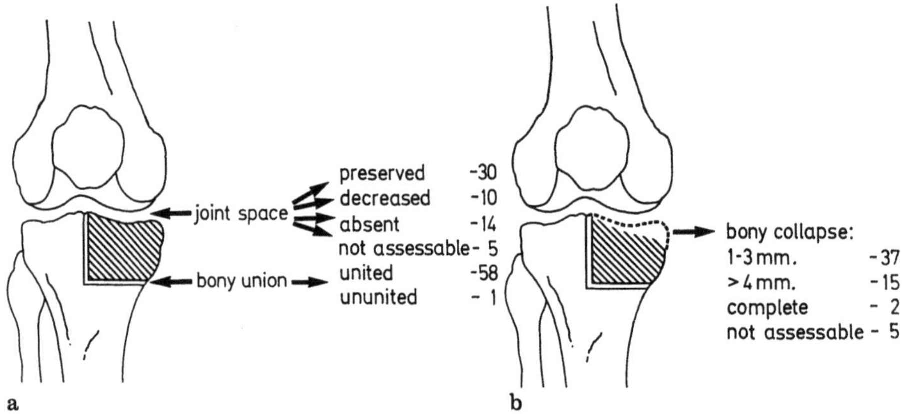

Fig. 5 a and b. Radiographic data

only 4 had an unsuccessful result. Of the 28 patients who received meniscal allografts 21 were successful. However, 7 of the 13 failures had an associated meniscal allograft.

The two patients who received allografts of the talus were considered as successes at 5- and 5.5-year follow-up, with diminution of pain and limp and improvement in function, including return to sports. The patient with a captellum replacement is doing well at 1.5 years, with no pain aqnd almost twice her preoperative range of motion. The patient who received the phalangeal allograft was considered a clinical failure within the first post-operative year, with X-ray evidence of graft resorption and non-union. This was related to technically inadequate graft fit and fixation.

Radiographic Review. Every attempt was made to standardize technique, but it was obvious during the course of this analysis that perfectly comparable views were the exception rather than the rule. This affects serial measurements of parameters such as height of the bone or cartilage.

Radiographic union was defined as establishment of structural continuity between host bone and allograft. A union occurred in 58 of the 59 grafts. This was usually present by 9–12 months. Restoration of normal bone density (of the allograft) was usually evident within 2–4 years.

Adequate X-rays for assessment of bony collapse and cartilage space were available in 54 patients (Fig. 5).

Joint space was seen to be well preserved in 30 patients, decreased in 10 and absent or arthritic in 14. Virtually all the grafts were at least 1–3 mm, and the majority did not collapse further. Fifteen grafts had evidence of collapse greater than 4–5 mm. Two grafts resorbed completely.

No actual fractures of grafts were seen. However, six grafts were fragmented adjacent to their articular surface. Whether this represents microfractures or mechanically induced degeneration remains unresolved.

Alignment of the knees was assessed on weight-bearing radiographs of the entire lower extremities. Forty-four patients had adequate X-rays for this. For a lateral compartment graft ideal alignment is considered to be a femoral-tibial axis

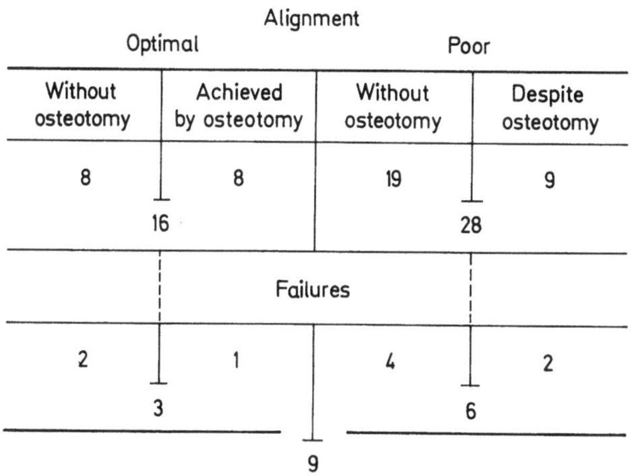

Fig. 6. Extremity alignment

of zero to a few degrees of varus. For a medial compartment replacement ideal alignment is 10 ° or more of femoral-tibial valgus. Sixteen patients were seen to be ideally aligned, eight of these by osteotomy (Fig. 6). In 28 patients alignment was judged to be suboptimal. Nine had undergone osteotomy with inadequate correction.

Clinical-Radiographic Correlation. Of the 16 well-aligned patients there were three failures. Only one of these three had had an osteotomy. Eliminating the other two where alignment correction was achieved by graft height alone, only one out of 14 patients with ideal alignment failed.

Of the 28 poorly aligned patients there were six failures. Only two of these six had had an osteotomy. One osteotomy was performed 3 years after allograft implantation, and the other 1 year after the graft with failure to adequately correct alignment.

Complications. Nine complications occurred in eight patients. Three knees required manipulations for stiffness early in the series when post-operative immobilization for 14–21 days was still being used. This complication was not seen following the introduction of CPM. One of these three cases was later diagnosed as reflex sympathetic dystrophy. Other complications included one wound haematoma which required evacuation and one intra-operative rupture of an already frayed patellar tendon which was successfully repaired immediately.

Three patients had complications related to the respiratory system. No documented deep vein thromboses or pulmonary emboli occurred. There were no infections. There were two late deaths unrelated to surgery, a 58-year-old man who had a myocardial infarction 2 years post-operatively and a 40-year-old alcoholic who committed suicide at 2 years post-operatively. The first was considered a failure and the second a successful allograft result at the time of death.

Subsequent Surgery. Five patients have undergone late "salvage procedures". The first patient was 21 years old when he received a left knee lateral compartment bipolar allograft. It functioned well for almost 7 years. However, collapse of the graft was noted beginning 3 years post-operatively with progressive development of tricompartmental osteoarthritis. The knee had not been realigned and was in excessive valgus, stressing the graft. He underwent arthrodesis at 8 years.

The next patient was 70 years old when she received a left lateral plateau graft. She underwent total knee arthroplasty 6 years later. In retrospect, it would seem that patient selection was a factor, as she was noted to have moderate to severe degenerative changes in all three compartments on her pre-operative X-rays.

The third patient was 35 years old when she received a left lateral plateau graft. In retrospect, the pre-operative clinical and radiographic picture indicate reflex sympathetic dystrophy. She was never satisfied with the procedure although her rating score increased 23 points. Her X-ray result was excellent at 1 year. She sought a multitude of opinions and underwent total knee arthroplasty 2 years following allograft.

The fourth patient was 27 years old when she received a left lateral plateau allograft. She did well for about 4 years, at one point having a score of 100. She was lost to follow-up after moving to the West Coast. Recently, correspondence with her current orthopaedic surgeon revealed that she is now on his waiting list for total knee arthroplasty.

The fifth patient was 27 years old when she underwent replacement of her right third middle phalanx. This was considered a technically inadequate procedure with respect to graft size and fixation and resulted in early failure. She is currently awaiting distal interphalangeal joint arthrodesis at 1.5 years.

Discussion

Long-term results of fresh small-fragment osteochondral allografts are encouraging (Fig. 7). The best indication is late reconstruction following traumatic loss of joint segment [27, 31]. However, patient selection remains a vital consideration. Best results have been seen in highly motivated patients who have no evidence of degenerative arthritis prior to allografting. Some of the unsuccessful results could be directly attributed to poor patient selection. This is especially true for Worker's

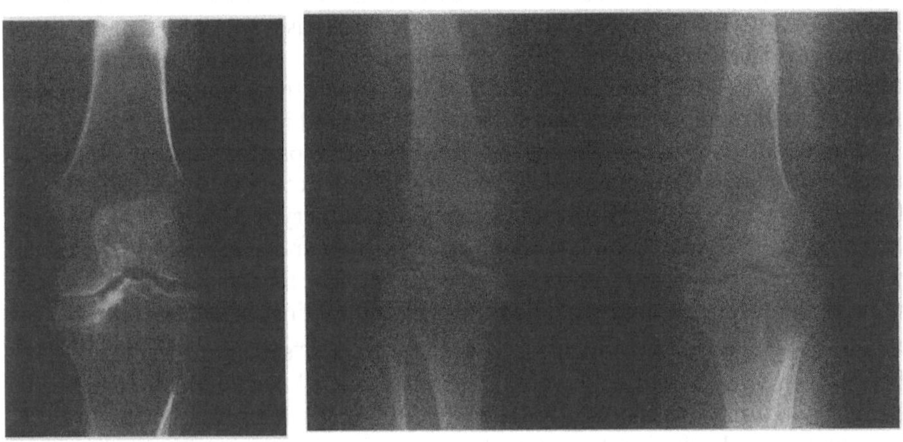

a b

Fig. 7 a, b. a Pre-operative anterioposterior X ray of 26-year-old woman, showing medial tibial plateau collapse following fracture. **b** Post-operative weight-bearing anterioposterior X ray of same patient showing successful result at 7-year follow-up

Compensation Board patients, where 7 out of 16 grafts failed. Although they comprised less than one-third of the total series, the WCB patients accounted for more than half of the failures. The incidence of failure for them was more than three times that for the rest of the patients.

The rationale for using fresh rather than stored allografts is clinical and experimental evidence supporting the maintenance of viability and function of chondrocytes after fresh transplantation. Currently, experimental work on cryopreservation techniques indicates that relatively high percentages of chondrocytes (50%) survive after freezing and thawing of cartilage in animal models [42, 44, 45]. However, as yet there is little objective evidence of prolonged survival of preserved cartilage following implantation in humans [33]. Few reports with histological evidence appear in the literature, and while these are often biopsies of failed cases, the cartilage is usually described as severely degenerated and "distinctly abnormal" [29, 30]. However, even in 12 out of 18 failed cases reported by Oakeshott et al. [35] hyaline cartilage survival and matrix production was seen as late as 9.5 years following transplantation of fresh grafts. This was demonstrated by staining techniques and electron microscopy. It is likely that in successful cases cartilage survival is even better.

While intact cartilage is considered immunoprivileged [22], the bony component of the graft is accepted to be immunogenic [5, 6, 39]. Antigenicity has been shown to be decreased significantly, although not completely eliminated, by freezing and freeze-drying (both of which adversely affect the cartilage) [21, 28]. A definite immune response following transplantation of fresh, frozen or freeze-dried bone has been well documented [13, 23, 24]. However, neither the presence nor the magnitude of this response correlates with clinical success or failures of the graft [37, 41]. Previous reviews of fresh bone and cartilage transplants have failed to reveal evidence of clinically significant or histologically detectable rejections [2, 8, 14, 20, 25, 26, 32].

In the literature, only the series of Volkov [47] reported the phenomenon of rejection, and this was with frozen grafts. However, clinical rejection has not been identified in 14 years of experience with over 130 fresh grafts at this institution.

Many authors have stated that the fate of the allograft depends heavily on mechanical factors [11, 29, 38, 43, 46]. Analysis of failed grafts from this centre revealed a high association of failure with poorly sized grafts, grafts less than 1 cm in thickness (resulting in fragmentation and fracture) and grafts where internal fixation was not used [35].

The present series illustrates the success of unipolar grafts in the knee and the talus. Although only a small number of bipolar grafts (four) are presented, they were all failures.

The role of osteotomy to realign the joint, especially in weight-bearing extremities, cannot be overemphasized. Of the 19 patients who underwent osteotomy – even when performed late – only 4 were in the failed group. The preferred relignment procedure to correct valgus deformity is a distal femoral varus osteotomy. Proximal tibial valgus osteotomy is used to correct varus deformity. Joint surface obliquity and site of the allograft must be taken into consideration. In the present series only 1 out of 14 grafts in well-aligned extremities failed. Best results can be achieved by adhering to the principles described, including correct sizing,

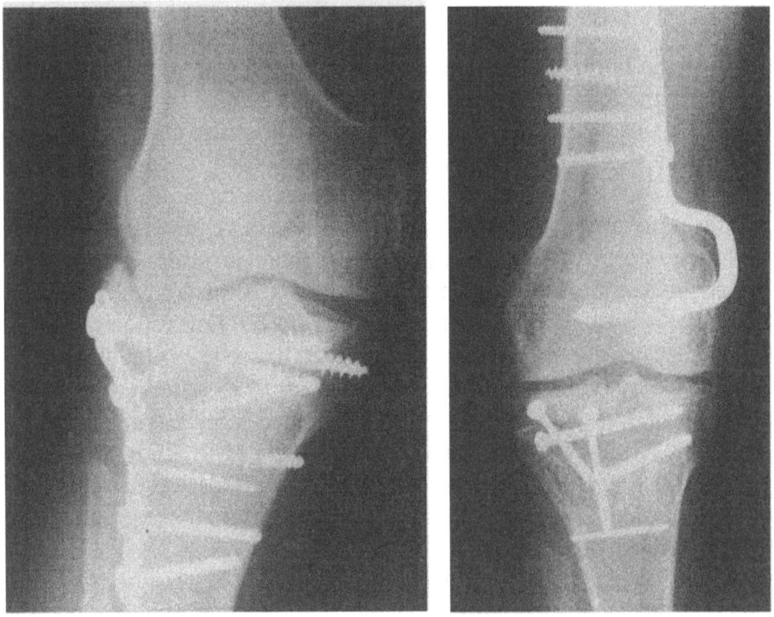

a b

Fig. 8 a, b. a Pre-operative anterioposterior X ray of 32-year-old man, showing collapse of lateral tibial plateau and 24° valgus deformity. **b** Post-operative X ray of same patient with successful result 3 years after lateral tibial plateau replacement and supracondylar varus osteotomy

realignment and fixation to achieve ideal mechanical conditions along with prompt implantation of fresh healthy cartilage to maximize cell viability (Fig. 8).

Patient selection remains a vital consideration. Best results have been seen in highly motivated patients who have no evidence of degenerative arthritis prior to allografting. Some of our unsuccessful results could be directly attributed to poor patient selection. This is especially true for Worker's Compensation Board patients where the incidence of failure was approximately three times that for the rest of the patients.

Substantial evidence in favour of meniscal allotransplantation has come from work with animal models [1]. Of the patients in this study, 28 had meniscal allografts, and 21 of these continue to do well. The failures were mainly on the basis of realignment or graft type, and none was directly attributable to the meniscus itself. None of the 28 patients has required re-operation because of meniscal tear or detachment.

The use of CPM post-operatively is beneficial. Cartilage nutrition is theoretically improved, helping to maintain cell viability. Perhaps better preservation of the matrix is also achieved, and since cartilage is immunologically privileged on the basis of an intact matrix [22], this would be advantageous. CPM has also eliminated stiffness as a complication in this series since its introduction as part of the post-operative protocol. The prompt return of range of motion is related to decreased intra-articular adhesions as seen in animal models [40].

The radiographic results are more difficult to interpret than the clinical results. Previous reviews of allograft series have illustrated that radiographic appearance and clinical result do not necessarily correlate – more specifically that good function is possible even with an obviously degenerated radiographic appearance [36, 46]. Radiographic appearance was worse in patients early in the series, when the grafts were used to correct alignment, and when internal fixation was often not used or was inadequate. With technical improvements such as realignment osteotomy to decompress the graft, rigid interfragmentary fixation, and better sizing, radiographic results have improved, at least in the short term.

A pattern of typical radiographic progression was identified. The first significant event is host-donor bony union, which is usually complete by 9–12 months and is accompanied by minimal setting of the bony portion (1–3 mm). Virtually all technically adequate grafts were seen to unite.

Grafts should be "decompressed" by realignment osteotomy either at the time of or prior to tranplantations. Perhaps consideration should be given to extending the period of protected weight bearing beyond 1 year (the interval currently used) to 2–3 years or until the bony portions returns to iso-density. Many of the early cases were performed prior to the recognition of the importance of these factors. Thus, long-term objective assessment of patients treated by adherence to the above principles is of considerable interest and is part of an ongoing study.

Complications in this series were relatively minor. As this is a relatively conservative procedure involving minimal bone resection, no "bridges are burned". Subsequent salvage surgery (i.e. arthroplasty or arthrodesis) certainly is not compromised and may even be facilitated because deficient bone stock has been replaced.

Summary

Long-term follow-up of fresh small-fragment osteochondral allograft reconstruction of traumatic joint surface defects revealed 76% to be clinically successful. Best results can be achieved by adhering to the principles described, including correct sizing, realignment and internal fixation to achieve ideal mechanical conditions, along with prompt implantation of fresh healthy cartilage to maximize cell viability.

Specific conclusions and recommendations include the following:

1. Traumatic loss of joint segment is the best indication for fresh osteochondral allografts.
2. Patient selection is a vital consideration.
3. Mechanical conditions seem more important to successful results than immunological factors.
4. Ideal alignment of the extremity to "unload" the graft is an absolute requirement and, if necessary, should be achieved by osteotomy prior to or simultaneous with allograft implantation.
5. Internal fixation of the allograft should be used.
6. Bipolar allografts should be avoided if at all possible.
7. Menisci can be implanted if the recipient's meniscus is absent or irreparably damaged.

8. CPM is a useful post-operative adjunct.
9. Fresh small-fragment osteochondral allografts can be used sucessfully to reconstruct joint surfaces following traumatic segmental loss.

References

1. Arnoczky SP, McDevitt CA, Cuzzell JZ, Warren RF, Kristinicz T (1985) Meniscal replacement using a cryopreserved allograft. An experimental study in the dog. Trans Orthop Res Soc 293
2. Aston JE, Bentley G (1986) Repair of articular surfaces by allografts of articular and growth-plate cartilage. J Bone Joint Surg [Br] 68:29
3. Bos GD, Goldberg VM, Gordon NH, Dollinger BM, Zika JM, Powell AE, Heiple KG (1985) The long-term fate of fresh and frozen orthotopic bone allografts in genetically defined rats. Clin Orthop 197:245
4. Brooks DB, Heiple KG, Herndon CH, Powell AE (1963) Immunological factors in homogenous bone transplantation. J Bone Joint Surg [Am] 45:1617
5. Brown KLB, Cruess RL (1982) Bone and cartilage transplantation in orthopaedic surgery. J Bone Joint Surg [Am] 64:270
6. Burchardt H (1983) The biology of bone graft repair. Clin Orthop 174:28
7. Burwell RG, Friedlander GE, Mankin HJ (1985) Current perspectives and future directions: the 1983 invitational conference on osteochondral allografts. Clin Orthop 197:141
8. Campbell CJ, Ishida H, Takahashi H, Kelly F (1963) The transplantation of articular cartilage. J Bone Joint Surg [Am] 45:1579
9. Czitrom AA, Axelrod T, Fernandes B (1985) Antigen presenting cells and bone allotransplantation. Clin Orthop 197:27
10. Czitrom AA, Langer F, McKee N, Gross AE (1986) Bone and cartilage allotransplantation: a review of 14 years of research and clinical studies. Clin Orthop 208:141
11. Depalma AF, Tsultas TT, Mauler GG (1963) Viability of osteochondral grafts as determined by uptake of 535. J Bone Joint Surg [Am] 45:1565
12. Friedlander GE, Mankin HJ (1979) Guidelines for the banking of musculoskeletal tissues. Am Assoc Tissue Banks Newsletter 3:2
13. Friedlander GE (1983) Immune responses to osteochondral allografts. Clin Orthop 174:58
14. Goldberg VM, Porter BB, Lance EM (1980) Transplantation of the canine knee joint on a vascular pedicle. J Bone Joint Surg [Am] 62:414
15. Gross AE, Lavoie MV, McDermott P, Marks P (1985) The use of allograft bone in revision of total hip arthroplasty. Clin Orthop 197:115
16. Gross AE, McKee NH, Pritzker KPH, Langer F (1983) Reconstruction of skeletal deficits at the knee. Clin Orthop 174:96
17. Gross AE, Langer F, Houpt J, Prizker KPH, Friedlander G (1976) Allotransplantation of partial joints in the treatment of osteoarthritis of the knee. Transplant Proc 8(2):129
18. Gross AE, Silverstein EA, Falk J, Falk R, Langer F (1975) The allotransplantation of partial joints in the treatment of osteoarthritis of the knee. Clin Orthop 108:7
19. Gross AE, McKee N, Farine I, Czitrom A, Langer F (1984) Reconstruction of skeletal defects following en bloc excision of bone tumours. In: Uhthoff HK, Stahl E (eds) Current concepts of diagnosis and treatment of bone and soft tissue tumours. Springer, Berlin Heidelberg New York, pp 163–174
20. Kandel RA, Gross AE, Ganel A, McDermott AGP, Langer F, Pritzker KPH (1985) Histopathology of failed osteoarticular shell allografts. Clin Orthop 197:103
21. Lance EM (1985) Some observations on bone graft technology. Clin Orthop 200:114
22. Langer F, Gross AE (1974) Immunogenicity of allograft articular cartilage. J Bone Joint Surg [Am] 56:297
23. Langer F, Czitrom AA, Pritzker KP, Gross AE (1975) The immunogenicity of fresh and frozen allogeneic bone. J Bone Joint Surg [Am] 57:216

24. Langer F, Gross AE, West M, Urovitz EP (1978) The immunogenicity of allograft knee joint transplants. Clin Orthop 132:155
25. Lexer E (1908) Substitution of joints from amputated extremities. Surg Gynecol Obstet 6:601
26. Lexer E (1925) Joint transplantation and arthroplasty. Surg Gynecol Obstet 40:782
27. Locht RC, Gross AE, Langer F (1984) Late osteochondral allograft resurfacing for tibial plateau fractures. J Bone Joint Surg [Am] 66:328
28. Malinin TI, Wagner JL, Pita JC, Lo H (1985) Hypothermic storage and cryopreservation of cartilage. Clin Orthop 197:15
29. Mankin HJ, Doppelt SH, Sullivan TR, Tomford WW (1982) Osteoarticular and intercalary allograft transplantation in the management of malignant tumours of bone. Cancer 50:613
30. Mankin HJ, Doppelt S, Tomford W (1983) Clinical experience with allograft implantation. Clin Orthop 174:69
31. McDermott AGP, Langer F, Pritzker KPH, Gross AE (1985) Fresh small fragment osteochondral allografts. Clin Orthop 197:96
32. Meyers MH (1985) Resurfacing of the femoral head with fresh osteochondral allografts. Clin Orthop 197:111
33. Mnaymneh W, Malinin TI, Makley JT, Dick HM (1985) Massive osteoarticular allografts in the reconstruction of extremities following resection of tumors not requiring chemotherapy and radiation. Clin Orthop 197:76
34. Oakeshott RD, Gross AE, Morgan DAF, Zukor DJ, Rudan JF, Brooks PJ (in press) Revision total hip arthroplasty with osseous allograft reconstruction. Clin Orthop
35. Oakeshott RD, Farine I, Pritzker KPH, Langer F, Gross AE (in press) A clinical and histological analysis of failed fresh osteochondral allografts.
36. Parrish FF (1973) Allograft replacement of all or part of the end of a long bone following excision of a tumour. J Bone Joint Surg [Am] 55:1
37. Prolo DI, Rodrigo JJ (1985) Contemporary bone graft physiology surgery. Clin Orthop 200:322
38. Rodrigo JJ, Sakovich L, Travis C, Smith G (1978) Osteocartilaginous allograft as compared with autografts in the treatment of knee joint osteocartilaginous defects in dogs. Clin Orthop 134:342
39. Rodrigo JJ, Block N, Thompson EC (1978) Joint transplantation. Vet Clin North Am 8:523
40. Salter RB, Simmonds DF, Malcolm BW, Rumble EJ, MacMichael D, Clements ND (1980) The biological effect of continuous passive motion on the healing of full-thickness defects in articular cartilage. J Bone Joint Surg [Am] 62:1232
41. Sedgwick AD, Moore AR, Al-Duaij AY, Edwards JCW, Willoughby DA (1985) Studies into the influence of carrageenan-induced inflammation on articular cartilage degradation using implantation into air pouches. Br J Exp Pathol 66:445
42. Schachar NS, McGann LE (1986) Investigations of low-temperature storage of articular cartilage for transplantation. Clin Orthop 208:146
43. Tanaka H, Inoue M, Suzuki M, Nojima M (1980) A study on experimental homocartilage transplantation. Acta Orthop Traumat Surg 96:165
44. Tomford WW, Duff GP, Mankin HJ (1985) Experimental freeze-preservation of chondrozytes. Clin Orthop 197:11
45. Tomford WW, Mankin HJ (1983) Investigational approaches to articular cartilage preservation. Clin Orthop 174:22
46. Urbaniak JR, Black KE (1985) Cadaveric elbow allografts. Clin Orthop 197:131
47. Volkov M (1970) Allotransplantation of joints. J Bone Joint Surg [Br] 52:49

Replacement of the Deficient Acetabulum by Bone Transplants in Total Hip Replacement

B. Radojevich, M. Zlatich, Z. Milinkovich, C. Lazovich, J. Nedeljkovich, N. Stankovich, and C. Abaidoo

Special Orthopedic Surgical Hospital Banjica, Belgrade, Yugoslavia

A good grip on the acetabular component of the replacing endoprothesis directly influences the duration of the replaced hip. In deficient acetabula, the causes of which could be dysplasia and dislocation, it is possible to compensate for the deficient part by means of an autogenous bone transplant from the femoral head and neck or by a homogenous transplant from a bone bank during total hip replacement. This makes it possible to solve this great source of invalidity satisfactorily by surgery.

The construction of the bone transplant actually influences the end result of the operation. The authors have used their own construction of a bone transplant from the resected head and neck. The bone transplant is modeled in such a way

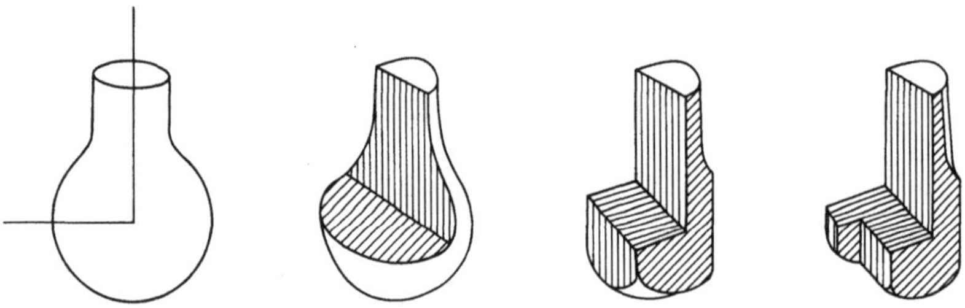

Fig. 1. Construction of a bone transplant. The resected head and neck are modeled in the shape of a letter "L." The longer part corresponds to the neck and the shorter one to the head

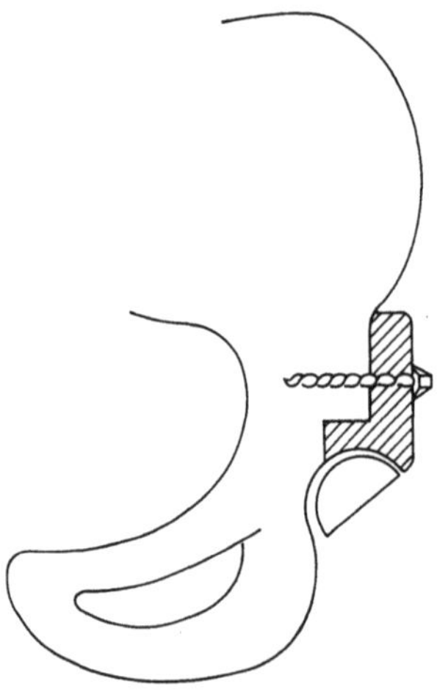

Fig. 2. The prepared graft is placed into the prepared beds with a shorter part in the upper part of the acetabulum and the longer one supraacetabularly in the refreshed iliac bone. The graft is well adapted and fixed with a single compressive screw with a washer vertically. Reconstructed acetabulum is ready for the usual preparation with reamers

Bone Transplantation
Eds.: M. Aebi, P. Regazzoni

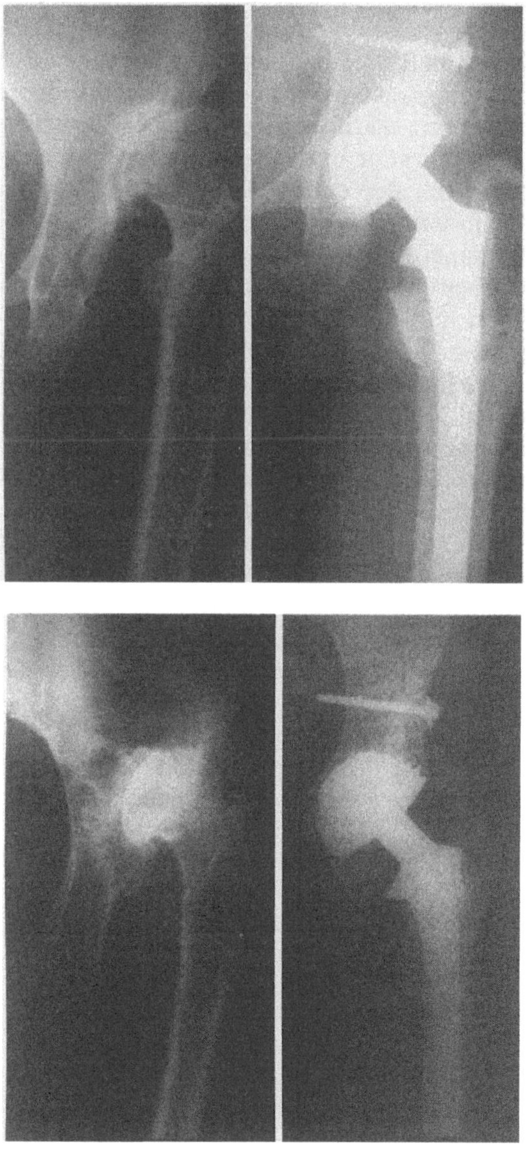

a

b

Fig. 3a, b. S.K., 37-year-old female. **a** High unreduced congenital dislocation. **b** Two years after the operation. Clinically and radiologically results

that it looks like the letter L, where the long branch corresponds to the cortical bone of the femoral neck and the shorter branch to the cancellous bone of the femoral head (Fig. 1). A corresponding bed must be made on the iliac bone so that it corresponds to the modeled bone transplant like a "jig and saw" (Figs. 2, 3). The bone transplant is fixed to the iliac bone by means of one compressive or bone screw, which is screwed vertically into the long branch of the transplant. The short branch of the transplant must be at least 10 mm long, with a thickness of at least 8 mm for the transplant to take the initial weight-bearing load. While preparing the bed on the iliac bone, one must insist on decortication so that the cancellous bone is reached. This makes early incorporation (union) of the bone transplant to the iliac bone possible. The authors used this method to operate on 207 patients and 237 hips. Of these, 164 hips were dysplastic with defective upper walls or with defective upper and anterior walls of the acetabulum. Of these hips, 72 were the result of high congenital dislocation of the hip, where only the rudimental acetabulum existed. In one patient, after traumatic dislocation of the hip and fracture of the acetabulum, the posterior wall was nonexistent.

A total of 215 autogenous transplants and 22 homogenous transplants from the bone bank were used. In the cases of the homogenous transplants, compatability was determined by blood group and Rh factor. All patients had postoperative physical therapy, and weight bearing on the operated hip was allowed after neurocirculatory equilibrium and muscular coordination were attained, which is often between 2–5 days postoperative.

Radiographic and clinical analyses showed that there was complete bony union 6–10 weeks postoperative in the cases where autografts were used. Radiographically, the bone structure of the grafts could not be differentiated from that of the surrounding bone tissues 3–7 months postoperative. In the 22 cases where homogenous bone grafts were used, union occurred between 8–24 months in 20 patients, as verified radiographically. In the remaining two cases destruction of the bone construction occurred in the second postoperative year (16–22 months), and these were reoperated. Histologic analyses in these two showed rejection of the incompatible foreign body.

This analysis shows that by this method it is possible to replace hips in cases of dysplasia and dislocation by placing the acetabular component of the replacing hip at its original location. This allows a nearly normal biomechanical relationship to be attained. This also allows cementless prosthesis to be used with excellent initial strength of the acetabulum. In rehabilitation, early weight bearing on the operated hip leads to better results. Autografts are better than homografts, as was seen in this study.

Fresh Bone Allograft in THR Revision Surgery

R. G. Ceroni, A. Pace, and M. Nicolosi
Istituto Ortopedico Galeazzi, Milan, Italy

Surgical procedures for reimplant in failed THR were performed up to 8 years ago at the Istituto Ortopedico Galeazzi in Milan without any bone allograft. Follow-up of this first group of patients usually showed no evidence of new bone formation in the medial wall of the acetabulum, even years after operation, and extremely slow bone remodeling of the diaphyseal cortical bone. Later, we started using massive bony allografts with or without internal fixation to get primary mechanical stability of the implant (mainly of the acetabular component). In control of this second group we often noticed a partial or total resorption of the graft, with consequent subsidence of the device.

Since November 1984 we have taken a different approach to the problem. Primary stability is achieved through the characteristics of the implant (cementless in any case): the acetabular component is fixed with pegs, and occasionally with screws, and the femoral component with press fit. A bony allograft is used to reconstruct the bone stock and to attain secondary stability, but without immediate mechanical effect. The graft is reamed out from the femoral head of other patients, carefully excluding cartilage and soft tissues. This may be obtained through a slow-speed reaming by means of a reamer of the acetabulum and not using a bone mill. The softer the bone, the easier it is for the reamer to bruise it. In this way the reamer is automatically rejected by the hard subchondral bone, therefore digging its way into the bone up to the formation of a thin shell of subchondral bone and cartilage. The resulting paste is scooped out from the reamer and put into a tea strainer to be washed out with Ringer's solution. This washing is done thoroughly and allows removal of most blood and fat tissue, as may be noticed in the washing liquid. Finally the paste is dried by pushing it into a gauze.

Usually the graft is used on the day of procurement, and for this reason cultures cannot be evaluated. Only clinical parameters are therefore taken into consideration: absence of infective diseases and cancer, normal erythrocyte sedimentation rate, and laboratory tests for hepatitis and AIDS. If the bone must wait a day to be used, the graft is wrapped in aluminum foil, put in a large sterile jar with air-proof lid, and preserved in a refrigerator at 4 °C. The paste is used to fill bone defects of the acetabulum and the femur.

We performed 47 surgical procedures according to this protocol. We checked the evolution of this graft by evaluating the X ray taken immediately postoperatively and at 4 months and at 1 year thereafter. In one case primary stability was not achieved, the acetabular component mobilized, the graft resorbed, and the patient required a new operation. In three cases, after 4 months, the graft in paste

Bone Transplantation
Eds.: M. Aebi, P. Regazzoni

put in the medial aspect of the acetabulum was seen to be resorbed. The implant is still stable, but the future looks uncertain. In the remaining 43 cases there was appearance of new bone formation in both the acetabular and femoral sides within the first 4 months. In the following year this new bone usually undergoes a remodeling that tends to reproduce the standard anatomical patterns. These results, compared with those of the two previous groups, encourage us to follow this procedure.

Use of Homologue Bone Graft Sterilized in Autoclave for Reconstruction in Loosening of Total Hip Prosthesis: A Series of 90 Reconstructions with Bone Graft and Cementless Hip Replacement CLW

D. Weill, M. Schroeder, and P. Fiore

Department of Orthopaedic Surgery, Hopital Belle Isle, Metz, France

We have been interested in the cementless fixation of total hip prostheses for over 11 years. Starting in 1982, we developed a new cementless total hip prosthesis, the acetabular component of which is now distributed in a great many countries, while the femoral implant is still in the experimental stage. Faced with a growing number of revisions, we have gradually chosen, wherever possible, cementless replacement with restitution of the bone stock by grafting.

The CLW cementless acetabular replacement is a self-tapping threaded ring made of pure titanium with a sand-blasted finish providing a surface phenomenon promoting bone union. The fixation is provided by four rows of self-tapping, cutting threads. The slightly ovoid truncated-cone shape is essential, as it is compatible with a hemispherical acetabulum, and it provides good primary and secondary stability, some freedom of orientation and maximum reduction of expulsion stresses. The absence of a bottom is essential as it reduces the rigidity of the implant and makes possible a peri-operative check of the positioning and the progress of the screwing. This absence of bottom is not prejudicial because the distribution of stresses mainly follows an elliptical path around the ring; the polyethylene insert is jammed by the tight truncated-cone fitting in the ring with a metal-back effect. The bottom of the insert may be covered with a metal net treated with titanium nitrite (sulmesh) to avoid contact between polyethylene and bone. These theoretical biomechanical considerations have been confirmed by the study of the finite elements and the biomechanical tests.

The femoral prosthesis CLW is a collarless stem made of a titanium alloy with a sand-blasted finish and a rotation-secured thread, a cone corresponding to the modular system, a longitudinal structure and a distal fissure. This prosthesis has staggered fixation and optimum stability and centering. Load-transmission is particularly smooth without hyperpressure or by-pass, as confirmed by study of the finite elements.

For graft material we use grafts sterilized in the autoclave, using all the femoral heads of the first arthroplasties. These heads are cleaned and sterilized two or three times; this gives us very plastic bone graft. After one sterilization, the osseous tissue seems perfectly in accord with histology and is normally mineralized. The intra-osseous spaces consist of a respected haemotopoietic tissue, the morphological appearance of which is largely comparable to that of osseous tissue

Bone Transplantation
Eds.: M. Aebi, P. Regazzoni

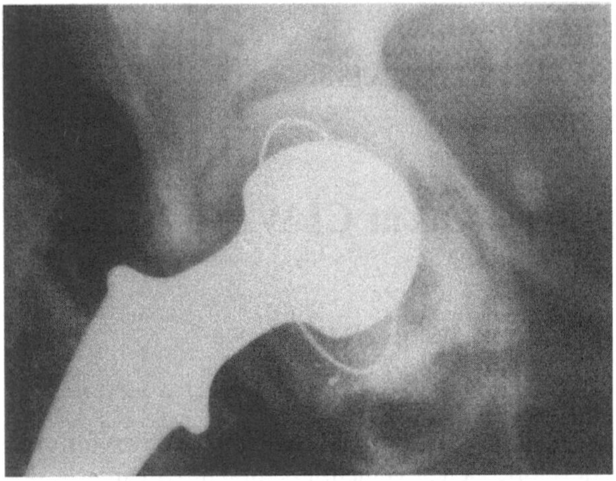

Fig. 1. THR loosening

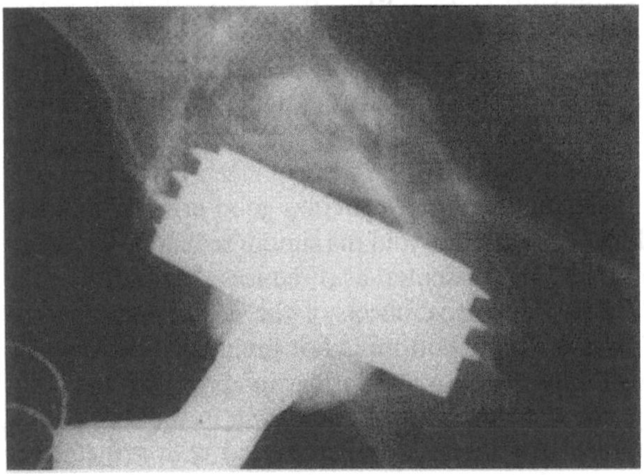

Fig. 2. X ray 24 months after revision (good result)

which has not been sterilized. After several sterilizations, the appearance of the osseous tissue is respected, but there is total necrotic coagulation of the medullary haemotopoietic elements.

Indication for this is wherever a firm fixation is possible; this is in seven or eight cases out of ten. This primary stability requires preservation or recuperation of the anterior wall by reaming. The stem must be stable. In infected prosthesis and septic loosening, we use the same method (Fig. 1).

Failures have included: one death, four failures at the acetabulum; one migration with secondary restabilization; and three instabilities because of insufficient primary fixation (technical error). At the femur, one recurrence of pre-operative infection. Apart from these failures, connected with the development of the method, results have been good on the whole: 90 rings, 29 stems; 67 good results on 73 cases with sufficient follow-up (Fig. 2).

In conclusion, CLW THR combined with homologous graft sterilized by autoclave gives good immediate results which must yet be confirmed.

References

1. Weill D (1986) Reconstruction du cotyle par greffe osseuse et anneau vissé autotaraudant non cimeté CLW. In: Poitout D (ed) Greffes de l'appareil locomoteur. Masson, Paris, pp 161–169
2. Weill D (1986) Cotyle vissé sans ciment CLW (et prothèse fémorale non cimentée espérimentale CLW) – Etude préliminaire. Ann Orthop Traumat 9(1):65–77
3. Weill D (1986) Reconstruction du cotyle par greffe osseuse et anneau vissé autotaraudant non cimenté CLW. Acta Belg Orthop 52(3):332–343
4. Kirschner P, Franz W (1987) Erste Erfahrungen mit dem neuen zementfreien Schraubring zum Hüftpfannenersatz nach D. Weill. Unfallchirurgie 13(1):27–31

Human Bone Morphogenetic Protein Augmentation Grafting of Segmental Defects of the Lower Extremity

E. E. Johnson and M. R. Urist

Bone Research Laboratory and the Division of Orthopaedic Surgery, University of California, Los Angeles Medical Center (UCLA), Los Angeles, California, USA

Nonunions or large segmental defects of long bones which have failed multiple surgical and conservative attempts at union are a significant problem and may be resistant to further standard surgical treatment. The implantation of a substance which induces primitive cells in the perinonunion area to undergo an osteogenetic pathway of development may represent a significant change in the management of the resistant nonunion or skeletal defects. This augmentation of the host healing response by the addition of human bone morphogenetic protein (hBMP) to cancellous autogeneic graft is the theoretical postulate used to definitively treat this series of resistant nonunions and skeletal defects.

A total of 26 patients with intractable nonunion or segmental defect of the femoral, tibial, or humeral shaft were successfully treated by a combination of débridement, internal or external fixation, autogeneic grafting (13/26 patients), and implantation of hBMP. There were 12 femoral nonunions, 6 tibial nonunions, 6 segmental tibial defects (3, 4, 5, 8, 13, 17 cm), and 2 humeral nonunions included in this study. Average preoperative duration of the nonunion or defect was 26.8 months (range, 5.1–68.3 months). In 23 patients 86 previous surgical procedures attempting union were performed (average, 3.7 per patient). Four patients were treated with cast immobilization. The hBMP was prepared in the form of an aggregate of bone matrix water-insoluble noncollagenous proteins (hBMP/iNCP). In the fracture gap 50–100 mg hBMP/iNCP was implanted as an intercalary implant in ultrathin gelatin capsules or incorporated in a strip of polylactic/polyglycolic acid (PLA/PGA) copolymer and placed as an onlay graft across the fracture gap.

In the 26 patients, 24 healed with the initial procedure; three initial failures healed with repeat hBMP implantation. The average time to union of the tibia nonunions was 3.7 months, femoral nonunions 4.4 months, humeral nonunions 2.3 months, and for the segmental tibial defects 5.7 months. Overall follow-up averaged 19.9 months (range, 5.4–45.2 months). In five of the six segmental tibial defects initial operation restored the bone continuity per primum, and by a second operation (repeat implantation of hBMP) in one. There were three failures under this protocol, all of which healed with repeat stabilization and hBMP grafting. The course of wound healing was remarkably uncomplicated in all patients without swelling, hyperemia, or evidence of immune reaction.

We feel that hBMP augmentation grafting favorably influenced healing in the majority of these resistant cases. Further clinical investigations should be designed to distinguish hBMP effect from the effects of new or improved methods of fracture fixation and autogeneic cancellous bone grafts. The problem to be

Bone Transplantation
Eds.: M. Aebi, P. Regazzoni

solved by further investigations is to measure the amount of new bone formation produced from preexisting host bone cells and to determine the amount new bone developed from bone marrow perivascular target cells that can be recruited to enter an osteogenetic pathway of development by augmentation with hBMP.

Sintered Bone: A New Type of Bone Graft

Yu Ueno

Department of Orthopaedic Surgery, Wakayama Medical College, Japan

One of the most pressing concerns among surgeons is to develop a new type of bone graft material. Additional surgery on the same patient is always necessary in procuring autograft, and there is often a limit to supply. Complications of autograft are also well-known. Allograft and xenograft cannot be totally free from immunological problems. Nowadays, serious infection such as AIDS or hepatitis and unknown infections must also be considered. To overcome these difficulties, in 1982 we developed sintered bone, termed True Bone Ceramics (Koken, Tokyo, Japan). This material is not synthesized but derived from mammalian bone.

Frozen bovine bones are treated in advance by boiling in water and immersing in a chemical solution for deproteinization. They are then sintered in a furnace in two stages at 600° and 1100°/1450 °C. These treatments result in complete deproteinization of bone and crystalization of bone minerals. No organic material remains; Ca 38.9%, P 21.3%, and a small amount of other minerals are found. Crylstalized bone apatite can be analysed by X-ray difraction. The anatomical structure is well preserved. Histological sections of sintered bone grafted into the bone of rabbits show good histocompatibility, new bone formation, and incorporation between the new bone and the graft. There is no foreign body reaction and a lack of intervening fibrous tissue between them. Furthermore, the villiform of bone matrix growing in between crystalline particles can be observed. New bone and bone marrow are formed in pores of the cancellous portion of sintered bone. Sintered bone was grafted in orthopaedic and facio-mandibular cases. Cubic cancellous blocks were grafted into cavities through surgical holes in tumor cases and into surgical defects or under decorticated spaces in pseudarthrosis. Supplementary autograft was carried out in some difficult cases.

Sintered bone grafting was carried out in 60 clinical cases up until March 1986. There were 38 men and 22 women. Age averaged 36.2 years (9–71). Supplementary autograft was done in 17 cases. Follow-up term averaged 9.6 months (2 weeks to 43 months). Aetiology of disease was: 7 cases of fracture, 8 of pseudarthrosis, 6 of osteomyelitis, 32 of tumour and tumourous conditions and 7 others. The grafts were totally or partially excised in two cases of malignancy and three of postoperative infection in the oral cavity. The others showed a good clinical course. No rejection of graft or persistent inflammation occurred, and normal serum data was observed. Incorporation between the graft and bone was observed by 5 months radiologically in most of the tumour cases. Grafted areas became gradually unclear due to new bone formation around grafts. Normal healing at the surgical holes, normal bone growth at the epiphyseal plate and remodelling were observed.

Bone Transplantation
Eds.: M. Aebi, P. Regazzoni

Sintered bone is a completely deproteinized bone, so that there are no risks of infection or immunological problems. The results of our work suggest that sintered bone has the potential for becoming a new bone graft instead of auto- and allograft. This encourages us to use sintered bone in some cases of revision arthroplasty and spinal surgery with or without supplementary autograft.

References

1. Ueno Y et al. (1985) Experimental studies of sintered bone implantation. Orthop Surg [Suppl] 8:85–88 (in Japanese)
2. Ueno Y, Shima Y, Akiyama T (1987) Development of a new biomaterial as a bone substitute; True Bone Ceramics. In: Ceramic in clinical applications. Elsevier, Amsterdam, pp 369–378 (Material science monographs, vol 39)

Massive Allografts in Non-tumorous Orthopaedic Conditions

W. Mnaymneh [1], T. Malinin [2], and W. Head [3]

[1] Department of Orthopaedics and Rehabilitation, University of Miami School of Medicine, Miami, Florida, USA
[2] Department of Surgery, University of Miami School of Medicine, Miami, Florida, USA
[3] Gaston Episcopal Hospital, Dallas, Texas, USA

Encouraged by our favourable results with the use of massive allografts in reconstructive surgery of bone tumors [1], we started a prospective clinical study in September 1982 to use massive osseous and osteo-articular allografts to replace destroyed, injured or diseased segments of the skeleton in non-tumorous orthopaedic conditions [2]. The purpose of this paper is to evaluate the results of this study.

A total of 90 patients operated upon at the University of Miami Medical Center in Miami, Florida, and the Gaston Episcopal Hospital in Dallas, Texas, between September 1982 and September 1984 were followed up for 2.5–4.5 years.

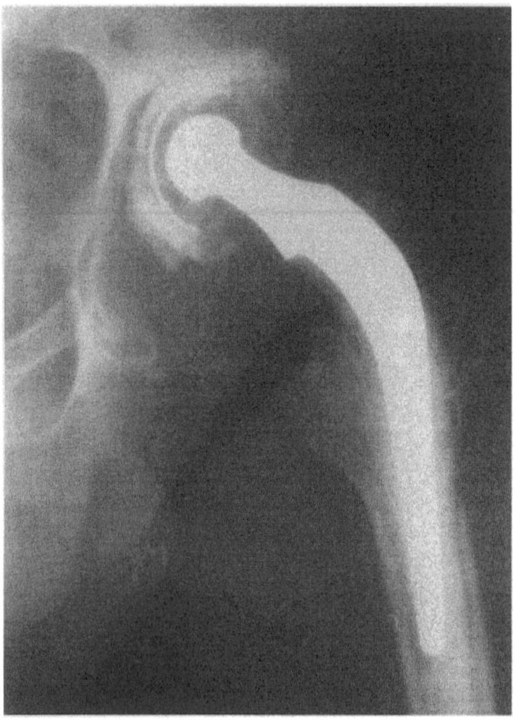

a

Fig. 1. a Grossly loose femoral prosthesis and acetabular cup with significant bone loss. **b** Illustration of the femoral and acetabular allografts. **c** Union of the graft-host junctions in the femur and acetabulum 2.5 years postoperative

Bone Transplantation
Eds.: M. Aebi, P. Regazzoni

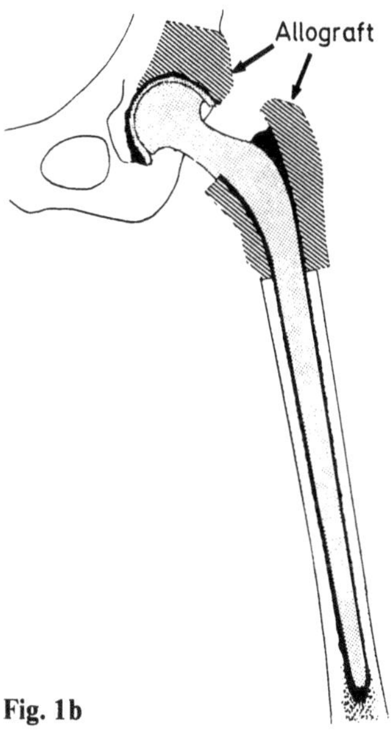

Fig. 1b

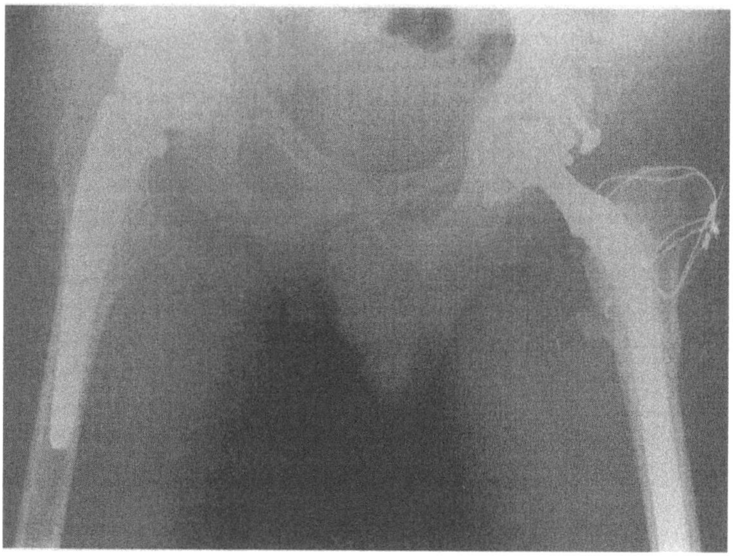

Fig. 1c

Three types of allografts were used: osteo-articular (35), intercalary (6) and graft-prosthesis composites (49). Of the osteo-articular allografts there were 18 whole joints, 13 hemijoints and 4 quarter joints. The clinical conditions included revision arthroplasty (54), trauma (6), osteo-arthritis (2), post-traumatic arthritis (6), rheumatoid arthritis (4), chondromalacia patella (10), osteonecrosis (4), femoral lengthening (3) and knee fusion after failed total knee replacement (1).

The initial overall results were 67% satisfactory and 33% unsatisfactory cases. The unsatisfactory results (30 cases) included cartilage failure in 18 cases (20%), non-union of the host-graft junction in 4 cases (4.4%), infection in 4 cases (4.4%), femoral stem loosening in 3 cases (3.3%), and femoral stem fracture in 1 case (1%). Over half of the unsatisfactory results were later salvaged and rendered satisfactory with subsequent surgery without causing serious disability to the patient. In terms of type of allografts, satisfactory results were obtained in 88% of graft-prosthesis composites, 83% of intercalary and only 35% of osteo-articular allografts.

Massive osseous and osteo-articular allografts provide a useful reconstructive alternative in selected non-tumorous orthopaedic conditions to replace lost, injured or diseased bone and joints of the extremities. The best results were achieved in allograft-prosthesis composites, especially in revisions of failed total hip [3, 4] and knee arthroplasties where there was deficient bone stock (Fig. 1). The worst results were in osteo-articular allografts, due mainly to articular cartilage failure (degeneration and conversion to fibrocartilage).

References

1. Mnaymneh W, Malinin T et al. (1985) Massive osteoarticular allografts in the reconstruction of extremities following resection of tumors not requiring chemotherapy or radiotherapy. Clin Orthop 197:876–878
2. Mnaymneh W, Malinin T et al. (1986) Massive osseous and osteoarticular allografts in non-tumorous disorders. Contemp Orthop 13:13–24
3. Borja F, Mnaymneh W (1985) Bone allografts in salvage of difficult hip arthroplasties. Clin Orthop 197:123–130
4. Head W, Malinin T (1987) Freeze dried proximal femur allografts in revision total hip arthroplasty. Clin Orthop 215:109–121

Our Experience with Frozen Allografts: First Short-Term Results

F. Handelberg, P. Yde, H. de Boeck, P. P. Casteleyn, and P. Opdecam

Department of Orthopaedics and Traumatology, Academic Hospital, Free University, Brussels, Belgium

Since revision arthroplasty of hip and knee came to be performed, and cases frequently present a lack of good bone stock, the necessity of having a bone bank became obvious.

In the first 18 months of experience, in our department we used frozen femoral heads as allografts. These femoral heads were obtained from patients undergoing hip arthroplasty for osteoarthritis or femoral neck fracture. A bacteriological sample was taken immediately thereafter. In most cases cartilage was removed and each femoral head was directly stored in a sterile box and quickly frozen to −25 °C in standard commericial deep freezer. Following a strict protocol, excluding infection, neoplasm or systemic disease of the donor, with control of hepatitis and syphilis serology, the bone grafts were considered ready for use after 3 weeks. They were discarded if the bacteriologic sample was positive, if postoperative infection of the donor (wound, urinary, etc.) occurred, and in any case after 3 months. The allografts were used either in toto or as bone chips, in combination or not with autologous grafts.

In all, 35 cases were reviewed. The major indications were: (a) reconstruction of the bone stock in revision arthroplasty of hip (8 cases) or knee (2 cases), and (b) multifragmentary fractures of lower limbs treated by internal fixation (9 femura, 4 tibiae, 1 calcaneum). Furthermore, frozen bone allografts were used in various indications, such as arthrodesis of foot and ankle (4 cases), filling up after curettage of tumors (2 fibrous dysplasia and 1 osteoblastoma of the talus), or osteomyelitis (1 case), and miscellaneous indications as one vertebral arthrodesis, one Leeds-Keio ligamentoplasty, and one Maquet osteotomy.

No major complications related to bone grafting occurred. Radiological ingrowth could be noticed in most cases. As an example, we show the complete ingrowth of mixed grafts 9 months after curettage of a fibrous dysplasia of the right distal humerus in a 15-year old girl (Fig. 1).

We found frozen femoral head allografts valuable, especially in the treatment of multifragmentary fractures of the lower limb and in revision arthroplasty, even without complex harvesting and storage techniques.

Bone Transplantation
Eds.: M. Aebi, P. Regazzoni

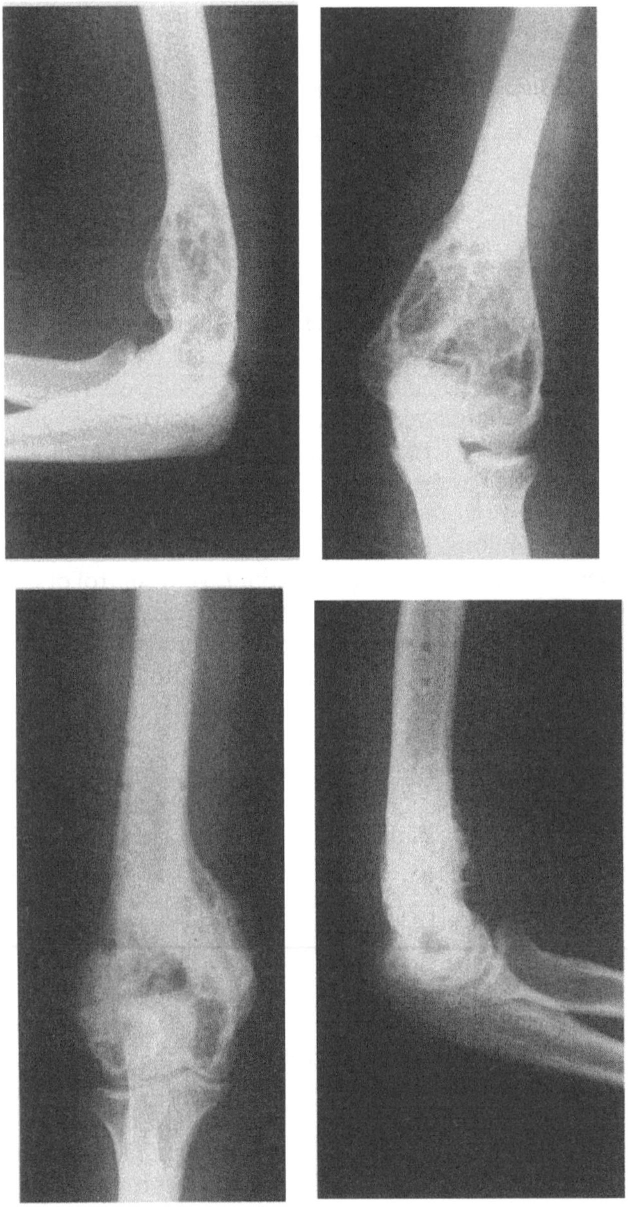

a
b

Fig. 1. a Fibrous dysplasia of the right distal humerus in a 15-year-old girl. **b** Complete ingrowth of mixed grafts 9 months after curettage

Our Experience with Massive Deep-Frozen Allografts in Limb Salvage Surgery and with Cryopreserved Osteoarticular Allografts in Joint Lesions

C. Delloye, P. de Nayer, L. Coutelier, and A. Vincent

Department of Orthopaedic Surgery, St-Luc University Clinics, 10 avenue Hippocrate, Brussels, Belgium

Massive bone allografting is particularly useful to restore skeletal continuity after tumor resection. The use of cryopreserved cartilage in joint allografting is still a matter of debate. The long-term fate of both is largely unknown. We present our experience of large bone allografts, three of them lasting more than 10 years, and the first results with cryopreserved osteoarticular allografts.

Twelve patients with massive deep-frozen (−80 °C) bone allografts after tumor resection were followed up from 14 months to 17 years. Most of the reconstructive procedures included a segmental bone allograft with knee or ankle fusion. The mean length of the dia/epiphyseal implants was 16 cm, and they were usually fixed with intramedullary nail. In nine other patients, an osteoarticular graft was transplanted for posttraumatic joint lesions (6 cases) or to preserve the joint after tumoral resection (3). The cartilage allograft was protected from freezing injury by dimethylsulfoxide during deep-freezing at −80 °C. The knee was concerned five times and shoulder, elbow, wrist, and hip once. The joint was totally replaced in two cases (elbow and knee).

Full loading was achieved at 8.5 ± 4 months (10) in total replacement. All the graft junctions healed primarily except one. Cancellous bone junctions were united within 6 months while cortical bone healed within 8–15 months.

Among the complications, graft infections (2) were the most critical as they finally required amputation in both cases. There were three stress fractures, treated surgically without further complications. Graft incorporation could be assessed by bone scintimetry in four cases. Tc diphosphonate (99m) uptake by the graft was found to be superior to control bone segments at only 15 years after surgery. By X-ray examination, 10 years are necessary to observe an extensive remodeling of the allografted bone. The two recovered allografts were studied by microradiography. It was found that in nailed massive deep-frozen allografts, creeping substitution was a very slow process and only located at the subperiosteal area of the cortex at 18 and 30 months after surgery.

Intracortical remodeling was characterized by large resorption cavities, incompletely filled with new lamellar bone. This creeping substitution was predominant in area where the implant was ensheathed by a new bone layer. New bone either along or within the graft was not fully mineralized. At the joint fusion side, new bone deposits on allograft trabeculae were observed up to 10 mm inside the implant. In the osteoarticular group, there was no nonunion. A functional mobil-

Bone Transplantation
Eds.: M. Aebi, P. Regazzoni

ity was rapidly restored when muscles were left intact. Full loading in knee replacements was obtained in 12 weeks.

Massive bone allografts are very slowly (> 10 years) revascularized by creeping substitution. They allow the preservation of a useful limb. Infection was the heaviest surgical complication. Critical factors in the fate of osteoarticular allograft appeared to be: a good fixation and stability to allow an early mobilization; the mechanical alignment and the fit of the new joint, which is difficult in partial replacement and especially in femoral condyles; and the preservation of the host synovial tissue to maintain chondrocyte viability, particularly in total joint.

Three-Years' Experience with Small Freeze-Dried Bone Implants used in Various Conditions

C. Delloye, N. Allington, E. Munting, B. Geulette, and A. Vincent

Department of Orthopaedic Surgery, St-Luc University Clinics, Brussels, Belgium

Since 1983, the authors have selected, prepared and used over 700 freeze-dried allogeneic bones in various orthopaedic conditions. In selected cases, an autograft can be substituted by an allograft, provided that the implant has a large and stable contact with a well-vascularized bone bed. These allografts were made available in order to spare the patient an additonal incision for autograft procurement in selected cases.

Bone samples are procured from young or middle-aged patients within 12 h of death. Potential donors are selected to avoid any transfer of disease. After skin preparation, bones are usually taken from lower limb epiphyses. Preparation includes soft tissue removal, thorough washing with distilled water, lipid extraction by immersion in a chloroform-methanol solution and distilled-water rinsing. Implants are freeze-dried and wrapped in two sterile packing systems and placed in a polyethylene bag. Processed bone are finally sterilized by gamma irradiation at a dose of 25 kGy. Before implantation, they are reconstituted in saline.

After 3 years, 222 patients had received over 500 freeze-dried allogeneic bones in 228 locations. The most frequent indications were: revision hip arthroplasty (20.6%), filling of cavities after removal of hardware or osteotomies (17.4%) and scoliosis (14.8%). Most patients received one implant (53.5%) while 9.6% were grafted with more than five implants, equivalent to about two or three femoral heads.

For this study, 64 cases were available in which X-ray assessment could be easily performed. In these cases, the implants were evident on X ray and well documented with a minimal 6-month follow-up. Based on graft union to host bed and graft volume preservation, 79.7% of implants gave a very good result (regular fusion within 6 months). A satisfactory course of healing was found in 9.4% of the grafts (irregular fusion but within 6 months and/or <25% decrease of the initial implant volume) while 10.9% were considered as failures (non-union at 6 months and/or >25% loss of the initial volume). Five of the seven failures were due to impaired graft implantation technique or improper indication that could be avoided. Clinically, allografts at 1 year, were assessed favourably by the surgeon in 90.5% of the cases.

As a preserved implant has only an osteoconductive property, successful incorporation relies critically on the osteogenic capacity of the bone bed. This grafting material appears reliable in its clinical results, as 89% of good or very good results were obtained when correctly implanted. Compared to sterile procured femoral heads, our processed acellular implant is less immunogenic (HLA and rhesus). It serves multiple purposes and increases the bone reconstruction possibilities.

Bone Transplantation
Eds.: M. Aebi, P. Regazzoni

Reference

Delloye et al. (1987) Acta Orthop Belg 53:2–11

Allogeneic Osteoarticular Grafts About the Knee

A. Alho [1], E.O. Karaharju [2], O. Korkala [2], E. Laasonen [2], T. Holmström [3], and G.P. Andersen [1]

[1] Ullevaal Hospital, University of Oslo, Oslo, Norway
[2] Töölö Hospital, Helsinki University Central Hospital, Helsinki, Finland
[3] Department of Pathology, Helsinki University, Helsinki, Finland

Osteoarticular resection of bone tumor results in a reconstruction problem which has not been solved satisfactorily. Allogeneic deep-frozen osteoarticular transplant is one of the alternatives.

We used osteoarticular allografts about the knee in 15 patients aged 17–63 years. Nine grafts were bicondylar femoral, three were unicondylar femoral, one was bicondylar tibial, and two were unicondylar tibial grafts. Thirteen transplantations were performed for bone tumor and two for incongruency after tibial condylar fracture. The transplants were harvested from donors between 16 and 50 years of age according to generally accepted criteria. The size of the allograft was the only decisive matching criterion. The tissue types were recorded, but not taken into consideration.

In the first nine cases the grafts were frozen at −70 °C for 2 days, and stored at −20 °C until used. In the last six cases, dimethylsulfoxide (DMSO) was used as chondrocyte preservative, with the storage temperature being −70 °C (freezing speed, 1 °C per h). Rapid thawing was utilized. The femoral grafts were fixed with AO plate osteosynthesis, the ligaments reconstructed, and a sleeve of autologous bone chips from iliac crest created over the host-graft junction. In the tibia, locking intramedullary nailing has lately replaced plate osteosynthesis.

Our present postoperative care consists of plaster cast for 3 weeks replaced by a hinged brace for 5 weeks. The patients did not bear weight for 3 months, and partial weight bearing was allowed according to radiographic controls during a further 3–8 months. The patients were followed once monthly during the 1st year, at 3- to 6-month intervals during the following 2 years, and each year thereafter. Scintigrams and computed tomograms were taken regularly. In ten cases biopsies were also taken.

The late result evaluation between 2 and 5 years and later was done according to the criteria of the Musculoskeletal Tumor Society, grading motion, pain, stability/deformity, strength, emotional acceptance/functional activities, and complications. The overall result was also graded according to Mankin [2] as excellent, good, fair, or poor. After shortening of the immobilization period, the knee motion improved significantly without any adverse effect on the joint stability.

Thirteen complications were experienced. Three grafts showed slow resorption. In one case graded as failure, the graft was replaced by hinged knee prosthesis. This was followed by a postoperative infection, and fusion was necessary. In two partial resorptions, where the joint surface was not affected, autografts were used. Three minor joint surface dissections were experienced. Three grafts fractured and were treated with osteosynthesis and autograft chips. One ligament in-

Bone Transplantation
Eds.: M. Aebi, P. Regazzoni

sufficiency was reconstructed, and one patellectomy performed due to subluxation. One giant cell tumor recurred and was treated by curettage and cementing. No infections complicating the grafting operation were experienced.

The scintigraphic patterns indicating osteogenesis, -conduction, and/or -induction varied, and we have not been able to find any clear-cut correlations to the clinical result. If any general conclusion can be drawn, it seems to be that a quick scintigraphic incorporation is consistent with a favorable clinical result.

The histologic picture corresponded to the scintigraphic findings, with varying rate and degree of incorporation. Accretion of living bone on dead trabeculae was the most common finding; in some cases total creeping substitution was observed. The computed tomograms also showed sclerotic accretion during several years. Without preservative the transplanted cartilage was obviously dead. The living cartilage seen in a specimen at 7 years was most probably fibrocartilage after regeneration. The survival of cartilage may be better using DMSO as preservative. Structurally, the chondrocytes looked normal in the early biopsies, but only partial survival seems to be the case. No clear correlation was found between radiographic and clinical results in individual cases, but a gradual deterioration in the whole series was obvious during the observation period. However, more recent cases start as excellent than was the case in the oldest transplantations.

At 2–5 years four results were excellent, six good, and five fair. At 9–16 years, no result was excellent, four were good, five fair, and one fusion was graded as failure.

We were interested in comparing our results with the reported results of allografting, resection arthrodesis, and prosthetic replacement of the knee. It seems that allografting and fusion are demanding for the patient due to several reoperations. The failure frequencies are similar, but the functional result after an allograft replacement is better. A 10% failure rate in the prosthesis series was obtained after salvaging the first failed prosthesis with a new one. But then, the same method may be used after a failed allograft replacement, which improves these results.

We conclude that osteoarticular allografting gives results which are comparable with the alternatives of arthrodesis and prosthesis replacement. However, at the present time, it does not represent a final solution due to the unpredictable problems of bone resorption and cartilage degeneration.

References

1. Alho A, Karaharju EO, Korkala O, Laasonen E (1987) Hemijoint allografts in the treatment of low grade malignant and aggressive bone tumours about the knee. Int Orthop (SICOT) 11:35–41
2. Mankin HJ (1983) Allograft replacement for the management of skeletal defects incurred in tumor surgery or trauma. In: Chao EYS, Ivins JC (eds) Tumor prostheses of bone and joint reconstruction: the design and application. Thieme-Stratton, New York, pp 23–24

Frozen Homologous Trabecular Bone Allografts: 12-Years' Experience with Banking and Clinical Use

G. U. Exner, A. R. Goldmann, M. Nottebaert, and A. Schreiber

Department of Orthopedics, Klinik Balgrist, University of Zurich, Forchstr. 340, 8008 Zurich, Switzerland

Frozen homologous trabecular bone (FHTB) is probably the most commonly used allogeneic material for biologic replacement of bone defects [1]. FHTB has been in use at the Klinik Balgrist since 1974. The results in cases of large defects are of interest in comparison with, for example, massive allografts.

Specimens stored and used consisted almost exclusively of material resected at implantation of hip endoprostheses. From a total of 423 samples taken for storage, 173 (40%) were rejected for use either because of pathologic findings in the donor patient (laboratory: ESR, CBC, SGOT, SGPT, or hepatitis, lues, or HIV

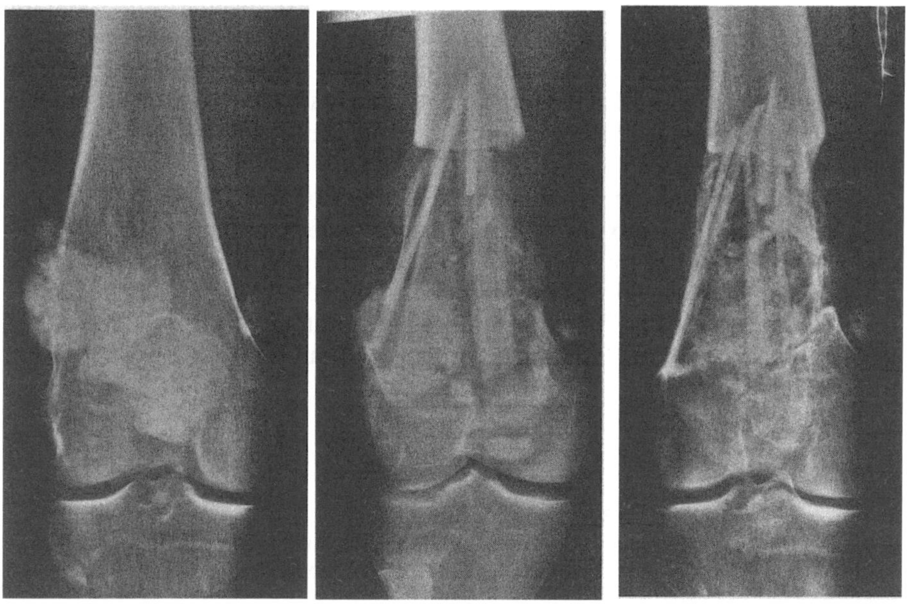

Fig. 1. Juxtacort. Chondrosarcoma distal right femur following repeated removal of multiple osteochondromas (*left*). On 31 January 1985 (*middle*) en bloc resection, stabilization with fixateur externe and fibular "spacer" transplants; filling of the defect centrally with four samples of banked trabecular bone impregnated with fibrin wrapped in a cuff of autologous iliac bone grafts taken bilaterally. Postoperatively arrosion of femoral artery by Steinmann pin, needing venous graft interposition and removal of the external fixator; leg cast until 22 July 1985. Mobilization with a splint until 28 January 1986 (*right*) with ischial weight bearing. Full weight bearing, apparatus-free, after 14 April 1986. Today, pain-free employment as plumber (50%). Because of still limited range of knee motion (F/E 70-0-0) open mobilization (Judet) planned

Bone Transplantation
Eds.: M. Aebi, P. Regazzoni

serology; wound infection, history of neoplasm, etc.), positive bacterial cultures from the bone sample, nonuse within 6 months of storage, or a defect of the freezer. Some of the remaining 250 units were given to other institutions. For the material used at the Klinik Balgrist the recipients were recorded in most cases ($n=60$). All charts of these 60 known recipients were reviewed. In almost every patient the FHTB was used in a mixture with autologous bone taken at surgery.

Eighteen patients received a total of 44 units FHTB mixed with autologous material at ratios ranging from 4:1 to 1:4 (average, 1:1) to fil defects after removal of benign tumors (fibrous dysplasia, nonossifying fibroma, juvenile cysts, aneurysmal bone cyst, chondroma, giant cell tumor). Follow-up ranged from 2 to 9 years (average, 6 years) and was uneventful except in three patients with reoperations because of recurrent giant cell tumors. Five patients received FHTB after local resections of malignant tumors (chondrosarcoma, osteosarcoma, giant cell tumor). One had a persistent pseudarthrosis after 5 years; the others died or had amputations because of local recurrence. Two patients had large bone resections, and each received 2 units of FHTB in combination with autologous bone at a ratio of 2:1; during a follow-up of 6 years no recurrence was noted.

Other applications of FHTB were in spinal fusion for scoliosis ($n=22$) with a follow-up of 1–10 years, in two reoperations because of pseudarthrosis, and for lumbal degenerative disease ($n=11$), in which the factor is difficult to assess. In the treatment of pseudarthrosis of long bones FHTB was used twice, successfully in one case. At present, FHTB is increasingly used to fill large bone defects during replacement of loosened hip alloarthroplasty; the duration of follow-up does not yet allow evaluation.

FHTB is thus useful in the replacement of large bone defects. Since FHTB has always been used in a mixture with autologous bone transplants, no interpretation as to its advantages over pure homologous transplantation is possible. The good results, however, of this empirically introduced mixture may find support from experimental data [2], and theoretically the autologous bone may add osteoblasts and in part replace bone-morphogeneic substances destroyed during freezing.

References

1. Orthopäde (1986) 15:1–58 (several articles)
2. Köhler P (1986) Reimplantation of bone after autoclaving. Reconstructions of large diaphyseal defects in the rabbit. Thesis, University of Stockholm (ISBN 91-7900-038-X)

Orthopedic Results of 87 Massive Allografts in Reconstructive Surgery for Bone Cancers

G. Delepine [1], P. Hernigou [2], D. Goutallier [2], and N. Delepine [3]

[1] Orthopedic Clinic Pre Gentil, 93110 Rosnyl Paris, France
[2] Service d'Orthopedie, Hôpital H. Mondor, 94000 Creteil, France
[3] Pediatric Oncologic Unit, Hôpital Herold, 75019 Paris, France

Since May 1984 we have used 87 bank allografts to reconstruct large (+7-cm) bone defects after en bloc resection for limb cancers. Average length of bone defect was 20 cm (range, 7–43). Allografts were conserved at −30 °C and preoperatively sterilized by beta irradiation. Synthesis of grafts used long-stem titanium prostheses in 55 cases and nail, plate, and cement in the others. Histology of tumors was: osteosarcoma in 40, chondrosarcoma in 13, Ewing's sarcoma in 9, fibrosarcoma in 10, bone metastasis in 8, and others in 7. According to Ennecking, staging was IA in 2, IB in 3, IIA in 2, IIB in 66, and IIIB in 14. Location of tumors was: distal femur in 26, upper femur in 13, upper humerus in 13, upper tibia in

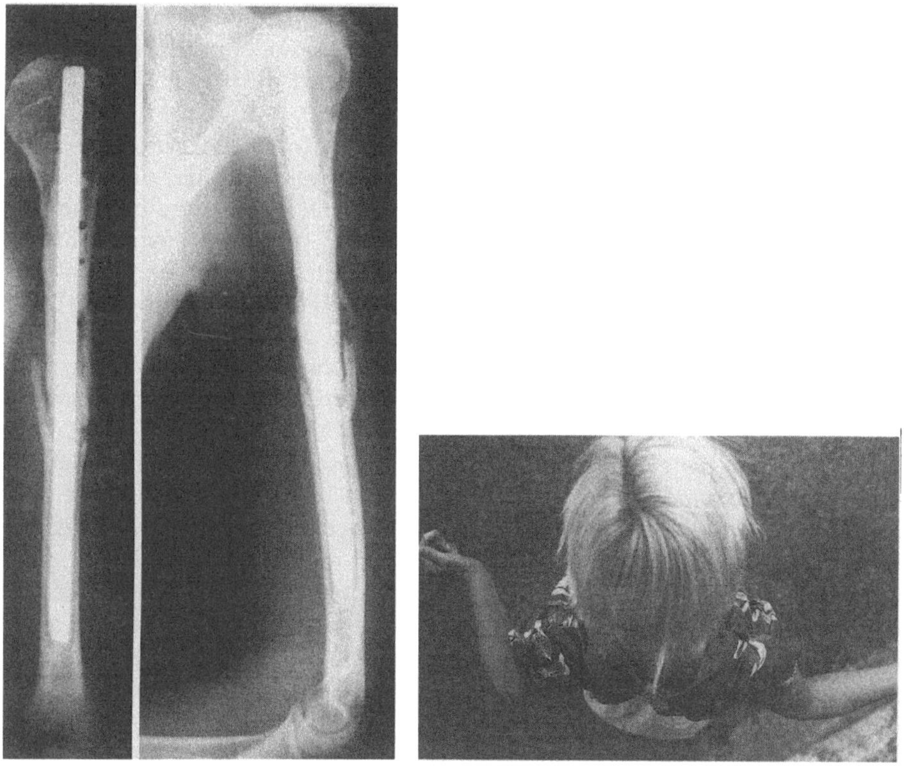

a b

Fig. 1. a Allograft replacement of upper humerus for chondrosarcoma. **b** Active external rotation obtained

Bone Transplantation
Eds.: M. Aebi, P. Regazzoni

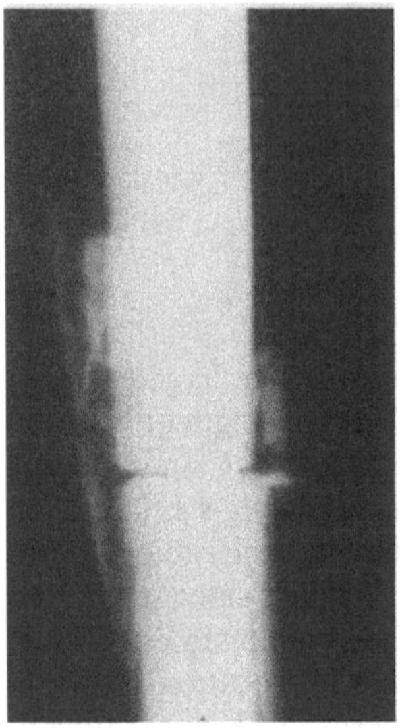

Fig. 2. High-grade osteosarcoma. TID protocol. Little peripheral ossification after 18 months

12, humeral diaphysis in 10, distal tibia in 4, others in 9. Local treatment was completed by radiotherapy in 62 and chemotherapy in 69. Weight bearing was immediate in 69 cases but postponed 3–6 months in 16 cases. For upper tibia and proximal humerus, active articular mobility was restricted during 45 days to help muscles reattachment.

All patients were followed by the same physician, for an average length of 16 months (range, 3–33). At last follow-up, 74 patients were still alive. Five local recurrences and three deep infections have been observed, leading to three amputations. Orthopedic complications included nine diaphyseal pseudarthrosis (seven cured by reoperation) and five secondary fractures (only one symptomatic). No bone resorption (except in one infection and one local recurrence), fracture of cement or of stem prosthesis, or radiological sign of loosening have been observed, in contrast with our former massive prostheses. Muscle reinsertion seems to be effective on clinical examination of all patients and on macroscopic findings of reoperated cases.

This reliable reattachment of tendons and muscles improves functional results. After proximal humerus resection replaced by allograft the rotator cuff reattachment improves active motion and allows active external rotation (Fig. 1). In proximal femur reconstruction, the reattached muscles stabilize the hip, preventing dislocation (Fig. 2). After proximal tibia reconstruction, the reinsertion of patellar tendon avoids extensor lag. For distal femur reconstruction the allograft decreases stress on the prosthesis stem and helps prevent future loosening, as shown by minimal radiographic changes around stem prosthesis compared to our former massive stainles steel prostheses.

Reconstructive surgery using sterilized allografts gives better functional results than massive prostheses. Immediate weight bearing and bone union are always obtained when allografts are combined with very strong titanium nail or long-stem prostheses. Such reconstructive procedure is indicated whenever life expectancy seems greater than 1 year.

Bone Union of Allografts and Chemotherapy Considerations About 55 Consecutive Cases

N. Delepine [1], G. Delepine [2], P. Hernigou [3], M. Hassan [4], and J. C. Desbois [1]

[1] Pediatric Oncologic Unit, Herold, 75019 Paris, France
[2] Orthopedic Oncologic Unit, Pre Gentil, 93110 Rosny/Paris, France
[3] Orthopedic Unit, Hôpital Henri Mondor, 940000 Creteil, France
[4] Radiologic Unit, Hôpital Herold, 75019 Paris, France

After conservative surgery for bone sarcoma reconstructive procedures can use massive prostheses or bank allografts. Both have their own advantages and drawbacks. Massive stainless steel protheses permit immediate weight bearing but do not permit reliable muscles reattachment and are threatened by secondary failures (progressive bone resoprtion, loosening, stem fracture). Bank allografts permit muscles reattachment and usually give better functional results and long-term tolerance but are threatened by fracture, infection, and nonunion, especially when chemotherapy is used. This study evaluates the risk of nonunion of massive bank allografts when chemotherapy is used. To avoid bias by mechanical complications we analyzed only masive allograft-coating long-stem prostheses.

Beginning in August 1984 we used 55 massive, bank allograft-coating, long-stem titanium protheses to reconstruct bone defects after en bloc resection for limb cancers. Histology was: osteosarcoma in 27, Ewing's sarcoma in 8, chondrosarcoma in 10, others in 10. Location was distal femur in 26, proximal femur in 13, upper tibia in 8, upper humerus in 8. Average length of bone defect was 22 cm (range, 15–43). Allografts were harvested in sterile conditions, cryocon-

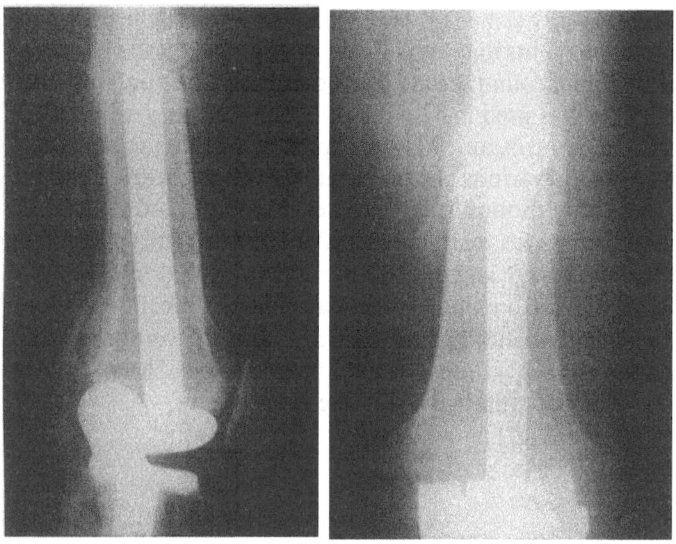

Fig. 1. Grade II chondrosarcoma. No chemotherapy. Peripheral bone healing after 3 months

Bone Transplantation
Eds.: M. Aebi, P. Regazzoni

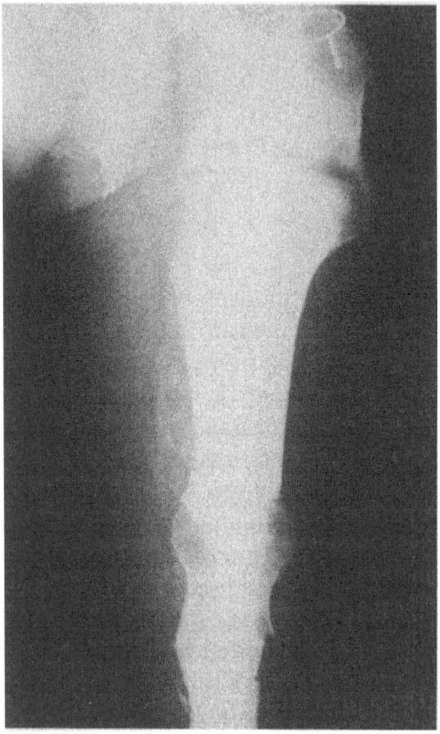

Fig. 2. Massive allograft-coating long-stem titanium prosthesis after resection of upper femoral Ewing's sarcoma. X-ray examination shows the effectiveness of trochanteric reattachment

served at −30 °C and preoperatively sterilized by beta irradiation. Prostheses were long-stem titanium prostheses, custom-made with individualized designs and sizes. Allografts were usually cemented on the prosthesis stem; the prosthesis was then cemented into the patients diaphysis. Fresh autogenous grafts harvested for opposite epiphysis was put around the allograft-diaphysis junction. Postoperative radiotherapy of 35 Gy was used in 42 patients. Chemotherapy included: 26 T 10 protocol (high-dose methotrexate), 9 Hayes's protocol (endoxan and adriamycin), 12 no chemotherapy, 8 various chemotherapies. Weight bearing was immediate in all cases, but active motion was restricted for 45 days in upper tibia and upper humerus to help muscles reattachment. All patients were followed up by the same surgeon for an average length of 14 months (range, 3–33).

Five patients were excluded from analysis for early death, infection, or local recurrence. The 50 others, had no mechanical problems, and an average duration of peripheral bone healing (ABHD) for each could be evaluated. The adverse effect of chemotherapy was evident; the ABDH in the groups were:

- No chemotherapy, 75 days (Fig. 1).
- Other chemotherapies, 160 days.
- Adriamycine-endoxan, 175 days.
- T 10 protocol, 246 days (Fig. 2).

We concluded that chemotherapy delays allograft bone union particularly when high-dose methotrexate is used. In such situation, allograft reconstruction should be protected by very strong synthesis or prosthesis, and fresh autogenous graft around junction seems mandatory.

The Influence of Pre- and Postoperative Polydrug Chemotherapy on Bone Healing in Tumor Surgery

W. Winkelmann [1] and H. Jürgens [2]

[1] University of Düsseldorf, Department of Orthopedic Surgery, Düsseldorf, FRG
[2] University of Düsseldorf, Department of Pediatric Oncology and Hematology, Düsseldorf, FRG

Combination chemotherapy in the treatment of most primary malignant bone tumors was introduced in the early 1970s, and it was expected that these highly potent drugs would have a negative effect on bone healing, particularly in cases of bone transplantation. Experimental investigations by Sauer et al. [3] on the influence of cyclophosphamide on bone healing and those by Burchardt et al. [1] on the influence of adriamycin and methotrexate on bone healing have confirmed this. In the literature there are until now no clinical results of bone healing after osteosynthesis or bone transplantation in patients under polydrug chemotherapy.

We could observe bone healing under chemotherapy in 32 patients with rotationplasty. In this procedure, osteosynthesis is done either between two diaphyseal or two dia/methaphyseal bones or between the distal femur and the ala of the ilium. Furthermore, since 1978 we have done 24 bone transplantations in patients under chemotherapy in the local treatment of malignant bone tumors. Overall, half the cases were operated on for small bone defects, such as tumor resection of the vertebral column, clavicle, wrist, or pelvis. After tumor resection 12 patients had large defects of the proximal humerus, the proximal or distal femur and the proximal tibia. These patients were either children or adolescents in whom an implantation of a tumor prosthesis was not possible or judicious. In most cases we used autologous bone material, such as cancellous bone, sliding bone grafts from the neighboring bone, free corticospongious tibial grafts, or free or vascularized fibula grafts. We required homologous bone grafts as an additional internal support in only four cases. Where necessary, an internal osteosyn-

Table 1. Average time required for bone union after osteosynthesis in patients with rotation plasty

	Age at surgery	
	To 16 years	Over 16 years
Osteosynthesis between femur and tibia: type A rotation plasty	7.9 months	16 months
Osteosynthesis between femur and the ala of the ilium: type B (hip) rotation plasty	11.4 months	15.7 months

In all cases polydrug chemotherapy was begun 2–3 weeks after surgery.

Bone Transplantation
Eds.: M. Aebi, P. Regazzoni

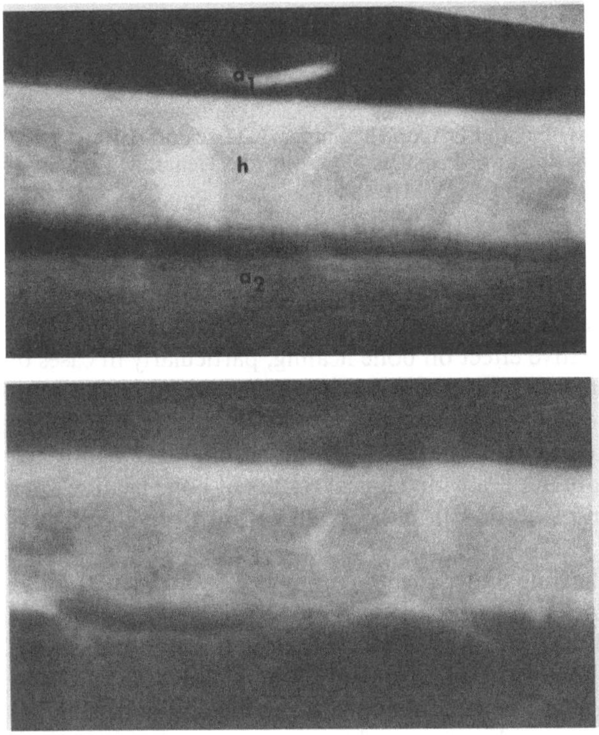

Fig. 1 a and b. X rays (sections) of a 12-year-old girl with an interposition plasty after resection of a femur osteosarcoma. Due to severe but superficial disturbances in postoperative wound healing and 8-week break in chemotherapy was necessary. **a** At 8 weeks postsurgery (May 1980, *05 80*) discrete signs of incorporation and repair of the transplanted autologous cancellous bone (*a1*), homologous (*h*), and autologous tibial grafts (*a2*) are seen. **b** At 18 months (August 1981, *08 81*) the repair processes are almost completed

thetic stabilization was undertaken. We used removable osteosynthetic material only, in most cases plates.

Bone healing after an osteosynthesis took twice or three times as long as a comparable osteosynthesis in patients not under chemotherapy (Table 1). None of the patients achieved a corresponding time interval for healing of the bone transplants. Of the 24 patients 16 had to be repeatedly operated on or are still under treatment, for their extremity is unable to be put under strain. The amount of repair and extent of incorporation processes of the transplanted cancellous or cortical bone grafts were better in those patients in whom chemotherapy was interrupted over a longer period of times due to problems with wound healing (Figs. 1, 2). Long-term control showed no difference between the healing process of homologous and autologous bone transplants. Vascularized bone grafts showed the best healing tendency.

It is known from patients not under chemotherapy that for bone transplantation in tumor surgery other standards must be applied for the length of time required for repair processes. Following segmental tumor resection, the bone trans-

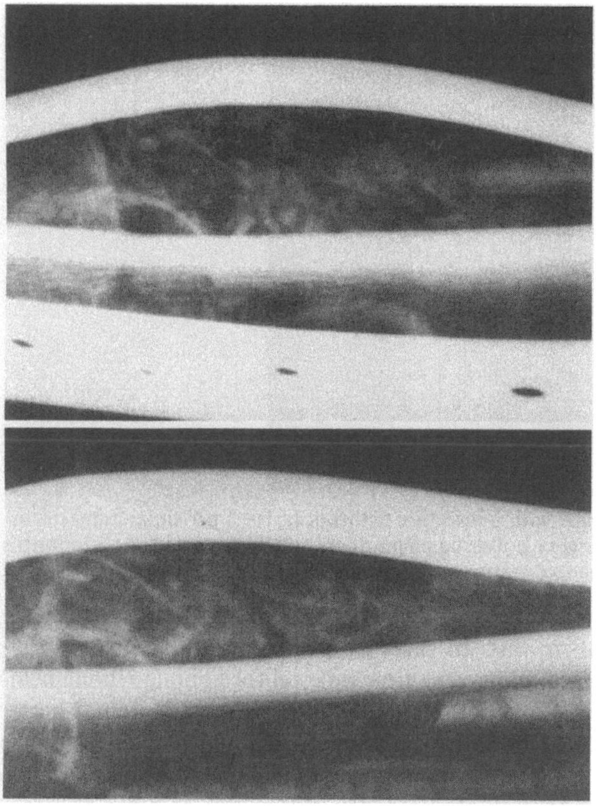

Fig. 2 a and b. X rays (sections) of a 12-year-old girl with a resection arthrodesis for a distal femur osteosarcoma. At 14 days postsurgery polydrug chemotherapy was restarted. **a** At 18 months postsurgery (May 1982, *05 82*) there are no notable reactions of the transplanted bone. **b** At 26 months (January 1983, *01 83*) one plate was removed and homologous cancellous bone and cortical bone grafts were transplanted additionally. Histological examination of the primary transplanted cancellous bone (multiple biopsies) shows no vascularization

plant is vascularized by the adjacent diaphysis and the surrounding soft tissue. Muscles, and not uncommonly subcutaneous tissue and skin, often have no immediate contact with the transplant and present a poor bed for transplantation, compared to those with an intact periosteum. Vascularization of a bone transplant is a deciding factor in the metaplasia and incorporation of the transplanted bone.

Burchardt et al. [1] showed in their experimental investigations a suppression of new bone formation within and about cortical segmental autografts when animals were treated with either adriamycin or methotrexate. Sauer et al. [3] showed that cyclophosphamide significantly retards the course of fracture reparation. The degree of retardation was directly dependent on the phase of fracture healing during cyclophosphamide treatment. The retarding effect was greatest with coincidence of the beginning of fracture healing and treatment with cyclophosphamide.

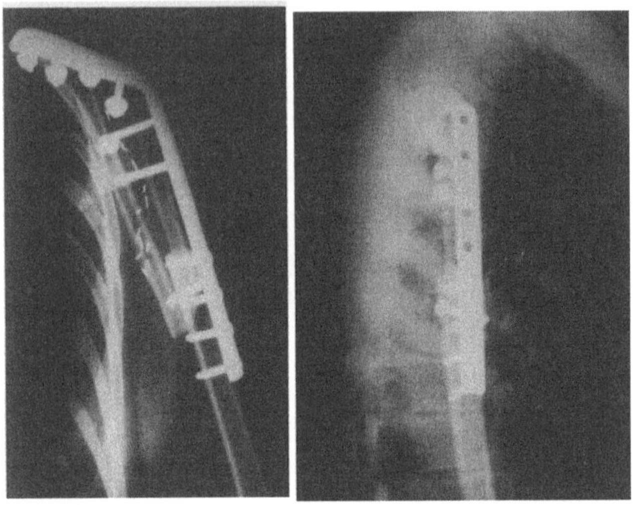

Fig. 3. X rays of a 19-year-old girl with a resection arthrodesis for a proximal humerus osteosarcoma. At 14 days postsurgery polydrug chemotherapy was restarted. At 13 months no signs of incorporation of the two transplanted fibula allografts

Our clinical results confirm this. In cases of an osteosynthesis of two diaphyseal or two dia/metaphyseal bones, the time interval for complete bone healing was much longer than in a comparable osteosynthesis in patients not under chemotherapy. In our cases of bone transplantation we had a high incidence (65%) of nonunion or fatigue fractures. In many cases in which the postoperative chemotherapy was restarted 14 days after surgery, there were no signs of incorporation of the transplanted bone within 12–18 months (Fig. 3). There was no difference in patients who had had an osteosarcoma and received postoperative chemotherapy according to the COSS protocol [4] or a Ewing's sarcoma and received postoperative chemotherapy according to the CESS protocol [2].

Therapeutic agents used in modern polydrug chemotherapy protocols prolong the time of bone healing and the time required for osseous graft-host union and inhibit new bone formation. Therefore, we regard bone transplantation after tumor resection in patients under chemotherapy as a temporary solution and point out to our patients that following completion of chemotherapy further reconstructive procedures are required.

References

1. Burchardt H, Glowczewskie FP, Enneking WF (1983) The effect of adriamycin and methotrexate on the repair of segmental cortical autografts in dogs. J Bone Joint Surg [Am] 65:103
2. Jürgens H et al. (1985) Die cooperative Ewing-Sarkom Studie CESS 81 der GPO – Analyse nach 4 Jahren. Klin Pädiatr 197:225
3. Sauer HD, Sommer-Tsilenis E, Borchers D, Schmidt H (1982) Die Beeinflussung der Knochenbruchheilung durch das Zytostatikum Zyklophosphamid. Z Orthop 120:783
4. Winkler K (1986) Zur Chemotherapie des Osteosarkoms. 9 Jahre kooperative Osteosarkomstudie (COSS) der GPO. Onkol Forum 3:1

Clinical, Metabolic, and Structural Studies on Large Osteoarticular Allografts in Bone Tumor Surgery

A. J. Aho, T. Ekfors, J. Eskola, and P. Jussila

Department of Surgery, Pathological Anatomy and Microbiology, University Central Hospital, Turku, Finland

In order to give answers to some questions in allograft surgery the clinical results of 14 patients after a long follow-up time were reviewed. The other objects of interest were: the incorporation and regeneration of the grafts, their metabolism, late radiological changes, and immunological aspects. Biochemical composition was studied in experiments on dogs.

Allografts consisting of meta/diaphyseal part and joint cartilage surface were obtained from young donors under 40 years of age. The bank bone was preserved for 1 week to 3 years in plastic bags according to a modification of Imamaliev's technique at a constant temperature of −70 °C. After resection of the total osteoarticular part with metaphysis a bank half joint was fixed to the host bone by means of AO plates. The collateral and cruciate ligaments of the knee in man were reconstructed utilizing the host's own ligaments by fixing subperiosteal insertions to the graft (Aho 1985). Autogenous iliac bone chips were transplanted to the osteosynthesis site in man. The clinical series consisted of 14 patients with malignant (osteosarcoma, chondrosarcoma), semimalignant (giant cell tumor), or large aggressive benign (aneurysmal bone cyst, etc.) bone tumors. Immunosuppression was not used. Two patients received preoperative radiotherapy. The follow-up time was 1.5–13 years (mean, 5.5 years). Weight bearing was gradually began at 6 months, being full at 8–10 months. The first transplantation operation was done in 1973 in man and in 1968 in dog. Methods used included: radiographs, isotopes, conventional histology, host lymphocyte transformation, cell-mediated immunity test, and biochemistry.

Metabolism and regeneration began early, at 2–3 weeks, indicated as positive isotope uptake of technetium DPD, especially at the osteosynthesis site lasting many years. Biopsies for histology showed the onset of weak new bone formation at 4–6 months, but typically areas of old dead bone and slight new bone were seen side by side.

The incorporation, consolidation of the graft at the osteosynthesis site illustrated in radiographs, began slowly from 3–5 months, continuing to bony union at 10–16 months. The grafts looked rather normal at 2 years, but later subchondral sclerotic cyst-like changes and mild joint surface degeneration was evident (Fig. 1). However, the joints were nearly painless in the knee region, too.

No changes were found in the mitotic response of lymphocytes to phytohemagglutinin (PHA) and concanavalin A (Con A) assessed by whole blood microculture. The lymphocyte transformation, reaction against the graft, showed in one patient only a transiently increased value. No patient showed evidence of clinical rejection or adverse reaction.

Bone Transplantation
Eds.: M. Aebi, P. Regazzoni

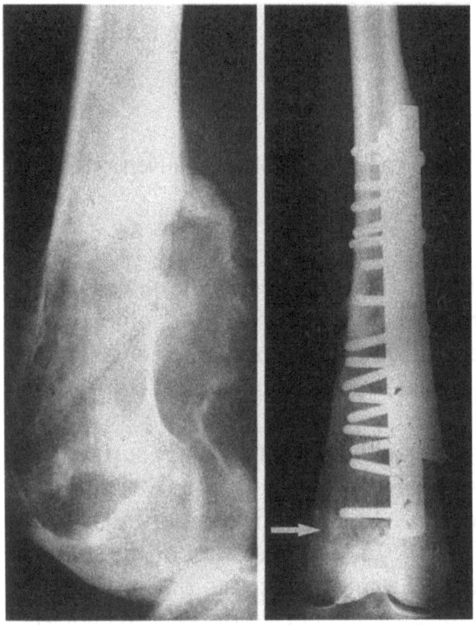

Fig. 1. A recurrent aneurysmal bone cyst involving the distal femur in an young woman (*left*). Some sclerotic and cystic changes (*arrow*) are seen 3 years after the massive osteoarticular allograft transplantation (*right*)

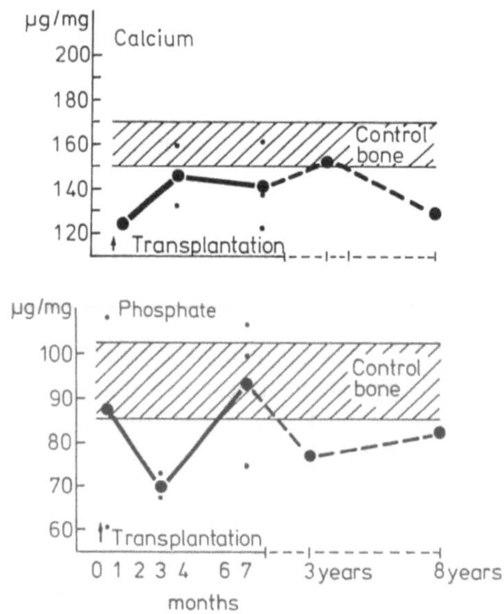

Fig. 2. Curves illustrating and phosphate concentrations (μg/mg) in osteoarticular allografts in dogs as function of age

The clinical results with 1–13 years observation time (mean, 5.5 years) were good in 9 out of 14 patients (64%). If two tumor failures are excluded, the results were good in 75%. Grading by Mankin's (1983) score was used.

Six patients had complications: deep infection, fatigue fractures, valgus deformation, resorption, ligament instability, peroneal palsy. Three infections healed after trepanation but resulted in a poor functional end result (e.g., arthrodesis). The other complications healed.

The organic components increased, remaining at an increased level for up to 3 years, suggesting a regeneration process of the organic matrix. The mineral components of calcium and phosphate, on the other hand, remained consistently lower than the control values (Fig. 2). The results will be published later in detail.

In principal, our results parallel those observed in larger series in man (Mankin et al. 1983; Mnaymneh et al. 1985). However, by a longer observation time sclerotic and degenerative changes can be seen in large knee allografts often beginning about 3 years after the transplantation. This finding has also been stated by Alho et al. (1987). In spite of the relatively low number of patients the absence of nonunion in our series is worth noticing, which means a good incorporation of the grafts. And, in spite of some data indicating a decreased activity and the risk of complications, the allograft technique is a biological substitute method for bone tumor surgery in young individuals without significant immunological reactions.

References

Aho AJ (1985) Half-joint allograft transplantation in human bone tumour. Int Orthop (SICOT) 9:77–87

Alho A, Karaharju EO, Korkala O, Laasonen E (1987) Hemijoint allografts in the treatment of low grade malignant and aggressive bone tumours about the knee. Int Orthop (SICOT) 11:35–41

Imamaliev AS (1969) The preparation preservation and transplantation of articular bone ends. In: Apley AG (ed) Recent advances in orthopaedics. Churchill, London, pp 209–263

Mankin HJ, Doppelt S, Tomford W (1983) Clinical experience with allograft implantation: the first ten years. Clin Orthop 174:69–86

Mnaymneh W, Malinin TJ, Makley JT, Dick HM (1985) Massive osteoarticular allografts in the reconstruction of extremities following resection of tumors not requiring chemotherapy and radiation. Clin Orthop 197:76–87

A Massive Vascularized Allograft of Femoral Shaft

P. Chiron, J. A. Colombier, J. L. Tricoire, J. Puget, G. Utheza, Y. Glock, and P. Puel

Centre Hospitalier Universitaire, Toulouse Rangueil, France

The allograft receiver was a 35-year-old male whose thigh was crushed by a train. Initial lesions were severe muscular defect, degloving syndrome of the entire thigh and pulverized femoral shaft. Such a lesion usually indicates amputation. In this particular case, however, both the superficial femoral vessels and the sciatic nerve were uninjured. This status allowed us to foresee a favorable result if reconstructive surgery was attempted. Open-site techniques are lengthy, committed, and are liable to produce a repeated complications. We therefore preferred a closed-site technique. The limb was immobilized by an external fixation bridging the femur; skin closure was effected by grafts and flaps. Multiresistant *Staphylococcus aureus* sepsis complicated the postoperative course.

In the 4th posttraumatic month, we were faced with a 27-cm long bone defect initially infected, but which eventually closed. The various techniques proposed to treat a bone defect were not very convenient in this case. Ilizarov's method would have meant neglecting the mobility of the hip, allowing only that of the head and neck. A free vascularized fibula autograft is well-known to survive in a septic locus, but it is not indicated in bone defects of over 20 cm. A massive allograft allows a stable assembly, but it is hazardous in the presence of sepsis.

We performed a vascularized massive allograft after initial endeavors to perfuse antibiotic agent. The donor was a man in a premortem coma. Procurement was separated from the graft operation by 3 h. The femoral shaft graft is an outstanding free graft because of its uniquely large pedicle. The graft is 27 cm long. Assembly is performed so as to favor stability. Arterial and venous vessels of the graft were anastomosed to femoral vessels (arterial end-to-end anastomosis on the deep femoral artery stump; and veinous end-to-side anastomosis on the femoral vein).

Upon 9-month follow-up the patient was walking with complete weight bearing, and hip flexion was 90°; the patient was back at home. Healing of junctions took 6 months.

Is the graft perfused? Intraoperative arteriography shows intraosseous circulation.

Did the graft remain perfused? Selective arteriographies in the 3rd week, 6th month, and 9th month showed perfusion of the large vessels. Stetho doppler allowed a good follow-up of patency. Scintiscanning demonstrated hyperfixation of the junctions, in contrast to normal fixation of the shaft. Isotopic transit measured the vascular pool of the shaft. There is no direct evaluation of intraosseous vascularization.

Bone Transplantation
Eds.: M. Aebi, P. Regazzoni

Was there rejection? We did not use immunnosuppressive therapy. The patient was compatible with the donor for ABO group and DR locus. The cortical bone showed no modification during the first 3 months. Afterwards, a few irregular prints appeared as bony layers surrounded the graft.

Was it mandatory to vascularize this graft? At the end of the 2nd month, an abscess was discovered in the muscles of the upper thigh, without osteitis. Has the bone graft been protect by antibiotic perfusion?

Massive allografts are being used increasingly in reconstructive surgery after tumorectomy; however, they remain very uncommon in traumatology. The rationale for massive vascularized allografts calls upon the following data: massive allografts allow a steady reconstruction, helping early rehabilitation, and preserved vascularization of the transplanted bone enhances the potential survival of the graft during infection, due to perfusion and antibiotics.

Collagen and Bone Formation After Metaphyseal Osteotomy and Gradual Distraction

J. Peltonen, E. Karaharju, K. Aalto, M. Vauhkonen, and I. Alitalo

Invalid Foundation Orthopedic Hospital, Helsinki; Department of Orthopedics and Traumatology,
University Central Hospital, Department of Medical Chemistry, University of Helsinki; and Department of Surgery, College of Veterinary Medicine, Helsinki, Finland

It has been shown that new bone is formed as a result of osteotomy and gradual distraction. The mode of bone formation and the role of collagen in this process is, however, obscure. In epiphyseal distraction, prior to bone formation, collagen is first organized according to the direction of the distraction [1]. The types and quantity of collagen in distractional bone healing has not been investigated earlier.

Transversal osteotomy of the distal radius was performed on 12 sheep. Distraction by external fixation was started 1 week after the osteotomy, at a rate of 0.3–0.5 mm per day. It was continued for 3–5 weeks, after which the fixation was kept as neutral until consolidation of the distraction area. Collagen types I, II, and III were determined by analysis of the cyanogen bromide peptides on sodium dodecyl sulfate polyacrylamide gel [2]. Quantitation of the collagen was based on the hydroxyproline content of the organic matrix. The mineralization was determined from sequential biopsies taken from the distraction area. Bone formation was studied radiologically and by means of oxytetracycline (OTC) labeling. Conventional histology using hematoxylin and eosin, and van Gieson stainings were undertaken.

The dominant type of collagen in the distraction area was type I, $\alpha1(I)_2\,\alpha2(I)_1$, throughout the distraction period and was qualitatively comparable to the collagen types of the control radius during the follow-up of 5 weeks. Histologically the collagen bundles were organized according to the direction of the distraction. The amount of the collagen increased up to 4 weeks after starting the distraction (Fig. 1). Bone formation occurred both endosteally and through periosteal callus formation, and into the organized collagen template. The most immature bone

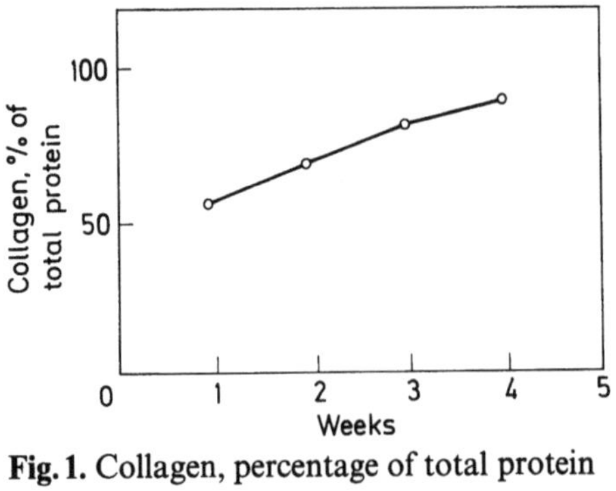

Fig. 1. Collagen, percentage of total protein

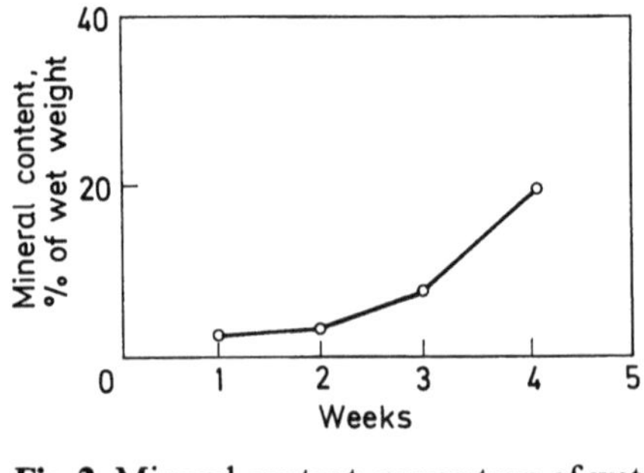

Fig. 2. Mineral content, percentage of wet weight

Bone Transplantation
Eds.: M. Aebi, P. Regazzoni

was observed in the center of the distraction gap. The mineralization increased clearly from 3 weeks after the distraction was started (Fig. 2), and it was more advanced near the osteotomized bone ends than in the center of the distraction area. Remodeling of the medullary canal occurred rapidly after consolidation (2–3 months) of the distraction area.

Type I collagen, characteristic of mature bone, is the principal protein component of the organic matrix formed in the distraction area. The collagen fibers obviously act as a template for the new bone, which is formed as a result of the distraction.

References

1. Monticelli G, Spinelli R, Bonucci E (1981) Distraction epiphysiolysis as a method of limb lengthening, II. Morphologic investigations. Clin Orthop 154:262–273
2. Bornstein P, Sage H (1980) Structurally distinct collagen types. Ann Rev Biochem 49:957–1003

Bone Lengthening Methods in the Treatment of Large Segmental Bone Defects

J. de Pablos [1], J. Cañadell [1], G. D. MacEwen [2], and J. R. Bowen [2]

[1] University Clinic of Navarra, 31080 Pamplona, Spain
[2] Alfred I. DuPont Institute, 19899 Wilmington, Delaware, USA

Ilizarov's concept of treating large segmental bone defects (LSBD) by means of bone transport along the defect is, in our opinion, an outstanding idea [3]. On the other hand, Ilizarov's circular external device used for this purpose has certain drawbacks due to its bulkiness, placement difficulties, postoperative management, and the transfixing system used. The Department of Orthopedic Surgery of the University of Navarra in collaboration with the Department of Orthopedics of the Alfred I. DuPont Institute (Wilmington, Delaware) experimented on this concept in animals, but using monolateral frames with which it was attempted to minimize the drawbacks involved in Ilizarov's apparatus while maintaining the advantages of his original idea. The objective was to assess the suitability of monolateral frames in the treatment of LSBD following Ilizarov's concept.

Five male mongrel dogs aged 6–12 months and five male merino lambs, 6 months old, were used. In all cases the experiment consisted in attempting the reconstruction of a 5-cm segmental bone loss of one of the femoral diaphyses of the

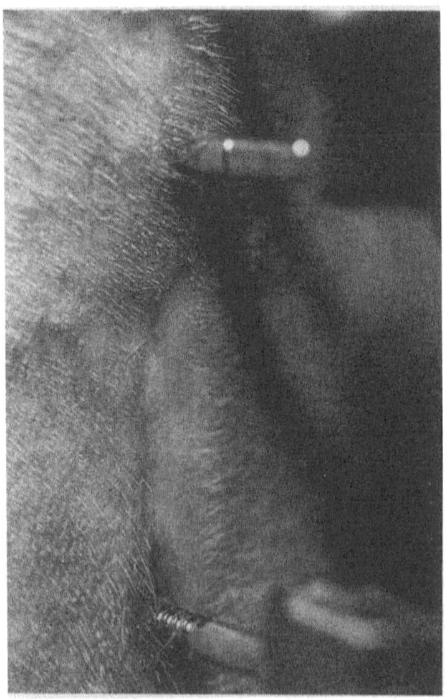

Fig. 1. Wound produced by descent of intermediate screws during bone transport

Bone Transplantation
Eds.: M. Aebi, P. Regazzoni

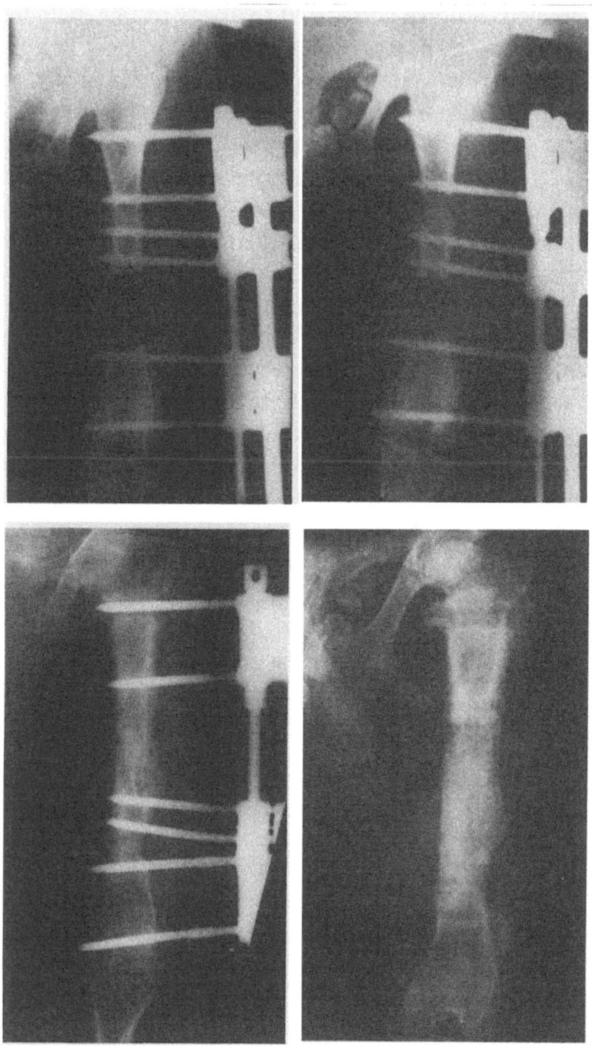

a b c d

Fig. 2 a–d. Radiological stages of the experiment. **a** Immediately postoperative. **b** At 10 days. **c** At 50 days. **d** At 4 months

animals. First, a diphyseal femoral segment was removed, and immediately afterwards three pairs of screws were inserted into the same femur. This was followed by the performance of a percutaneous osteotomy between the proximal and intermediate pairs of screws, with which a small fragment of the proximal femoral segment was detached. The monolateral frame was then placed and adjusted. Two types of monolateral frame were used, both allowing placement of three pairs of screws and the independent longitudinal mobilization of each pair of screws with respect to the other two. Starting on the first postoperative day, progressive distraction (1 mm/day) was carried out until transport of this small bone cylinder along the bone loss was completed. Studies performed to assess results included X rays, bone and muscle histology, and specimen measurements.

Clinically, the distraction stage until bone transport was completed presented no problems worthy of mention. We observed that, on advancing, the screws inserted in the transported piece of bone were cutting the skin and producing a longitudinal wound which healed proximally as the screws passed (Fig. 1). The radiological study showed that from the very first stages of distraction, the space produced between the proximal femoral segment and the transported bone cylinder was gradually occupied by an increasingly dense, calcified tissue. At the end of bone transport, and particularly 3 months later, this space showed a quite satisfactory reconstruction – consolidation and remodeling (Fig. 2). Histologically, the repair of the space produced during distraction followed a pattern similar to that observed in bone lengthening by means of diaphyseal percutaneous osteotomy [1, 2]. Muscle histology showed that there was apparently no injury to muscles and nerves at the level of distraction significant enough as to prevent an easy bone transport.

These results show that the treatment of LSBD by means of Ilizarov's concept can be accomplished experimentally using monolateral frames. With them we can minimize several of the Ilizarov's device drawbacks while maintaining the advantages of his original idea.

References

1. Arrien A (1986) Estudio comparativo de la osteotomía a cielo abierto y percutánea en la elongación de las extremidades. Thesis, Universidad de Navarra, Pamplona
2. Cañadell J, Arrien A, de Pablos J (1986) Ossification after bone lengthening. In: Meeting on recent advances in external fixation. Riva del Garda
3. Ilizarov GA (1971) The main principles of transosseous compression and distraction osteosynthesis. Orthop Travnmatol Protez 11:7–15

The Promising Application of Special Plastics as a Substitute for Bone Tissue

P. Korbelář

Orthopedic Clinic, Charles University, Prague 5, Czechoslovakia

In spite of the rapid development of various natural and artificial implants of bone tissue, bones, or whole joints, no material has yet been found which maximally resembles the structure of bone tissue and is also maximally compatible with it. In the 1960s insoluble hydrophilic gels were introduced for clinical purposes, and these have successfully been applied in various branches of medicine ever since. However, they have not yet attracted sufficient attention in orthopedic surgery, in spite of the fact that their inertness, biocompatibility, easy processibility, controllable swelling, ability to bind other compounds (antibiotics, cytostatics), and in some cases biodegradability make them very well suited indeed for just this purpose. The following questions here were to be answered:

1. How does the hydrogel behave in the bone tissue with respect to biocompatibility?
2. How does biocompatibility of the hydrogel depend on its porosity?
3. In what way does methacrylic acid added to gel affect biodegradability of the implant?
4. How does the hydrogel behave in spongious and compact bone?

(2-Hydroxyethyl)methacrylate (polyHEMA), cross-linked with a small quantity of glycoldimethacrylate, was used, where – by merely changing the monomer : water ratio – it is possible to obtain a polymer structure varying from homogenous to macroporous. A special treatment allowed a sintered gel structure to be prepared, possessing double porosity, which was further surface-modified. The implants were prepared in the form of cylinders, 3.5 mm in diameter in eight different modifications (samples A–H). These were implanted into the subtrochanteric and supracondylic part of rabbit femur. In all, 42 animals were operated upon. The preparations thus obtained were macroscopically evaluated and histologically treated by the half-thin cuts method. The total was of 124 samples. Some polymers were X-ray contrast. No complications due to a wrong operative technique, postoperative infect, or poor healing have been recorded. The rabbits were killed after an interval of 1–6 months (32–193 days).

The hydrogel modifications used are highly biocompatible, and the compatibility improves with increasing porosity. Nonporous and microporous hydrogel (samples A–C) are not compatible and are limited by fibrous capsule. The sintered macroporous gel is surrounded only by a thin fibrin membrane, which reflects the high degree of compatibility with the bone tissue (samples D–H). Addition of methacrylic acid on the hydrogel surface brings about a marked rise in the adhesiveness of macrophages and destruction of the polymer, quite pronounced in the spongious bone (samples F, G). The gel is actively degraded in the

Bone Transplantation
Eds.: M. Aebi, P. Regazzoni

bone marrow, even though direct phagocytosis could not be proved. During degradation in the compact bone the activity of macrophages was delayed; when the gel without methacrylic acid was used, no activity was observed even after 193 days of implantation, and the implant was growing through the bone. Degradation occurs only if methacrylic acid is added.

In view of the fact that, according to the available literature, these problems (implantation of sintered hydrogel into the bone) have not yet been studied in such an extensively conceived experiment, our conclusions cannot be adequately compared with those by other authors. However, macroporous sintered insoluble gel designed by us for application in bone surgery has clearly shown in this long-term experiment that the material involved is highly biocompatible.

Future Directions in Research: Outlook

M. Aebi and R. Ganz

Department of Orthopedic Surgery, University of Berne, Inselspital, CH-3010 Berne, Switzerland

In the last two decades it has become apparent – and this symposium has confirmed – that osteoarticular allograft transplantation has gone beyond the stage of laboratory trials and experimental animal models to become a useful tool in the management of patients suffering from orthopedic disorders.

Although knowledge of bone and cartilage biology, biomechanics and immunology has increased significantly, these remain some fundamental problems that must be solved if osteoarticular allotransplantation is to become a routine procedure in orthopedic surgery. This is especially true if we intend to perform genuine transplantation – orthotopic transfer of a viable tissue complex or organ from a donor to a recipient with maintenance of the blood supply and morphologic integrity of the tissue system. This definition makes it clear that most of the so-called bone or joint transplantations reported in a myriad of scientific papers in the past 100 years are in fact no transplantations at all. The transfer of bone as usually carried out is only possible because bone is a privileged tissue system with an enormous capacity to completely remodel its tissue structure over a certain time, to adapt to new mechanical conditions, and to offer a certain stability and support, even when dead. We usually transfer only parts of a bone. As long as we only reconstruct segmental defects of bone it is not mandatory to perform a viable bone transfer, except in cases with an extensive defect and a bad tissue bed. This problem may be solved by means of a vascularized fibular transplant. However, as soon as we contemplate transplanting joints the need for viable allogenic bone and consequently cartilage is of utmost importance. The remodeling of the subchondral bone in an avascular joint transplant due to necrosis may initiate damage to the cartilage. This has been demonstrated clearly by the clinical experience with massive osteochondral allografting, which eventually results in secondary arthrosis.

This consideration leads to the conclusion that in future research, efforts must be made to differentiate between the needs for joint transplantation and for segmental defect transplantation (Fig. 1). To bridge a diaphyseal segmental defect of 6 cm or more several alternative techniques have been proposed:

1. Nonvascularized cancellous or cortical autograft or combined corticocancellous autograft
2. Vascularized autograft (pedicled fibular graft)
3. Nonvascularized allografts
4. Filling of the defect with bone morphogenetic protein in combination with bone, or other biodegradable bone substitutes alone or in combination with bone

Bone Transplantation
Eds.: M. Aebi, P. Regazzoni

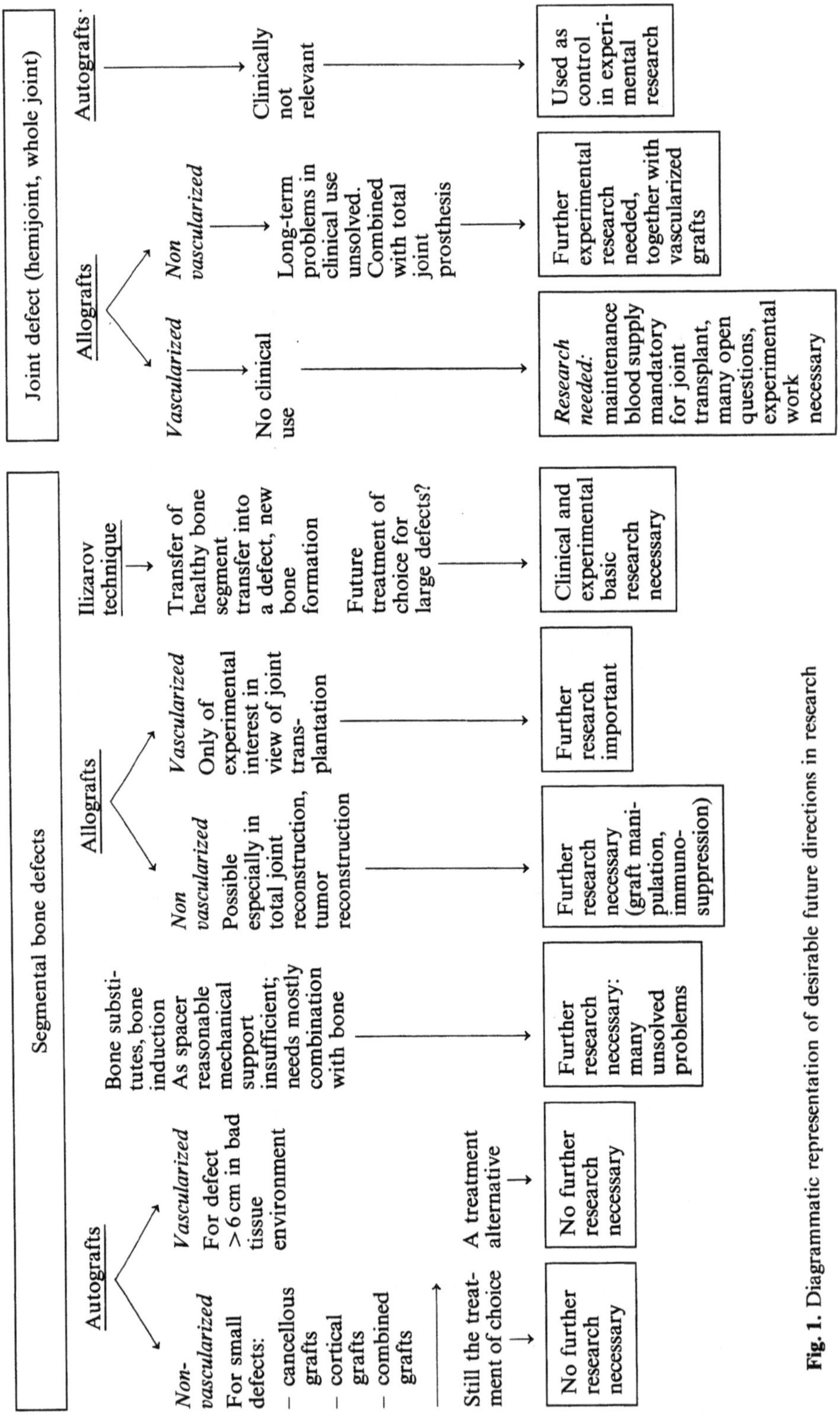

Fig. 1. Diagrammatic representation of desirable future directions in research

5. Bone lengthening according to Ilizarov, transferring healthy bone into the defect
6. Artificial prostheses

The biology of graft incorporation is broadly clear and is widely determined by the mechanical conditions under which the graft has been implanted. Stable fixation by means of appropriate osteosynthesis is a prerequisite for graft incorporation. Immediate revascularization of the graft, a second prerequisite, can only be achieved optimally by microsurgical anastomosis of the feeding vessels. Only by this procedure can the viability of a large number of osteoblasts and osteocytes within the graft be maintained. This has never been possible in a nonvascularized autograft, except to some extent by special preservation techniques in the presence of an optimal graft bed, and of course is not feasible in segmental allografts. To extend this knowledge to allografts is a most important step, especially for working toward osteoarticular allografting although the vascularized segmental allograft may be useless for clinical purposes. However, it has become obvious that once allogenic bone is perfused with the recipient's blood, the immunologic response is that of a transplanted organ and differs from the response long postulated for nonvascularized bone allografts. Therefore, we have arrived at a point – which kidney and heart transplantation surgery reached several years ago – where the main task is preventing immunologic incompatibility.

Although classical immunosuppressive agents may never be used to keep segmentally transplanted bone allografts viable, due to the inherent problems of the adverse effects, experimental bone transplantation with immediate revascularization and immunosuppression is of great importance to increase our knowledge, which can then be applied for joint transplantation. To maintain viability, and thus unimpaired function, immediate and lasting revascularization of the joint is mandatory. This can only be achieved by suppression or by omission of the immunologic reaction. Future research, therefore, has to address the question of whether the graft can be manipulated and prepared so that it is no longer immunogenic without killing osteoblasts and osteocytes of osteaoarticular transplants, whether the host response can be suppressed or even eliminated by more specific immunosuppressive agents with less severe or no adverse effects, or both in combination. Tolerance induction by pretreatment of the host may not be of importance, as it has not proved useful in renal transplants. The same is true for the use of monoclonal antibodies for purposes of long-term immunosuppression.

Conditioning or manipulation of graft or donor in order to modify the antigenicity of the transplant has so far been relatively unsuccessful. The basic idea is to modify the antigen-presenting cells, such as dendritic cells or macrophages, either chemically or by physical methods, so that they lose their efficiency. This concept has only recently attracted renewed interest in the field of bone transplantation research (see chapter by Czitrom in this volume).

Ex vivo perfusion, although it has not been very successful in organ transplants, may be of great interest for osteochondral allografts, where prolonged graft preservation in culture media or in an appropriate perfusion system seems to be possible: an exciting research field of our own!

Renal and heart transplants from polytransfused donors have a better 1-year graft survival than those from nontransfused donors; whether this is also true for osteochondral allografts has not been evaluated. However, is may be possible for the donor, and therefore the graft, to be conditioned in such a way before transplantation. This would mean a weaker immune response by the recipient, who would then require smaller quantities of immunosuppressive agents.

It is clear that the prospects for joint transplantation are not the same as for segmental transplantation, but since joint prostheses represent a strong and rapidly developing alternative to biologic materials, further research into joint transplantation seems necessary. However, the protheses surgery currently still has the inherent problem of loosening and many other complications. Biologic joint replacement therefore remains, especially in younger patients, a valuable option, so that joint survival has to be assured by immediate surgical revascularization, stable fixation, and suppression of the immunologic reaction.

As long as the primary aim of transferring bone is merely to bridge a defect, induce incorporation, and maintain mechanical stability, it may be best to use the patient's own bone. However, this is often not available in sufficient amounts.

The new Ilizarov technique seems to enable a completely new approach to the bone defect problem. By means of compactotomy and progressive transfer of autogenous bone, the original defect is filled with mechanical intact bone. The new defect which originates from this bone transfer is filled with "self-produced" bone. This method has not yet been widely applied even in experimental work in the western world, but some clinical examples at our institutions and elsewhere encourage us to see in this technique a very promising alternative to bone grafting.

Of course, the ideal material for filling a segmental defect would be one which is sufficiently available and which will induce formation of new bone in situ which may be incorporated by mechanical adaption in the course of time. The very promising bone morphogenetic protein (BMP) cannot yet meet these demands and needs to be combined with sufficient bone, so that other solutions are still needed for large, mechanically important defects, as well as for joint replacement. BMP and the related substances are far from being understood completely.

Those dealing with bone transplantation have been becoming more and more concerned about legal aspects, especially since AIDS is a significant threat to graft recipients. This disease will make the banking and procurement procedures more complicated and may divert research away from bone allografting toward autogenous solutions or artificial substitutes, just at a time when it seemed that biological transplants were about to have a future in joint replacement.

In conclusion, whatever the future brings, as long as biologic material continues to be grafted, especially in the form of joint transplants, the following criteria are of fundamental significance and will determine the form taken by future research programs:

1. Stable internal fixation of the transplant to maintain graft viability mechanically
2. Immediate revascularization of the transplant to keep cells viable, especially in subchondral bone and cartilage in joint transplants
3. The control of immunologic reaction

In order to fulfill these demands enormous efforts will be necessary to improve microsurgical vascular techniques and better to understand the ideal conditions for revascularization. Against the background of stable internal fixation and immediate revascularization, the prerequisites for the success of any allografting surgery, the following points must be researched and elucidated:

- Donor graft conditioning
- Graft preservation
- Selective immunosuppression aimed at precise events during induction of the immune response, combined with refined monitoring
- Antigen-specific immunosuppression with the aim of inducing a tolerant state necessitating only limited multidrug immunosuppression

All of these are beyond the scope of an orthopedic surgeon. Therefore multidisciplinary transplantation research groups should become the standard, together with an orthopedic department policy which reflects the needs and clinical applications of transplantation biology in and outside of orthopedic surgery. The orthopedic surgeon who plans, organizes, performs, and analyzes the results of a transplant without assistance from others belongs to the past.

Subject Index

B.-D. Katthagen, University of Homburg/Saar

Bone Regeneration with Bone Substitutes

An Animal Study

1987. 101 figures. 15 tables. X, 159 pages. Soft cover.
ISBN 3-540-17425-7

Contents: Introduction and Scope of the Study. - Bone Matrix. - Bone Transplants. - Bone-Replacement Materials. - Experimental Section. - Discussion of the Experimental Results. - Summary. - Subject Index.

Congenital and acquired bone defects constitute a central problem of traumatology and orthopedics. In order to cure these defects it is often necessary to fill up the bones operatively with suitable substances. Recently, so-called bone substitutes (collagen, gelatine, bone matrix, calcium phosphate, hydorxyapatite) have also been recommended.
Following an introductory presentation of bone regeneration and transplants, these substitutes are discussed here in a comprehensive survey of the literature. Particular attention is given to the significance of mineral substance such as hydroxyapatite, which will undoubtedly find a place in bone surgery owing to its outstanding bioactivity and biotolerance. The implants examined are also of significance for maxillofacial surgery and dentistry. The histologic techniques in the staining of undecalcified bone preparations and in histomorphometry are presented in a special chapter.

Springer-Verlag
Berlin Heidelberg New York
London Paris Tokyo Hong Kong

MIX
Papier aus verantwortungsvollen Quellen
Paper from responsible sources
FSC® C105338

If you have any concerns about our products,
you can contact us on
ProductSafety@springernature.com

In case Publisher is established outside the EU,
the EU authorized representative is:
Springer Nature Customer Service Center GmbH
Europaplatz 3, 69115 Heidelberg, Germany

Printed by Libri Plureos GmbH
in Hamburg, Germany